Multiple Sclerosis

Guest Editor

EMMANUELLE L. WAUBANT, MD, PhD

NEUROLOGIC CLINICS

www.neurologic.theclinics.com

Consulting Editor
RANDOLPH W. EVANS, MD

May 2011 • Volume 29 • Number 2

SAUNDERS an imprint of ELSEVIER, Inc.

W.B. SAUNDERS COMPANY
A Division of Elsevier Inc.

1600 John F. Kennedy Boulevard • Suite 1800 • Philadelphia, Pennsylvania 19103-2899

http://www.theclinics.com

NEUROLOGIC CLINICS Volume 29, Number 2
May 2011 ISSN 0733-8619, ISBN-13: 978-1-4557-0469-9

Editor: Donald Mumford
Developmental Editor: Eva Kulig

Neurologic Clinics (ISSN 0733-8619) is published quarterly by Elsevier Inc., 360 Park Avenue South, New York, NY 10010–1710. Months of issue are February, May, August, and November. Periodicals postage paid at New York, NY, and additional mailing offices. Subscription prices are $264.00 per year for US individuals, $441.00 per year for US institutions, $130.00 per year for US students, $332.00 per year for Canadian individuals, $530.00 per year for Canadian institutions, $368.00 per year for international individuals, $530.00 per year for international institutions, and $184.00 for Canadian and foreign students/residents. To receive student/resident rate, orders must be accompanied by name of affiliated institution, date of term, and the *signature* of program/residency coordinator on institution letterhead. Orders will be billed at individual rate until proof of status is received. Foreign air speed delivery is included in all *Clinics* subscription prices. All prices are subject to change without notice. **POSTMASTER:** Send address changes to *Neurologic Clinics*, Elsevier Health Sciences Division, Subscription Customer Service, 3251 Riverport Lane, Maryland Heights, MO 63043. **Customer Service: Telephone: 1-800-654-2452 (U.S. and Canada); 314-447-8871 (outside U.S. and Canada). Fax: 314-447-8029. E-mail: journalscustomerservice-usa@elsevier.com (for print support); journalsonlinesupport-usa@elsevier.com (for online support).**

Reprints. For copies of 100 or more of articles in this publication, please contact the Commercial Reprints Department, Elsevier Inc., 360 Park Avenue South, New York, New York, 10010-1710; Tel.: (+1) 212-633-3812; Fax: (+1) 212-462-1935, and E-mail: reprints@elsevier.com.

Neurologic Clinics is also published in Spanish by Nueva Editorial Interamericana S.A., Mexico City, Mexico.

Neurologic Clinics is covered in *Current Contents/Clinical Medicine, MEDLINE/PubMed (Index Medicus), EMBASE/Excerpta Medica, and PsycINFO, and ISI/BIOMED.*

Printed and bound by CPI Group (UK) Ltd, Croydon, CR0 4YY

Transferred to Digital Print 2011

Contributors

CONSULTING EDITOR

RANDOLPH W. EVANS, MD
Clinical Professor, Department of Neurology, Baylor College of Medicine, Houston, Texas

GUEST EDITOR

EMMANUELLE L. WAUBANT, MD, PhD
Associate Professor, Department of Neurology, Director, UCSF Regional Pediatric MS Center, University of California, San Francisco, San Francisco, California

AUTHORS

ENRIQUE ALVAREZ, MD, PhD
Neuroimmunology Fellow, Division of Multiple Sclerosis, Department of Neurology, Washington University, St Louis, Missouri

ERIK BEALL, PhD
Mellen Imaging Center, Imaging Institute, Cleveland, Ohio

PALLAB BHATTACHARYYA, PhD
Mellen Imaging Center, Imaging Institute, Cleveland, Ohio

ALLEN C. BOWLING, MD, PhD
Medical Director, MS Service; Colorado Neurological Institute (CNI), Englewood; Director, Complementary and Alternative Medicine Service, CNI; Clinical Associate Professor, Department of Neurology, University of Colorado, Denver, Colorado

DOROTHEE CHABAS, MD, PhD
Department of Neurology, UCSF Regional Pediatric MS Center, University of California, San Francisco, San Francisco, California

JACQUELINE T. CHEN, PhD
Department of Neurosciences, Cleveland Clinic, Cleveland, Ohio

TANUJA CHITNIS, MD
Assistant Professor in Neurology, Harvard Medical School; Director, Partners Pediatric Multiple Sclerosis Center, Massachusetts General Hospital for Children, Boston, Massachusetts

VITA DI RENZO, MD
Department of Neurological and Psychiatric Sciences, University of Bari, Bari, Italy

MARIANGELA D'ONGHIA, MD
Department of Neurological and Psychiatric Sciences, University of Bari, Bari, Italy

ROBERT J. FOX, MD
Mellen Center for Multiple Sclerosis, Neurological Institute; Cleveland Clinic Lerner
College of Medicine, Cleveland, Ohio

BARBARA S. GIESSER, MD
Clinical Professor of Neurology, David Geffen University of California, Los Angeles School
of Medicine, Los Angeles, California

GAVIN GIOVANNONI, MBBCh, PhD, FCP(SA), FRCP, FRCPath
Professor of Neurology, Neuroscience and Trauma Centre, Blizard Institute of Cell
and Molecular Science, Barts and The London School of Medicine and Dentistry,
Queen Mary University of London, London, United Kingdom

ANDREW D. GOODMAN, MD
Professor, Department of Neurology, University of Rochester School of Medicine
and Dentistry, Rochester, New York

KATHLEEN HAWKER, MD
Eli Lilly and Company, Lilly Corporate Center, Indianapolis, Indiana

PIERO IAFFALDANO, MD
Department of Neurological and Psychiatric Sciences, University of Bari, Bari, Italy

LAURA J. JULIAN, PhD
Assistant Professor of Medicine, Department of Medicine, University of California San
Francisco, San Francisco, California

MARIKO KITA, MD
Virginia Mason Multiple Sclerosis Center; Department of Neurology, University
of Washington School of Medicine, Seattle, Washington

LAUREN KRUPP, MD
Department of Neurology, National Pediatric MS Center, SUNY Stony Brook,
Stony Brook, New York

NANCY KUNTZ, MD
Associate Professor of Pediatrics and Neurology, Department of Pediatric Neurology,
Northwestern Feinberg School of Medicine, Children's Memorial Hospital, Chicago, Illinois

FRED D. LUBLIN, MD
Director, Corinne Goldsmith Dickinson Center for Multiple Sclerosis; Saunders
Family Professor of Neurology, Department of Neurology, Mount Sinai Medical Center,
New York, New York

GUGLIELMO LUCCHESE, MD
Department of Neurological and Psychiatric Sciences, University of Bari, Bari, Italy

RUTH ANN MARRIE, MD, PhD
Assistant Professor of Internal Medicine and Community Health Sciences,
University of Manitoba, Winnipeg, Manitoba, Canada

JAMES J. MARRIOTT, MD, FRCPC
Assistant Professor, Section of Neurology, University of Manitoba, Health Sciences
Centre, Winnipeg, Manitoba, Canada

JOSEPH P. MCELROY, PhD
Postdoctoral Researcher, Department of Neurology, School of Medicine,
University of California San Francisco, San Francisco, California

ELLEN M. MOWRY, MD, MCR
Assistant Professor of Neurology, Multiple Sclerosis Center, University of California
San Francisco, San Francisco, California

JAYNE NESS, MD, PhD
Associate Professor of Pediatrics, University of Alabama at Birmingham; Director,
Center for Pediatric Onset Demyelinating Disease, Children's Hospital of Alabama,
Birmingham, Alabama

PAUL W. O'CONNOR, MD, MSc, FRCPC
Professor, Division of Neurology, University of Toronto; Director, Department of
Neurology, MS Clinic and MS Research, St Michael's Hospital, Toronto,
Ontario, Canada

JORGE R. OKSENBERG, PhD
Professor in Residence, Department of Neurology, School of Medicine, University of
California San Francisco, San Francisco, California

DAMIANO PAOLICELLI, MD
Department of Neurological and Psychiatric Sciences, University of Bari, Bari, Italy

SREERAM V. RAMAGOPALAN, D. Phil
Wellcome Trust Centre for Human Genetics; Department of Clinical Neurology, University
of Oxford, Oxford, United Kingdom

CHRISTEL RENOUX, MD, PhD
Department of Medicine, Center for Clinical Epidemiology, Jewish General Hospital,
McGill University, Montreal, Quebec, Canada

PAVLE REPOVIC, MD, PhD
Neurologist, Multiple Sclerosis Center, Swedish Neuroscience Institute,
Seattle, Washington

MOSES RODRIGUEZ, MD
Mayo Clinic Pediatric Multiple Sclerosis Center, Mayo Clinic, Rochester, Minnesota

JENNIFER RUBIN, MD
Assistant Professor in Pediatrics, Department of Pediatric Neurology, Northwestern
Feinberg School of Medicine, Children's Memorial Hospital, Chicago, Illinois

A. DESSA SADOVNICK, PhD
Department of Medical Genetics, Faculty of Medicine; Division of Neurology,
University of British Columbia, Vancouver, Canada

KEN SAKAIE, PhD
Mellen Imaging Center, Imaging Institute, Cleveland, Ohio

LAWRENCE M. SAMKOFF, MD
Associate Professor, Department of Neurology, University of Rochester
School of Medicine and Dentistry, Rochester, New York

NANCY L. SICOTTE, MD
Associate Professor of Neurology, David Geffen School of Medicine at UCLA; Director,
Multiple Sclerosis Program, Cedars-Sinai Medical Center, Los Angeles, California

S. SIMPSON Jr, MPH
PhD Student, Menzies Research Institute, University of Tasmania, Hobart,
Tasmania, Australia

J. STANKOVICH, PhD
Research Fellow, Menzies Research Institute, University of Tasmania, Hobart,
Tasmania, Australia

JONATHAN B. STROBER, MD
Director, Pediatric Muscular Dystrophy Association Clinic; Associate Clinical Professor,
Neurology and Pediatrics UCSF, Division of Child Neurology, Department of Neurology,
University of California, San Francisco, San Francisco, California

B.V. TAYLOR, MD
Associate Professor of Neurology, Menzies Research Institute, University of Tasmania,
Hobart, Tasmania, Australia

CARLA TORTORELLA, MD
Department of Neurological and Psychiatric Sciences, University of Bari, Bari, Italy

MARIA TROJANO, MD
Department of Neurological and Psychiatric Sciences, University of Bari, Bari, Italy

I.A.F. VAN DER MEI, PhD
Research Fellow, Menzies Research Institute, University of Tasmania, Hobart,
Tasmania, Australia

EMMANUELLE L. WAUBANT, MD, PhD
Associate Professor, Department of Neurology; Director, UCSF Regional Pediatric MS
Center, University of California, San Francisco, San Francisco, California

BIANCA WEINSTOCK-GUTTMANN, MD
Associate Professor of Neurology, SUNY University of Buffalo; Director,
Baird MS Center and Pediatric MS Center of Excellence, Jacobs Neurological
Institute, Buffalo, New York

GREGORY F. WU, MD, PhD
Assistant Professor, Division of Multiple Sclerosis, Department of Neurology,
Washington University, St Louis, Missouri

ANN YEH, MD
Assistant Professor of Neurology and Pediatrics, Co-Director, Pediatric MS Center of
Excellence, Jacobs Neurological Institute, Buffalo, New York

Contents

promoting inflammatory damage of the central nervous system, B-cell involvement, and inflammatory damage of axons and neurons. This article preferentially focuses on MS rather than animal models of the disease, such as experimental autoimmune encephalomyelitis.

disease-modifying therapies and changes in specific health behaviors, in the broad context of coexisting health issues. Such information can facilitate appropriately adjusted comparisons within and between populations. Elucidation of these factors will require careful study of well-characterized populations in which the roles of multiple factors are considered simultaneously.

Magnetic Resonance Imaging in Multiple Sclerosis: The Role of Conventional Imaging   343

Nancy L. Sicotte

Magnetic resonance imaging (MRI) of the brain and spinal cord plays a central role in establishing the diagnosis of multiple sclerosis (MS), in monitoring disease activity, and as a key outcome measure in clinical trials of new MS therapies. Conventional MRI continues to evolve, reflecting advances in imaging hardware and software. These advances have led to important new insights into MS disease pathophysiology and can be used to improve patient management. Despite these improvements, standard MRI continues to capture only a small portion of the underlying changes that occur during the course of the disease.

Advanced MRI in Multiple Sclerosis: Current Status and Future Challenges   357

Robert J. Fox, Erik Beall, Pallab Bhattacharyya, Jacqueline T. Chen, and Ken Sakaie

MRI has rapidly become a leading research tool in the study of multiple sclerosis (MS). Conventional imaging is useful in diagnosis and management of the inflammatory stages of MS but has limitations in describing the degree of tissue injury and cause of progressive disability seen in later stages. Advanced MRI techniques hold promise for filling this void. These imaging tools hold great promise to increase understanding of MS pathogenesis and provide greater insight into the efficacy of new MS therapies.

Diagnosis of Multiple Sclerosis   381

Barbara S. Giesser

There is no pathognomonic symptom, sign, or paraclinical result that provides an unfailingly accurate diagnosis of multiple sclerosis (MS), and hence, MS remains largely a clinical diagnosis. However, being a clinical diagnosis does not mean that the diagnosis of MS is one of exclusion. Increasingly sophisticated guidelines and objective paraclinical findings are generally sufficient to allow the clinician to confirm or rule out the diagnosis with confidence. This article presents the most recent guidelines for using clinical, radiological, and other paraclinical information and the red flags that should alert the clinician to investigate other diagnostic possibilities.

Treatment of Multiple Sclerosis Exacerbations   389

Pavle Repovic and Fred D. Lublin

The understanding of the mechanisms that lead to MS exacerbations continues to produce novel treatments for patients with relapsing forms of MS. However, even with the most potent agents available, the exacerbations remain a distinct possibility and a source of concern for patients and clinicians. Therefore, the treatment of acute MS exacerbations remains an indispensable element of MS care. Reviewed here are the available treatment options, their implementation, side effects, and evidence supporting their efficacy in promoting recovery from MS relapses.

Relapsing-remitting multiple sclerosis is highly variable in its presentation and disease course. The approach to initiating first-line preventative therapies must focus on individualizing treatment strategies. Careful discussion of available treatment options and appropriate expectations regarding outcomes is important to ensure a successful start. Early treatment is recommended, as is on-going monitoring of patients who may choose to forego therapy.

Conventional disease-modifying agents are only moderately effective, so breakthrough disease activity is commonly seen. The evidence from randomized clinical trials and real-world observational data supporting the use of the second-line agents natalizumab, mitoxantrone, and cyclophosphamide are reviewed. Potential future treatment options are also discussed. Management algorithms for breakthrough disease are outlined.

Progressive multiple sclerosis (MS) consists of 3 phenotypic subtypes: secondary progressive MS, primary progressive MS, and progressive relapsing MS. There has been a paucity of approved treatments for these subtypes possibly driven by irreversible neurodegeneration within the central nervous system and not amenable to drugs that target inflammation. This article reviews magnetic resonance imaging and clinical data that show that progression may occur early in the course of MS and specific subsets of progressive patients may respond to disease modifying drugs.

Until recently, interferon beta and glatiramer acetate were the only licensed disease-modifying therapies for relapsing forms of multiple sclerosis. These agents have a modest effect on reducing relapse rates. The licensing of two more effective agents, mitoxantrone and natalizumab, provided alternatives. These agents are associated with potentially life-threatening or serious side effects. In addition, none of these licensed agents has been shown to be effective in primary progressive MS. There is a large unmet need, with several promising new therapies in the pipeline. This article reviews the proposed mechanisms of action of the anticipated treatments, their efficacy, and risks associated with their use.

FORTHCOMING ISSUES

RECENT ISSUES

RELATED INTEREST

THE CLINICS ARE NOW AVAILABLE ONLINE!

Access your subscription at:
www.theclinics.com

Preface
Multiple Sclerosis in the 21st Century

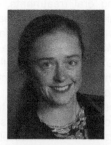

Emmanuelle L. Waubant, MD, PhD
Guest Editor

The face of multiple sclerosis (MS) has changed considerably over the past 10 years; thus, a special issue focusing on the disease was in order. Several conceptual shifts have occurred in the past decade that have resulted in improved understanding of disease processes that in turn have ultimately advanced patient care.

The consistent increase in MS incidence reported in various regions of the world in the past 50 years has triggered a renewed interest in the quest for susceptibility risk factors, as such a rapid change in incidence is unlikely explained by genetic risk factors. Large collaborative genetic studies have also thrived and accelerated the pace of discovery. The list of genetic polymorphisms that increase MS risk has considerably lengthened in the past 5 years and has opened new avenues of development for promising therapies. The understanding of risk factors and their complex interactions has been a flourishing research area that might result in implementing strategies for disease prevention in the future. The recognition that up to 5% of MS cases have their onset before the age of 18 years has led to new efforts to dissect specificities of disease phenotype in the younger age group. These efforts have directly resulted in improved diagnosis and broader use of adult-approved disease-modifying therapies in children, which will contribute to a better outcome. The understanding of the underlying molecular mechanisms that modify MS phenotype in very young patients may also in turn be important clues to disease processes.

In contrast with previously accepted paradigms, a neurodegenerative component of MS, even in relapsing forms and early after disease onset, has been consistently demonstrated in the past few years. This paradigm shift is the result of improved quantification of tissue loss with state-of-the-art imaging technology. Meanwhile, evidence for axonal and neuronal loss has strengthened, not only in MS lesions but also to a lesser extent in "normal-appearing white matter" as defined by conventional imaging. Furthermore, the concept of MS as a demyelinating disorder electively affecting the

Neurol Clin 29 (2011) xiii–xiv
doi:10.1016/j.ncl.2011.02.001
0733-8619/11/$ – see front matter © 2011 Elsevier Inc. All rights reserved.

neurologic.theclinics.com

deep white matter has progressively evolved as it is now obvious that the gray matter, both in the cortex and in the deep nuclei, is also undergoing tissue damage. Intriguingly, the pathophysiology of gray matter injury might be, at least in part, different from the one recognized for white matter injury.

Animal models and clinical trials have both contributed to unravel the critical role of B cells in disease processes, thus opening new avenues for treating our patients. Additional highly effective therapeutic strategies, including oral treatments, have been developed that target various critical discrete biological mechanisms leading to the recent and anticipated approval of three or more drugs. With the availability of these new effective disease-modifying therapies for MS, concerning rare side effects have emerged. Neurologists are thus now facing the relatively new challenge of balancing benefit and risk when treating their patients with MS and have to actively educate them so they can be involved in therapeutic decisions.

In parallel to clinical trials, several epidemiological studies have contributed to our understanding of factors that may worsen disease course such as low vitamin D status and smoking. Some of these factors, such as 25(OH) vitamin D serum level, are amenable to adjustment and have in turn developed into clinical trials that will confirm whether inexpensive supplementation strategies can decrease disease activity.

Finally, the increased recognition of disabling MS symptoms including fatigue, cognitive, and emotional problems has contributed to the development of multidisciplinary care for patients with MS. In this 21st century model of care, patients play a more active role in the management of their disease, and their continuous education by the team of care providers becomes central to the effectiveness of the delivered care and to their overall quality of life.

Emmanuelle L. Waubant, MD, PhD
Department of Neurology
UCSF School of Medicine
350 Parnassus Avenue
San Francisco, CA 94117, USA

E-mail address:
Emmanuelle.waubant@ucsf.edu

Epidemiology of Multiple Sclerosis

Sreeram V. Ramagopalan, D. Phil[a,b], A. Dessa Sadovnick, PhD[c,d],*

KEYWORDS

- Multiple sclerosis • Risk factors • Sex ratio • Birth cohort
- Gene-environment interactions

Multiple sclerosis (MS) is the most common disease of the central nervous system that causes permanent disability in young adults.[1] Based on strong circumstantial evidence, MS is considered to be an organ-specific autoimmune disorder,[1,2] but much remains to be understood about the initiation of the disease. It seems unlikely that MS results from a single causative event, but rather the disease develops in a genetically susceptible population as a result of environmental exposures. Epidemiologic studies have been highly informative in trying to understand the nature, contribution, and interaction of genetic and environmental factors in MS. Reproducibility of results is most dependent on avoiding nonrandom ascertainment. As a general note, the method of sampling cases, controls, and families (ascertainment) in epidemiologic studies is critical. Ascertainment through hospitals[3] or volunteer appeals is easier but often results in overrepresentation of increased severity, women, and relatives concordant for the disease.[4] Correcting for bias is difficult.[5] Valid conclusions require population-based studies.[6]

RISK FACTORS FOR MS
Genetic

The development of MS starts in individuals who are genetically susceptible. Studies such as the US Veterans series that controlled for confounding factors showed lower prevalence of MS in certain races such as African American (African American men were shown to have an approximate 40% lower MS risk than white men), Native

[a] The Wellcome Trust Centre for Human Genetics, University of Oxford, Roosevelt Drive, Oxford OX3 7BN, UK
[b] Department of Clinical Neurology, John Radcliffe Hospital, University of Oxford, Level 3 West Wing, Oxford OX3 9DU, UK
[c] Department of Medical Genetics, Faculty of Medicine, University of British Columbia, VCHA-UBC Hospital, S113-2211 Wesbrook Mall, Vancouver, British Columbia V6T 2B5, Canada
[d] Division of Neurology, University of British Columbia, VCHA-UBC Hospital, S113-2211 Wesbrook Mall, Vancouver, British Columbia V6T 2B5, Canada
* Corresponding author. Department of Medical Genetics, Faculty of Medicine, University of British Columbia, VCHA-UBC Hospital, S113-2211 Wesbrook Mall, Vancouver, British Columbia V6T 2B5, Canada.
E-mail address: sadovnik@infinet.net

Neurol Clin 29 (2011) 207–217
doi:10.1016/j.ncl.2010.12.010
0733-8619/11/$ – see front matter © 2011 Elsevier Inc. All rights reserved.

American, Mexican, Puerto Rican Japanese, Chinese, and Filipino.[7] This race effect is almost certainly genetically determined.

The importance of genetic factors in MS susceptibility has been demonstrated by genetic epidemiologic studies.[8] Family studies assessing risks to relatives of patients with MS have revealed a marked familial aggregation of the disease. First-degree relatives are generally at a 15 to 35 times greater risk of developing MS than the general population. This risk correlates with the degree of kinship, that is, the amount of sharing DNA identical by descent (**Fig. 1**).[9,10] Nevertheless, familial clustering of a disease is not sufficient to infer the importance of genetics because environmental influences also aggregate in families.

Several strategies have been used to dissect the environmental from the genetic components underlying MS susceptibility. Studies of MS in conjugal pairs[11,12] have shown that spouses of patients with MS develop MS no more often than the background general population. Together with data from half siblings raised together or apart,[13] step siblings,[14] and adoptees,[15] these studies provide no evidence for environmental factors operative within the familial microenvironment, either in childhood or adulthood. Thus, genetics is responsible for most, if not all, of the familial aggregation of MS.

Several small studies have suggested that patients with MS and their first-degree relatives are at an increased risk of other autoimmune diseases, implicating common genes between autoimmune disorders[16]; but this hypothesis has not been proven in a large population-based study.[17]

Genetic variation in the major human histocompatibility system (HLA being an acronym for human leukocyte antigens), a region on chromosome 6, exerts the strongest genetic effect in MS. However, the association is not straightforward with complex gene-gene interactions at play.[18] Genome-wide association studies, which have subsequently been replicated,[19,20] have uncovered several other genes of modest effect (odds ratios [ORs] in the range of 1.2) in MS, including the interleukin 7 receptor alpha and interleukin 2 receptor alpha genes.[19]

The half sibling studies found that the risk for maternal half siblings was 2.35% compared with 1.31% for paternal half siblings. These findings are taken to implicate

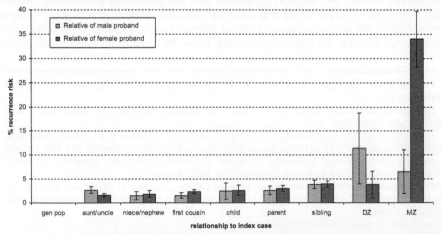

Fig. 1. Age-adjusted percentage recurrence risks for relatives of probands with MS. (*Data from* Willer CJ, Dyment DA, Risch NJ, et al. Twin concordance and sibling recurrence rates in multiple sclerosis. Proc Natl Acad Sci U S A 2003;100:12877–82.)

a maternal effect in disease susceptibility, despite the mothers not having MS.[13] This finding has since been confirmed in a Dutch extended pedigree,[21] a study of avuncular pairs,[22] and an investigation of interracial matings.[23] The maternal effect in MS is substantial. The risk for MS in siblings who share only a mother does not differ significantly (2.35% vs 3.11%, $P = .1$) from the risk for full siblings, indicating that maternal effects might even be the major component of familial aggregation. The mechanism of the increased risk conferred maternally remains to be elucidated but epigenetic mechanisms (DNA and chromatin alterations, including DNA methylation of C-G dinucleotides and histone modifications, that regulate genomic function[24]) are strongly implicated.[25]

Environmental

Although genes are needed for MS to develop, genetic epidemiologic studies clearly illustrate the predominant role of the environment in determining MS risk. Some environmental risk factors for MS must act at a very early period because some factors at the beginning of life are determinants of MS risk.

Latitude

Within regions of temperate climate, MS incidence and prevalence increases with latitude.[26] The clearest example of this effect is seen in Australia.[27] The prevalence of MS in Hobart is 75.6 per 100,000 compared with a prevalence of 11 per 100,000 in northern Queensland.[27] However, more complex patterns of disease distribution do exist. In Norway, for example, MS prevalence does not increase with latitude; prevalence here correlates with proximity to coastal fishing areas and subsequent fish consumption.[28] Some of the geographic distribution of MS can be explained by ethnicity and genetic factors,[29] but latitude remains the strongest risk for risk after controlling for ethnicity.[30] However, the latitude effect does seem to be decreasing to some extent over the last few decades[30] (relative risk of MS of 2.02 when comparing residence in northern US states with southern US states for Vietnam veterans; this risk was 2.64 for the earlier-born World War II veterans). Recent studies have clearly shown that the prevalence of MS in low-risk regions in areas nearer the equator is increasing. To illustrate, this finding has been clearly shown in South America[31–33] and Spain.[34]

Place of birth

The effects of migration between high- and low-risk geographic regions for MS have been examined in several populations. Although there is potential for migration bias, these studies consistently show that MS risk is influenced at least to some extent by the migrant's country of origin.[35] Despite the limits of small sample sizes, a critical age has been hypothesized; immigrants who migrate before adolescence acquire the risk of their new country, whereas those who migrate after adolescence retain the risk of their home country.[36] However, the Australian data have suggested that this critical age may extend into adult life.[37] The influence of the place of birth is further highlighted by the fact that first-generation Afro-Caribbean and Asian immigrants to Britain have a much lower incidence of MS than their second-generation counterparts born in the United Kingdom.[38] Additional support comes from space-time cluster analysis on the location of a cohort of patients with MS in Sardinia, revealing that patients were significantly more likely to live near one another between the ages of 1 and 3 years.[39]

Sex

Observed temporal increases in prevalence/incidence of MS virtually worldwide[31] have been reported, but whether this finding represents true increases or artifacts associated with improved and earlier diagnosis has long been questioned. A female-specific increase in the incidence of MS has been documented.[30,40,41] A recent Canadian study showed that this increase was real and not an artifact related to changes in ascertainment.[42] The year of birth was shown to be a significant predictor of the female:male sex ratio of MS over the period 1931 to 1980, with the ratio increasing from 1.9 to 3.2 during this time (**Fig. 2**).[42] Although sex ratio data do not identify reasons for these changes, they are useful in addressing various theories. For example, any short-term fluctuations caused by putative sex-specific delays in diagnosis should be serially washed out in the Canadian study because of the length of the observations and the use of a year-of-birth analytical approach.[42] Furthermore, although women have a slightly earlier onset than men, their time from clinical onset to diagnosis in Canada is identical (mean of 3 years in each group). The extent of the change in sex ratio, its progressive nature, and use of year of birth as the predicting variable make it unlikely that the findings could be explained by any artifact related to ascertainment. This female-specific increasing incidence of MS has since been confirmed in several other populations.[43–45]

Month of birth

The relative risk of developing MS north of the equator for people born in May is 1.18 (95% confidence interval [CI], 1.10–1.30) compared with 0.89 (95% CI, 0.81–0.98) for

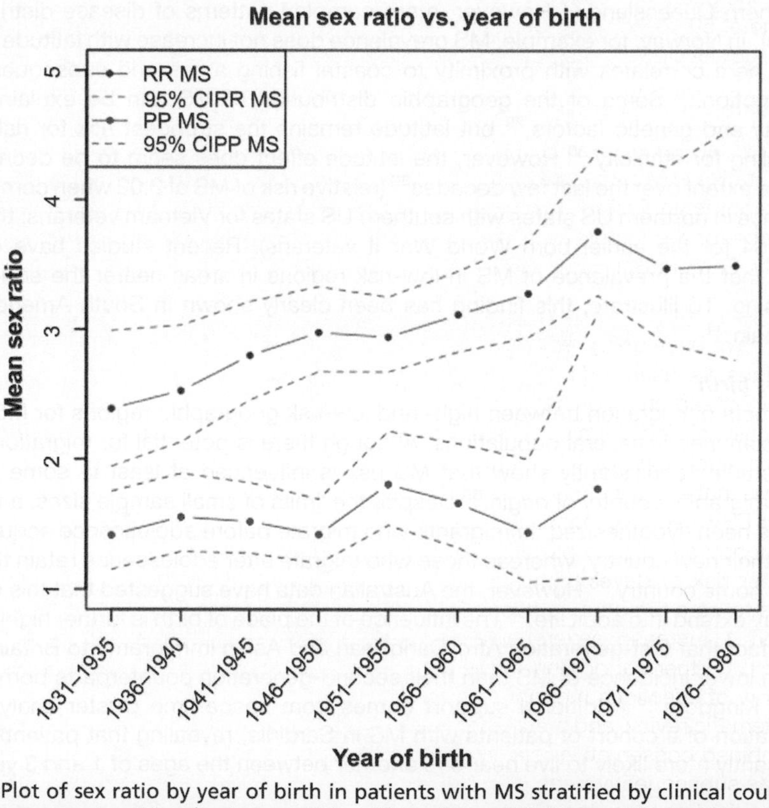

Mean sex ratio vs. year of birth

Fig. 2. Plot of sex ratio by year of birth in patients with MS stratified by clinical course. PP, primary progressive; RR, relapsing remitting. (*From* Orton SM, Herrera BM, Yee IM, et al. Sex ratio of multiple sclerosis in Canada: a longitudinal study. Lancet Neurol 2006;5(11):933; with permission.)

those born in November.[46] Variation in the deviation pattern of MS births by latitude supports an ultraviolet effect. Indeed, this effect was observed in Sicily[47] and in individuals born in the southern hemisphere,[46] but conflictingly, the month-of-birth effect in Sardinia was similar to that of northern Europeans.[48] The month-of-birth effect is more pronounced in Scotland, with 31% more MS births in April and 20% fewer births in November ($P = .001$).[49]

Hygiene hypothesis

In developed countries, strong evidence of steady increases in incidence of allergic and some autoimmune diseases parallels a decreasing incidence of childhood infections. Antibiotics, vaccination, or improved hygiene and better socioeconomic conditions have been credited. The hygiene hypothesis proposing that early-life infections downregulate allergic and autoimmune disorders[50] was not supported for MS, that is, siblings with MS are not more likely to be born early in birth order.[51]

Later-acting environmental factors

Because the average age of onset of MS is approximately 30 years, there is a long period from birth to MS diagnosis for the environment to act. Migration data highlight adolescence as being important, further illustrated by associations of the age of menarche and adolescent obesity with MS.[52,53] Other epidemiologic studies (eg, occupational data) suggest influences of the environment extending into adult life.[54] The chances of developing MS is age-related and decrease precipitously after the age of 50 years[55]; so, whatever risk factors that do play a role must be unable to incite the development of MS after a certain time point.

Candidate Environmental Risk Factors in MS

Although the earlier-mentioned data point to when environmental factors are likely to be operative in MS, the authors still do not have unequivocal evidence for the identity of environmental factors involved. In the following sections, the authors summarize the evidence for the factors with the strongest evidence for involvement in MS etiology, namely, Epstein-Barr virus (EBV), vitamin D, and smoking.

EBV

There have been many reports suggesting an association between 1 or more of these infectious diseases and MS,[56,57] but the epidemiologic data associating EBV infection with MS stand on its own for replication.

Virtually all individuals with MS (>99%) are infected with EBV compared with approximately 94% of age-matched control individuals.[58] The corollary to this observation is that MS is very rare in adults who are not infected with EBV; the relative risk of MS for EBV-negative individuals is very low (OR, 0.06; 95% CI, 0.03–0.13).[58,59] Levels of antibody are also important. People with high titers of anti-EBV antibodies have a higher risk of developing MS compared with subjects with low titres.[60,61] There seems to be a temporal relationship, plasma antibody titers against the EBV nuclear antigen 1 increase several years before the onset of neurologic symptoms of MS.[60,61] Further supporting a role for EBV in MS is the finding that individuals with a history of infectious mononucleosis (IM) have an increased risk of developing MS. A systematic review and meta-analysis of 14 case-control and cohort studies reported a combined conservative relative risk of MS after IM of 2.3 (95% CI, 1.7–3.0).[55] This risk has subsequently been confirmed in large population-based studies.[62,63]

In pediatric cases, there is a weaker association between EBV infection and the development of MS. In a North American study, 108 (86%) of the children with MS were seropositive for remote EBV infection compared with only 61 (64%) of matched controls.[64] In a European seroprevalence study of 147 pediatric patients, 99% with MS had detectable antibody against EBV compared with only 72% of age-matched controls.[65] The observation that the EBV seroprevalence rate in the American pediatric cohort with MS is not 100% is a strong argument against the association between EBV and MS being causative. However, it is more difficult to diagnose MS in children, and there remains some uncertainty about the nosology of MS in this group. Therefore, it is critical to establish with long-term follow-up if EBV-seronegative children with a diagnosis of MS turn out to have typical MS seen in adults. There is also an apparent paradox in that EBV infection in pediatric patients with MS increases risk, whereas in adult-onset MS, delayed infection, as manifested by IM, is associated.

Vitamin D

Sunlight exposure and associated vitamin D status are potential explanations for the link between geography, in particular latitude, and the incidence of MS.[66] Levels of past sun exposure are inversely related to MS susceptibility (adjusted OR for high summer sun exposure [2–3 hours per day] during childhood and adolescence is 0.31 (95% CI, 0.16–0.59).[67] Questionnaire-based studies are prone to recall bias, but a confirmation of an effect of sun exposure on MS was seen when using the objective measure of actinic damage. Greater actinic damage is associated with a decreased risk of MS (OR, 0.32; 95% CI, 0.11–0.88 for grades 4–6 of damage); however, the timing of damage could not be determined in this retrospective study.

Experimental and epidemiologic data suggest that vitamin D is the mediator of the sunlight effect. There has also been the suggestion that in animal models, sun exposure immunomodulates dendritic cell/antiphospholipid syndrome, a pathway that could possibly be vitamin D independent.[68]

It was noted many years ago that the consumption of fatty seafood and cod liver oil in Norway, both rich sources of vitamin D, provided protection against the risk of MS,[28] although this outcome may also arise from the biologic effects of omega-3 fatty acids. A prospective cohort study found that taking vitamin supplementation that included vitamin D was associated with an approximate 40% reduction in the risk of developing MS,[69] but the amounts of vitamin D[69] taken are thought to be insufficient to make much change in circulating vitamin D levels, and effects of multivitamin intake may be confounded by behavioral differences. The strongest evidence for a role for vitamin D comes from a prospective nested case-control study in military personnel in the United States, who had serum samples stored, which showed that a lower risk of MS was associated with high serum 25-hydroxyvitamin D levels.[70] In whites, the risk of developing MS decreased significantly with increasing levels of 25-hydroxyvitamin D (OR for a 50-nmol/L increase in 25-hydroxyvitamin D is 0.59 (95% CI, 0.36–0.97).[71]

Smoking

A recent retrospective meta-analysis gave a pooled relative risk estimate for developing MS of 1.51 (95% CI, 1.24–1.83) for ever versus never smoking,[72] and earlier studies showed a dose-dependent (ie, number of cigarettes smoked) relationship to MS risk.[73] Swedish snuff use does not increase the risk of MS (OR, 0.3; 95% CI, 0.1–0.8), suggesting factors present in smoked tobacco or the route of administration as being important.[74]

SUMMARY

The cause of MS is still unclear, but it is now recognized that the degree of complexity of MS is beyond what was believed even up to 10 to 15 years ago. The complexity arises because the expression of the phenotype cannot be predicted from knowledge of the individual effects of the single factors considered alone. Genes, environment, postgenomic modifications, and chance all interact.

The associated risk factors for MS seem to delineate a putative causal cascade. Factors largely defined from birth (ie, sex, HLA antigen status, place of birth) need inciting environmental factors (vitamin D deficiency, late EBV exposure) to develop the abnormalities required, which subsequently can lead to MS. The latitude effect (early life) and IM associations (adolescence) support the notion that vitamin D deficiency precedes EBV infection,[75] but the Australian migration data and the evidence for vitamin D related influences on risk during adult life (eg, outdoor occupations decrease MS risk)[76] suggest that vitamin D has the potential to play a role over a wider period. It is not yet clear whether MS susceptibility is a result of a chain of adverse factors that need to occur in a specific order and are dependent on one another (ie, a domino effect) or whether risk factors are independent of each other but each acting in either an additive/multiplicative manner to push an individual closer to the threshold of developing MS. The fact that no factor has yet to be shown to be present in all patients with MS, with the possible exception of EBV in adult-onset MS, suggests that causal pathways likely differ in individuals and support the latter hypothesis.

Although some progress has been made, our understanding of the stages involved in the development of MS is still limited. Further study is required to understand the causal pathway of MS to prevent this often devastating disease.

REFERENCES

1. Noseworthy JH, Lucchinetti C, Rodriguez M, et al. Multiple sclerosis. N Engl J Med 2000;343(13):938–52.
2. Giovannoni G, Ebers G. Multiple sclerosis: the environment and causation. Curr Opin Neurol 2007;20(3):261–8.
3. Torgersen S. Genetics of neurosis. The effects of sampling variation upon the twin concordance ratio. Br J Psychiatry 1983;142:126–32.
4. Bundey S. Uses and limitations of twin studies. J Neurol 1991;238(7):360–4.
5. Olson JM, Cordell HJ. Ascertainment bias in the estimation of sibling genetic risk parameters. Genet Epidemiol 2000;18(3):217–35.
6. Ellsworth DL, Manolio TA. The emerging importance of genetics in epidemiologic research II. Issues in study design and gene mapping. Ann Epidemiol 1999;9(2): 75–90.
7. Kurtzke JF, Beebe GW, Norman JE Jr. Epidemiology of multiple sclerosis in U.S. veterans: 1. Race, sex, and geographic distribution. Neurology 1979;29(9 Pt 1): 1228–35.
8. Dyment DA, Ebers GC, Sadovnick AD. Genetics of multiple sclerosis. Lancet Neurol 2004;3(2):104–10.
9. Sadovnick AD, Baird PA, Ward RH. Multiple sclerosis: updated risks for relatives. Am J Med Genet 1988;29(3):533–41.
10. Willer CJ, Dyment DA, Risch NJ, et al. Twin concordance and sibling recurrence rates in multiple sclerosis. Proc Natl Acad Sci U S A 2003;100(22): 12877–82.
11. Robertson NP, O'Riordan JI, Chataway J, et al. Offspring recurrence rates and clinical characteristics of conjugal multiple sclerosis. Lancet 1997;349(9065): 1587–90.

12. Ebers GC, Yee IM, Sadovnick AD, et al. Conjugal multiple sclerosis: population-based prevalence and recurrence risks in offspring. Canadian Collaborative Study Group. Ann Neurol 2000;48(6):927–31.
13. Ebers GC, Sadovnick AD, Dyment DA, et al. Parent-of-origin effect in multiple sclerosis: observations in half-siblings. Lancet 2004;363(9423):1773–4.
14. Dyment DA, Yee IM, Ebers GC, et al. Multiple sclerosis in stepsiblings: recurrence risk and ascertainment. J Neurol Neurosurg Psychiatry 2006;77(2):258–9.
15. Ebers GC, Sadovnick AD, Risch NJ. A genetic basis for familial aggregation in multiple sclerosis. Canadian Collaborative Study Group. Nature 1995;377(6545): 150–1.
16. Broadley SA, Deans J, Sawcer SJ, et al. Autoimmune disease in first-degree relatives of patients with multiple sclerosis. A UK survey. Brain 2000;123(Pt 6): 1102–11.
17. Ramagopalan SV, Dyment DA, Valdar W, et al. Autoimmune disease in families with multiple sclerosis: a population-based study. Lancet Neurol 2007;6(7): 604–10.
18. Ramagopalan SV, Ebers GC. Epistasis: multiple sclerosis and the major histocompatibility complex. Neurology 2009;72(6):566–7.
19. De Jager PL, Jia X, Wang J, et al. Meta-analysis of genome scans and replication identify CD6, IRF8 and TNFRSF1A as new multiple sclerosis susceptibility loci. Nat Genet 2009;41(7):776–82.
20. Hafler DA, Compston A, Sawcer S, et al. Risk alleles for multiple sclerosis identified by a genomewide study. N Engl J Med 2007;357(9):851–62.
21. Hoppenbrouwers IA, Liu F, Aulchenko YS, et al. Maternal transmission of multiple sclerosis in a Dutch population. Arch Neurol 2008;65(3):345–8.
22. Herrera BM, Ramagopalan SV, Lincoln MR, et al. Parent-of-origin effects in MS. Observations from avuncular pairs. Neurology 2008;71:799–803.
23. Ramagopalan SV, Yee IM, Dyment DA, et al. Parent-of-origin effect in multiple sclerosis. Observations from interracial matings. Neurology 2009;73:602–5.
24. Handel AE, Ebers GC, Ramagopalan SV. Epigenetics: molecular mechanisms and implications for disease. Trends Mol Med 2010;16(1):7–16.
25. Chao MJ, Ramagopalan SV, Herrera BM, et al. Epigenetics in multiple sclerosis susceptibility: difference in transgenerational risk localizes to the major histocompatibility complex. Hum Mol Genet 2009;18(2):261–6.
26. Kurtzke JF. Geographic distribution of multiple sclerosis: an update with special reference to Europe and the Mediterranean region. Acta Neurol Scand 1980; 62(2):65–80.
27. Hammond SR, McLeod JG, Millingen KS, et al. The epidemiology of multiple sclerosis in three Australian cities: Perth, Newcastle and Hobart. Brain 1988;111(Pt 1): 1–25.
28. Kampman MT, Brustad M. Vitamin D: a candidate for the environmental effect in multiple sclerosis—observations from Norway. Neuroepidemiology 2008;30(3): 140–6.
29. Weinstock-Guttman B, Jacobs LD, Brownscheidle CM, et al. Multiple sclerosis characteristics in African American patients in the New York State Multiple Sclerosis Consortium. Mult Scler 2003;9(3):293–8.
30. Wallin MT, Page WF, Kurtzke JF. Multiple sclerosis in US veterans of the Vietnam era and later military service: race, sex, and geography. Ann Neurol 2004;55(1): 65–71.
31. Christiano E, Patrucco L, Rojas JI. A systematic review of the epidemiology of multiple sclerosis in South America. Eur J Neurol 2008;15(12):1273–8.

32. Cristiano E, Patrucco L, Rojas JI, et al. Prevalence of multiple sclerosis in Buenos Aires, Argentina using the capture-recapture method. Eur J Neurol 2009;16(2): 183–7.
33. Abad P, Pérez M, Castro E, et al. Prevalence of multiple sclerosis in Ecuador. Neurologia 2010;25(5):309–13.
34. Otero S, Batlle J, Bonaventura I, et al. Multiple sclerosis epidemiological situation update: pertinence and set-up of a population based registry of new cases in Catalonia. Rev Neurol 2010;50(10):623–33.
35. Dean G, Elian M. Age at immigration to England of Asian and Caribbean immigrants and the risk of developing multiple sclerosis. J Neurol Neurosurg Psychiatry 1997;63(5):565–8.
36. Dean G. Annual incidence, prevalence, and mortality of multiple sclerosis in white South-African-born and in white immigrants to South Africa. Br Med J 1967; 2(5554):724–30.
37. Hammond SR, English DR, McLeod JG. The age-range of risk of developing multiple sclerosis: evidence from a migrant population in Australia. Brain 2000; 123(Pt 5):968–74.
38. Elian M, Nightingale S, Dean G. Multiple sclerosis among United Kingdom-born children of immigrants from the Indian subcontinent, Africa and the West Indies. J Neurol Neurosurg Psychiatry 1990;53(10):906–11.
39. Pugliatti M, Riise T, Sotgiu MA, et al. Evidence of early childhood as the susceptibility period in multiple sclerosis: space-time cluster analysis in a Sardinian population. Am J Epidemiol 2006;164(4):326–33.
40. Barnett MH, Williams DB, Day S, et al. Progressive increase in incidence and prevalence of multiple sclerosis in Newcastle, Australia: a 35-year study. J Neurol Sci 2003;213(1/2):1–6.
41. Grytten N, Glad SB, Aarseth JH, et al. A 50-year follow-up of the incidence of multiple sclerosis in Hordaland County, Norway. Neurology 2006;66(2): 182–6.
42. Orton SM, Herrera BM, Yee IM, et al. Sex ratio of multiple sclerosis in Canada: a longitudinal study. Lancet Neurol 2006;5(11):932–6.
43. Hirst C, Ingram G, Pickersgill T, et al. Increasing prevalence and incidence of multiple sclerosis in South East Wales. J Neurol Neurosurg Psychiatry 2009; 80(4):386–91.
44. Alonso A, Hernan MA. Temporal trends in the incidence of multiple sclerosis: a systematic review. Neurology 2008;71(2):129–35.
45. Debouverie M, Pittion-Vouyovitch S, Louis S, et al. Increasing incidence of multiple sclerosis among women in Lorraine, Eastern France. Mult Scler 2007; 13(8):962–7.
46. Willer CJ, Dyment DA, Sadovnick AD, et al. Timing of birth and risk of multiple sclerosis: population based study. BMJ 2005;330(7483):120.
47. Salemi G, Ragonese P, Aridon P, et al. Is season of birth associated with multiple sclerosis? Acta Neurol Scand 2000;101(6):381–3.
48. Sotgiu S, Pugliatti M, Sotgiu MA, et al. Seasonal fluctuation of multiple sclerosis births in Sardinia. J Neurol 2006;253(1):38–44.
49. Bayes HK, Weir CJ, O'Leary C. Timing of birth and risk of multiple sclerosis in the Scottish population. Eur Neurol 2009;63(1):36–40.
50. Bach JF. The effect of infections on susceptibility to autoimmune and allergic diseases. N Engl J Med 2002;347(12):911–20.
51. Sadovnick AD, Yee IM, Ebers GC. Multiple sclerosis and birth order: a longitudinal cohort study. Lancet Neurol 2005;4(10):611–7.

52. Ramagopalan SV, Valdar W, Criscuoli M, et al. Age of puberty and the risk of multiple sclerosis: a population based study. Eur J Neurol 2009;16(3): 342–7.
53. Munger KL, Chitnis T, Ascherio A. Body size and risk of MS in two cohorts of US women. Neurology 2009;73(19):1543–50.
54. Freedman DM, Dosemeci M, Alavanja MC. Mortality from multiple sclerosis and exposure to residential and occupational solar radiation: a case-control study based on death certificates. Occup Environ Med 2000;57(6):418–21.
55. Paty DW, Ebers GC. Multiple sclerosis. Philadelphia: Davis; 1998.
56. Pekmezovic T, Jarebinski M, Drulovic J. Childhood infections as risk factors for multiple sclerosis: Belgrade case-control study. Neuroepidemiology 2004;23(6): 285–8.
57. Tarrats R, Ordonez G, Rios C, et al. Varicella, ephemeral breastfeeding and eczema as risk factors for multiple sclerosis in Mexicans. Acta Neurol Scand 2002;105(2):88–94.
58. Ascherio A, Munger KL. Environmental risk factors for multiple sclerosis. Part I: the role of infection. Ann Neurol 2007;61(4):288–99.
59. Thacker EL, Mirzaei F, Ascherio A. Infectious mononucleosis and risk for multiple sclerosis: a meta-analysis. Ann Neurol 2006;59(3):499–503.
60. Sundstrom P, Juto P, Wadell G, et al. An altered immune response to Epstein-Barr virus in multiple sclerosis: a prospective study. Neurology 2004;62(12): 2277–82.
61. Levin LI, Munger KL, Rubertone MV, et al. Temporal relationship between elevation of Epstein-Barr virus antibody titers and initial onset of neurological symptoms in multiple sclerosis. JAMA 2005;293(20):2496–500.
62. Nielsen TR, Rostgaard K, Nielsen NM, et al. Multiple sclerosis after infectious mononucleosis. Arch Neurol 2007;64(1):72–5.
63. Ramagopalan SV, Valdar W, Dyment DA, et al. Association of infectious mononucleosis with multiple sclerosis. A population-based study. Neuroepidemiology 2009;32(4):257–62.
64. Banwell B, Krupp L, Kennedy J, et al. Clinical features and viral serologies in children with multiple sclerosis: a multinational observational study. Lancet Neurol 2007;6(9):773–81.
65. Pohl D, Krone B, Rostasy K, et al. High seroprevalence of Epstein-Barr virus in children with multiple sclerosis. Neurology 2006;67(11):2063–5.
66. Acheson ED, Bachrach CA, Wright FM. Some comments on the relationship of the distribution of multiple sclerosis to latitude, solar radiation, and other variables. Acta Psychiatr Scand Suppl 1960;35(147):132–47.
67. van der Mei IA, Ponsonby AL, Dwyer T, et al. Past exposure to sun, skin phenotype, and risk of multiple sclerosis: case-control study. BMJ 2003; 327(7410):316.
68. Simon JC, Tigelaar RE, Bergstresser PR, et al. Ultraviolet B radiation converts Langerhans cells from immunogenic to tolerogenic antigen-presenting cells. Induction of specific clonal anergy in CD4+ T helper 1 cells. J Immunol 1991; 146(2):485–91.
69. Munger KL, Zhang SM, O'Reilly E, et al. Vitamin D intake and incidence of multiple sclerosis. Neurology 2004;62(1):60–5.
70. Vieth R, Cole DE, Hawker GA, et al. Wintertime vitamin D insufficiency is common in young Canadian women, and their vitamin D intake does not prevent it. Eur J Clin Nutr 2001;55(12):1091–7.

71. Munger KL, Levin LI, Hollis BW, et al. Serum 25-hydroxyvitamin D levels and risk of multiple sclerosis. JAMA 2006;296(23):2832–8.
72. Hawkes CH. Smoking is a risk factor for multiple sclerosis: a metanalysis. Mult Scler 2007;13(5):610–5.
73. Hernan MA, Olek MJ, Ascherio A. Cigarette smoking and incidence of multiple sclerosis. Am J Epidemiol 2001;154(1):69–74.
74. Hedstrom AK, Baarnhielm M, Olsson T, et al. Tobacco smoking, but not Swedish snuff use, increases the risk of multiple sclerosis. Neurology 2009;73(9):696–701.
75. Goodin DS. The causal cascade to multiple sclerosis: a model for MS pathogenesis. PLoS One 2009;4(2):e4565.
76. Ascherio A, Munger KL. Environmental risk factors for multiple sclerosis. Part II: noninfectious factors. Ann Neurol 2007;61(6):504–13.

Multiple Sclerosis Genetics 2010

Joseph P. McElroy, PhD*, Jorge R. Oksenberg, PhD

KEYWORDS

• Multiple sclerosis • Genetics • Review
• Genome-wide association

Extensive epidemiologic data in the form of familial disease aggregation and differential disease incidence across ancestral groups suggested that genetic variation is an important determinant of susceptibility to multiple sclerosis (MS) (**Box 1**). A broad consensus has since emerged clustering MS with the so-called complex genetic disorders, a group of relatively frequent diseases characterized by moderate heritability, the involvement of common DNA variants each with modest effects on the total risk, and multifaceted gene–environment interactions (**Fig. 1**). Although the polygenic model of MS genetics provided for many years a useful conceptual framework to study the disease, classical genetic techniques were largely ineffective when searching for susceptibility genes because of underpowered datasets, disease heterogeneity, and the absence of large extended families showing a clear and homogeneous mode of transmission. The singular exception is the human leukocyte antigen (*HLA*) gene cluster in chromosome 6p21.3. *HLA* represents by far the strongest MS susceptibility locus genome-wide, and was unambiguously identified by candidate gene association and linkage approaches (**Fig. 2**). The primary signal arises from the *HLA-DRB1* gene in the class II segment of the locus, with hierarchical allelic and haplotypic effects, complex epistatic interactions across the locus, and independent protective signals in the class I region.[1,2]

Large, multicenter DNA collections have prospered as the development of new laboratory and analytical approaches has matured at a remarkable pace, allowing the pursuit of comprehensive "agnostic" genome-wide association studies (GWAS) to identify and characterize the non-*HLA* genetic component of MS. This article summarizes the new knowledge gained from this experimental approach.

THE AGE OF THE MS GWAS

The objective of GWAS is to identify DNA variants located across the genome that are unevenly distributed between a group of unrelated individual carriers of a quantifiable

The authors have nothing to disclose.
Department of Neurology, School of Medicine, University of California at San Francisco, 513 Parnassus Avenue, San Francisco, CA 94143, USA
* Corresponding author.
E-mail address: Joseph.McElroy@ucsf.edu

Neurol Clin 29 (2011) 219–231
doi:10.1016/j.ncl.2010.12.002
0733-8619/11/$ – see front matter © 2011 Elsevier Inc. All rights reserved.

Box 1
Epidemiologic evidence for genetic effects on MS

- Prevalence of MS differs by ethnic group[3]
- MS aggregates in families[4–7]
- Adopted (not genetically related) relatives living with a patient with MS do not have a corresponding increase in risk for developing MS[8]
- No difference in risk exists between half-siblings of patients with MS raised with or apart from the patient[9]
- Monozygotic twins have a higher concordance rate than dizygotic twins (25%–30% and 2%–5%, respectively)[10–12]

---

trait and an unrelated group of unrelated controls. Assay miniaturization allows these screens to be performed rapidly for large number of markers in large number of individuals. The arrays typically contain probes for polymorphisms selected based on frequency and linkage disequilibrium parameters to efficiently capture large portions of common variation across the genome. Thus, the selected polymorphisms act as surrogate markers of the broad genomic loci putatively associated with the trait of interest. Given the very large number of simultaneous tests in each study (>10^6 with

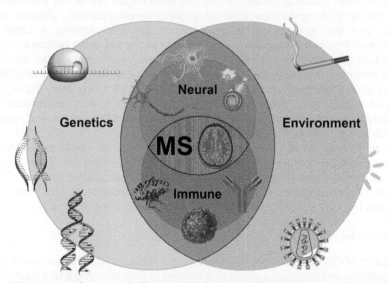

Fig. 1. MS as a complex genetic disease. MS shares much in common with other complex genetic disorders, defined as those with a polygenic heritable component, epistatic interactions, either programmed or stochastic, of two or more genes, several of postgenomic DNA changes, and multifaceted interactions, with environmental factors. This category includes most of the common diseases (cancer, cardiovascular diseases, behavior disorders, allergies, autoimmunity; the so-called diseases of civilization). In MS, genetically susceptible individuals (with genetic variants resulting in differences in gene expression and/or protein conformation from nonsusceptible individuals) exposed to a ubiquitous environmental factor or factors have corresponding changes in the neural and immune compartments that perpetuate inflammation leading to tissue injury, neurodegeneration, and neurologic deficits.

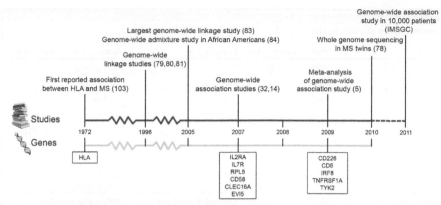

Fig. 2. Timeline of genetic research into MS. Modeling the available data predicts that the MS-prone genotype results from multiple interacting polymorphic genes, each exerting a small or at most a moderate effect to the overall risk. Early success in identifying the role of *HLA* was followed by intense, yet mostly ineffective efforts in the search of additional susceptibility genes. The recent publication of genome-wide association studies and identification of novel true disease genes has ignited the field with considerable drive. High-powered laboratory technologies will now allow the full array of genes, molecules, and pathways operating in MS to be defined. This goal can only be achieved if sufficient knowledge exists to distinguish disease variants, reliably classify therapeutic outcomes, and capture key individual molecular profiling variables.

current arrays), stringent *P* value thresholds are used to assess the statistical significance of associations. However, the gold standard for defining a true association is its replication in independent studies. Replication is important because even statistically significant associations can occur by chance alone, and within a single study it is possible that non MS related factors (such as genotyping errors) create artificial associations.

To date, seven GWAS have been reported for MS susceptibility, all in populations of European descent (**Table 1**), including data from an early study that only genotyped nonsynonymous coding single nucleotide polymorphisms (SNPs), and recent scans of a high-risk isolate from Finland and a Sardinian cohort.[13,14] The classic *HLA-DRB1* risk locus stood out in all studies with remarkably strong statistical significance, reflecting the robust statistical power embedded in the datasets. Replication and meta-analysis[15] efforts provided strong evidence for 11 novel non–major histocompatibility complex (MHC) loci affecting disease susceptibility (**Table 2**). The associated markers might not necessarily represent the causal disease variant themselves, partly explaining the modest independent odds ratios for each allele. Additional follow-up experiments refined some of the association signals, identified additional risk loci,[16,17] and provided early mechanistic insights into the functional consequences of the identified gene variants, such as an increase in the soluble to membrane-bound ratio for the interleukin (IL)-2 and IL-7 receptors.[18,19]

FIRST-GENERATION MS GWAS–ASSOCIATED GENES
CD58

Several studies have identified an association between *CD58* (chromosome 1p13) and MS susceptibility.[15,16,20–26] The original associated marker[24] is rs12044852 (*P* = 1.90×10^{-5}; odds ratio [OR], 1.24) and is located in an intron (noncoding region) of

Table 1 Genome-wide studies in MS				
Study	Year	Study Type	Population	Number of Individuals
Haines et al[89]	1996	Linkage	United States	52 families
Sawcer et al[90]	1996	Linkage	United Kingdom	129 families
Ebers et al[91]	1996	Linkage	Canada	61 families
Kuokkanen et al[92]	1997	Linkage	Finland	21 families
International Multiple Sclerosis Genetics Consortium[93]	2005	Linkage	Australia/Scandinavia/ United Kingdom/ United States	730 multiplex families
Reich et al[94]	2005	Admixture	African Americans	605 patients/1043 controls
Burton et al[42]	2007	Association	United Kingdom	975 patients/1466 controls
International Multiple Sclerosis Genetics Consortium[24]	2007	Association	United Kingdom/ United States	931 trios
Comabella et al[43]	2008	Association	Spanish	242 patients/242 controls
ANZgene[20]	2009	Association	Australia/New Zealand	1618 patients/3413 controls
Baranzini et al[41]	2009	Association	United States/Holland/ Switzerland	960 patients/862 controls
De Jager et al[15]	2009	Association	Meta-analysis	2624 patients/7220 controls
Jakkula et al[13]	2010	Association	Finland	68 patients/136 controls
Sanna et al[14]	2010	Association	Sardinia	882 patients/872 controls

the gene. The protein from *CD58* is localized to the plasma membrane and is involved in cell adhesion, T-cell receptor signaling, and T-lymphocyte activation. The G allele of the marker rs2300747 seems to be protective and associated with increased expression of *CD58* mRNA.[22] *CD58* expression is increased in patients with MS during remission and may have an effect on MS through enhancing the function of regulatory T cells.[22] Other variation in the *CD58* gene is associated with rheumatoid arthritis risk.[27]

RPL5

Ribosomal protein L5 (*RPL5*: chromosome 1p22) was found to be associated with MS in several studies.[15,16,20,24,26] The original associated marker[24] is rs6604026 ($P = 7.94 \times 10^{-5}$; OR, 1.15) and is located in an intron of the gene. RPL5 binds 5SRNA, is required for rRNA maturation, and is required for the formation of the 60S ribosomal subunits. It is the only gene in this list that is not obviously associated with immune function. This gene is associated with Diamond-Blackfan anemia, a disease in which the bone marrow is deficient in producing red blood cells.

EVI5

The association between ecotropic viral integration site 5 gene (*EVI5*: chromosome 1p22) and MS has also been shown in many studies.[15,16,20,23,24,28–30] The original associated marker[24] is rs6680578 ($P = 5.00 \times 10^{-4}$; OR, 1.11) and is located in an intron of the gene. This gene is involved in cell cycle, cell proliferation, and cell division.

Table 2
Genes indentified in GWAS for which there is strong evidence for an association with MS

Gene Symbol	Location	Gene Function	References
CD58	1p13	Cell adhesion, T-cell receptor signaling; T-lymphocyte activation	15,16,20–26
RPL5	1p22	5S rRNA chaperone; rRNA maturation; formation of 60S ribosomal subunits	15,16,20,24,26
EVI5	1p22	Cell cycle; cell proliferation; cell division; retroviral integration in T-cell lymphomas	15,16,20,23,24,28–30
IL7R[a]	5p13	Lymphocyte development; T-cell receptor gamma accessibility by STAT5; apoptosis; activation of T lymphocytes	15–18,23–25,32–34
HLA-DRB1	6p21	Immune response; pathogen defense; antigen presentation	95–102
IL2RA	10p15	Elimination of self-reactive T cells	15,16,20,23–26,32,52–56
CD6	11q13	Cell adhesion; T-cell activation	15,16,30,64
TNFRSF1A	12p13	Apoptosis; cytokine signaling	15,30,64
CLEC16A	16p13	Glycoprotein uptake for dendritic cell presentation; dendritic cell distinguishing between self and non-self antigens	15,16,23–26,30,68
IRF8	16q24	Regulation of interferon major histocompatibility complex class I genes; regulation of immune cells	15,16
CD226	18q22	Tumor suppression; T-cell differentiation and proliferation; monocyte migration; antigen presentation; cell adhesion	76–79
TYK2	19p13	Amino acid phosphorylation; type I IFN signaling; phosphorylates the IFN-alpha receptor chain	17,20,34,83

[a] First identified through candidate gene approach.

EVI5 is a common site of retroviral integration in T-cell lymphomas[31] and, if there is allelic preference for the integration, it is possible that the associations with MS may have arisen from retroviruses, disruption of the region affecting other genes, or disruption of the EVI5 gene itself. EVI5 was found to interact with HLA-DRB1*15.[20,30]

IL7R

Much evidence exists for the association between the IL-7 receptor and MS susceptibility (IL7R [CD127]: chromosome 5p13).[15–18,23–25,32–34] The original associated marker[24] is rs6897932 ($P = 2.94 \times 10^{-7}$; OR, 1.18), and the variation results in a nonsynonymous missense (amino acid changing) alteration in the IL7R protein. IL7R is involved in lymphocyte development, T-cell receptor gamma accession by STAT5, apoptosis, B-cell proliferation, and activation of T lymphocytes. IL7R is differentially expressed in patients with MS and controls,[35,36] and the increase of the expression of the non–membrane-bound form of the receptor, resulting from the skipping of exon 6, is what increases MS risk.[18] IL7R expression is also upregulated in response to interferon beta, which is the most common drug used to treat MS,[37] is upregulated in patients with psoriasis,[38] and the soluble form of IL7R was found to be upregulated and inhibiting IL-7 activity in people who were HIV-positive.[39] Because genes that influence MS susceptibility are, by definition, involved in biologic pathways influencing the disease risk, variation in other genes involved in these pathways may also be involved in MS susceptibility. Following this reasoning, variations in genes functionally related to *IL7R* were tested, and *IL7* and *SOCS1* were identified as MS susceptibility genes.[17]

HLA-DRB1

The predominant association with MS susceptibility in the HLA is with the class II *DR*15* (subset of DR*2) haplotype (*DRB5*01:01, DRB1*15:01, DQA1*01:02, DQB1*06:02*).[40] Highly significant associations for markers near or within the *DR*15* haplotype were identified in most of the GWAS with odds ratios of 2.0 to 3.4 and P values as low as 10^{-225},[13,15,20,24,41–43] including the marker rs3135388, which is a proxy for the *DRB1*15:01* allele. However, high linkage disequilibrium (LD) between the *DR*15* genes in the populations studied (ie, individuals of European descent[44–47]) is an obstacle to determining which of these genes is actually responsible for the association. Because *HLA* LD structure differs across ethnic groups, studying non–European-descended populations can facilitate identification of independent effects among genes in high LD within individuals of European descent. In a study of African American patients with MS and controls, the effect of *DRB1*15:01* was found to be independent of *DQB1*06:02*[48] and a *DRB1* effect was identified in the absence *DRB5*,[49] indicating that the *DRB1*15:01* allele is likely responsible for the major MS association in the HLA.[50,51]

IL2RA

An association between the IL-2 receptor-alpha gene (*IL2RA/CD25*: chromosome 10p15) and MS is one of the most replicated non–HLA gene/MS associations identified to date.[15,16,20,23–26,32,52–56] The original associated marker[24] is rs12722489 ($P = 2.96 \times 10^{-8}$; OR, 1.25) and is located in an intron of the gene. The protein produced by this gene is a receptor for IL-2 and is involved in the elimination of self-reactive T cells. Different independent associations have been identified between MS and markers within the *IL2RA* gene.[15,55] Although independent marker associations hint that multiple mutations within the gene may affect MS susceptibility, the markers could be independently tagging a single rare variant responsible for the effect.[57] *IL2RA* associations with several other autoimmune diseases (eg, Graves's disease,[58] juvenile idiopathic arthritis,[59] rheumatoid arthritis,[60] type 1 diabetes[61]) have been identified.[62] As with the associations with MS, whether multiple causative mutations exist or if different markers are tagging the same causative mutation in different populations is unclear. In a network-based analysis combining results from multiple studies within disease and comparing the genetic relatedness between diseases, *IL2RA* was identified as a strong factor relating MS to type 1 diabetes.[63]

CD6

An association between *CD6* (chromosome 11q13) and MS susceptibility has been identified and replicated in independent studies.[15,16,30,64] The original associated marker[15] is rs17824933 ($P = 3.79 \times 10^{-9}$; OR, 1.18) and is located in an intron of the gene. CD6 is a glycoprotein that is involved in cell adhesion and T-cell activation and is expressed on thymocytes, T cells, and B cells. Soluble CD6 may also downregulate proinflammatory cytokines,[65] and could be involved in MS susceptibility as a response to a pathogen.[64]

TNFRSF1A

Another gene strongly associated with MS is tumor necrosis factor receptor super-family, member 1 (TNFRSF1A: chromosome 12p13).[15,30,64] The original associated marker[15] is rs1800693 (P = 1.59×10^{-11}; OR, 1.20) and is located in an intron of the gene. TNFRSF1A is involved in apoptosis and cytokine signaling. A mutation in this gene is associated with tumor necrosis factor receptor–associated periodic syndrome (TRAPS), which is a recurrent autoimmune disease. In TRAPS, plasma levels of TNFRSF1A are lower than normal between attacks, but receptors for the TNFRSF1A protein on leukocytes are abnormally high.[66] This gene may also be associated with recurrent pericarditis.[67] Therefore, it would be interesting to test whether TNFRSF1A levels fluctuate with recurrences in relapsing remitting MS, pointing to a possible mechanism to explain the difference between relapsing and progressive disease.

CLEC16A

The association between the C-type lectin domain family 16, member A gene (CLEC16A: chromosome 16p13) and MS has been confirmed by many studies.[15,16,23–26,30,68] The original associated marker[24] is rs6498169 (P = 3.83×10^{-5}; OR, 1.14) and is located in an intron of the gene. C-type lectin receptors are important for the uptake of glycoprotein antigens by dendritic cells for presentation on MHC class I and II molecules, and for distinguishing between self and non-self anti-gens by dendritic cells.[69] In addition to MS, CLEC16A has been associated with other autoimmune diseases, such as Crohn's disease,[70] Addison's disease,[71] autoimmune thyroid disease,[72] rheumatoid arthritis,[73] and juvenile idiopathic arthritis.[73]

IRF8

Two studies have identified an association between interferon regulatory factor 8 (IRF8: chromosome 16q24) and MS.[15,16] The original associated marker[15] is rs17445836 (P = 3.73×10^{-9}; OR, 1.25). IRF8 plays a role in the differentiation of myeloid cells, regulation of myeloid lineage progression, B-cell lineage specification, and the rearrangement of the immunoglobulin light chain.[74] Mice lacking the IRF8 gene are immunodeficient,[75] implicating the gene as a major player in immune regulation.

CD226

The association between CD226 (chromosome 18q22) and MS susceptibility was identified in four studies.[76–79] The original associated marker[77] is rs763361 (P = 4.54×10^{-4}; OR, 1.13), and the variation results in a nonsynonymous missense alter-ation in the CD226 protein. This gene produces a receptor found on the surface of cytotoxic T cells, platelets, monocytes, dendritic cells, mast cells, and natural killer (NK) cells.[80] The CD226 protein is involved in tumor suppression, dendritic cell matu-ration, T-cell differentiation and proliferation, monocyte migration, antigen presenta-tion, and cell adhesion.[80] Anti-CD226 delays onset and reduces severity of experimental autoimmune encephalomyelitis (EAE),[81] and CD226 expression is down-regulated on NK T cells from active systemic lupus erythematosus.[82]

TYK2

Four studies have identified an association between tyrosine kinase 2 (TYK2: chromo-some 19p13) and MS susceptibility.[17,20,34,83] The original associated marker[34] is rs34536443 (P = 2.70×10^{-6}; OR, 1.32), and the variation results in a nonsynonymous missense alteration in the TYK2 protein. TYK2 is a member of the Janus kinase family, and is involved in the initiation of type I interferon signaling and IL-6, IL-10, IL-12, IL-13, and IL-23 signaling, indicating a possible role in immune functioning. In addition, a missense mutation in *TYK2* was recently shown to confer resistance to EAE.[84] Alternatively, the gene has also been shown to affect central nervous system repair in Theiler's virus–induced demyelination in mice,[85] suggesting that its function in MS susceptibility may be via myelin repair.

CONCLUDING REMARKS

Despite the success of GWAS in identifying novel susceptibility alleles, MS genetics is still a work in progress. Some models predict that available data from GWAS explain approximately 3% of the total variance in MS risk.[86] A GWAS comprising 10,000 cases and high-density SNP/copy number variation (CNV) platforms is near completion by the International Multiple Sclerosis Genetics Consortium. This study is expected to be adequately powered to identify common risk alleles with odds ratios of 1.2 or more. In addition, CNVs have yet to be reported for MS susceptibility. CNVs are duplications or deletions of sections of the genome and have been identified and shown to be associated with several diseases.[87]

Finally, new technologies, such as large-scale whole genome sequencing, are nearing feasibility for disease studies. A recent experiment that sequenced a pair of identical twins discordant for MS susceptibility[88] provides an idea of what is to come. This study also examined genome-wide methylation differences within the twin sets, highlighting recently developed epigenetic analyses now available, which shift the paradigm of what is considered "genetics." Future studies will sequence and contrast the complete genomes of many patients and controls, possibly identifying rare variants with large effects in subsets of the patients. Within the next few years, the availability of unique, large, and well-characterized cohorts, coupled with state-of-the-art laboratory and analytical methods, will facilitate discovery of key genetic pathways and networks operating in MS. Combining these results with data from epigenetic, environmental, and metabolic studies will produce a more refined representation of the genetic contributions to disease pathogenesis. The rapid advance in technology and decrease in costs, combined with analyses that amalgamate the multiple data types (eg, genetic, epigenetic, environmental, metabolic) will help bring to fruition the overall goal of MS research, which is to generate methods to prevent or treat this serious and debilitating disease.

REFERENCES

1. Oksenberg JR, Baranzini SE, Sawcer S, et al. The genetics of multiple sclerosis: SNPs to pathways to pathogenesis. Nat Rev Genet 2008;9(7):516–26.
2. Yeo TW, De Jager PL, Gregory SG, et al. A second major histocompatibility complex susceptibility locus for multiple sclerosis. Ann Neurol 2007;61(3): 228–36.
3. Rosati G. The prevalence of multiple sclerosis in the world: an update. Neurol Sci 2001;22(2):117–39.
4. Carton H, Vlietinck R, Debruyne J, et al. Risks of multiple sclerosis in relatives of patients in Flanders, Belgium. J Neurol Neurosurg Psychiatry 1997;62(4): 329–33.
5. Robertson NP, Fraser M, Deans J, et al. Age-adjusted recurrence risks for relatives of patients with multiple sclerosis. Brain 1996;119(Pt 2):449–55.
6. Sadovnick AD. Familial recurrence risks and inheritance of multiple sclerosis. Curr Opin Neurol Neurosurg 1993;6(2):189–94.

7. Sadovnick AD, Baird PA, Ward RH. Multiple sclerosis: updated risks for relatives. Am J Med Genet 1988;29(3):533–41.
8. Ebers GC, Sadovnick AD, Risch NJ. A genetic basis for familial aggregation in multiple sclerosis. Canadian Collaborative Study Group. Nature 1995; 377(6545):150–1.
9. Sadovnick AD, Ebers GC, Dyment DA, et al. Evidence for genetic basis of multiple sclerosis. The Canadian Collaborative Study Group. Lancet 1996; 347(9017):1728–30.
10. Mumford CJ, Wood NW, Kellar-Wood H, et al. The British Isles survey of multiple sclerosis in twins. Neurology 1994;44(1):11–5.
11. Sadovnick AD, Armstrong H, Rice GP, et al. A population-based study of multiple sclerosis in twins: update. Ann Neurol 1993;33(3):281–5.
12. Jersild C, Fog T. Histocompatibility (HL-A) antigens associated with multiple sclerosis. Acta Neurol Scand Suppl 1972;51:377.
13. Jakkula E, Leppa V, Sulonen AM, et al. Genome-wide association study in a high-risk isolate for multiple sclerosis reveals associated variants in STAT3 gene. Am J Hum Genet 2010;86(2):285–91.
14. Sanna S, Pitzalis M, Zoledziewska M, et al. Variants within the immunoregulatory CBLB gene are associated with multiple sclerosis. Nat Genet 2010;42(6):495–7.
15. De Jager PL, Jia X, Wang J, et al. Meta-analysis of genome scans and replication identify CD6, IRF8 and TNFRSF1A as new multiple sclerosis susceptibility loci. Nat Genet 2009;41(7):776–82.
16. International MS. Genetics Consortium. Comprehensive follow-up of the first gonome-wide association study of multiple sclerosis identifies KIF21B and TMEM39A as susceptibility loci. Hum Mol Genet 2010;19(5):953–62.
17. Zuvich RL, McCauley JL, Oksenberg JR, et al. Genetic variation in the IL7RA/IL7 pathway increases multiple sclerosis susceptibility. Hum Genet 2010;127(5): 525–35.
18. Gregory SG, Schmidt S, Seth P, et al. Interleukin 7 receptor alpha chain (IL7R) shows allelic and functional association with multiple sclerosis. Nat Genet 2007; 39(9):1083–91.
19. Maier LM, Anderson DE, Severson CA, et al. Soluble IL-2RA levels in multiple sclerosis subjects and the effect of soluble IL-2RA on immune responses. J Immunol 2009;182(3):1541–7.
20. ANZgene. Genome-wide association study identifies new multiple sclerosis susceptibility loci on chromosomes 12 and 20. Nat Genet 2009;41(7):824–8.
21. Arthur AT, Armati PJ, Bye C, et al. Genes implicated in multiple sclerosis pathogenesis from consilience of genotyping and expression profiles in relapse and remission. BMC Med Genet 2008;9:17.
22. De Jager PL, Baecher-Allan C, Maier LM, et al. The role of the CD58 locus in multiple sclerosis. Proc Natl Acad Sci U S A 2009;106(13):5264–9.
23. D'Netto MJ, Ward H, Morrison KM, et al. Risk alleles for multiple sclerosis in multiplex families. Neurology 2009;72(23):1984–8.
24. International MS Genetics Consortium. Risk alleles for multiple sclerosis identified by a genomewide study. N Engl J Med 2007;357(9):851–62.
25. Hoppenbrouwers IA, Aulchenko YS, Janssens AC, et al. Replication of CD58 and CLEC16A as genome-wide significant risk genes for multiple sclerosis. J Hum Genet 2009;54(11):676–80.
26. Rubio JP, Stankovich J, Field J, et al. Replication of KIAA0350, IL2RA, RPL5 and CD58 as multiple sclerosis susceptibility genes in Australians. Genes Immun 2008;9(7):624–30.

27. Raychaudhuri S, Thomson BP, Remmers EF, et al. Genetic variants at CD28, PRDM1 and CD2/CD58 are associated with rheumatoid arthritis risk. Nat Genet 2009;41(12):1313–8.

28. Alcina A, Fernandez O, Gonzalez JR, et al. Tag-SNP analysis of the GFI1-EVI5-RPL5-FAM69 risk locus for multiple sclerosis. Eur J Hum Genet 2010;18(7): 827–31.

29. Hoppenbrouwers IA, Aulchenko YS, Ebers GC, et al. EVI5 is a risk gene for multiple sclerosis. Genes Immun 2008;9(4):334–7.

30. Johnson BA, Wang J, Taylor EM, et al. Multiple sclerosis susceptibility alleles in African Americans. Genes Immun 2009;11(4):343–50.

31. Liao X, Buchberg AM, Jenkins NA, et al. Evi-5, a common site of retroviral integration in AKXD T-cell lymphomas, maps near Gfi-1 on mouse chromosome 5. J Virol 1995;69(11):7132–7.

32. Akkad DA, Hoffjan S, Petrasch-Parwez E, et al. Variation in the IL7RA and IL2RA genes in German multiple sclerosis patients. J Autoimmun 2009;32(2):110–5.

33. Alcina A, Fedetz M, Ndagire D, et al. The T244I variant of the interleukin-7 receptor-alpha gene and multiple sclerosis. Tissue Antigens 2008;72(2): 158–61.

34. Ban M, Goris A, Lorentzen AR, et al. Replication analysis identifies TYK2 as a multiple sclerosis susceptibility factor. Eur J Hum Genet 2009;17(10):1309–13.

35. Bomprezzi R, Ringner M, Kim S, et al. Gene expression profile in multiple sclerosis patients and healthy controls: identifying pathways relevant to disease. Hum Mol Genet 2003;12(17):2191–9.

36. Ramanathan M, Weinstock-Guttman B, Nguyen LT, et al. In vivo gene expression revealed by cDNA arrays: the pattern in relapsing-remitting multiple sclerosis patients compared with normal subjects. J Neuroimmunol 2001;116(2):213–9.

37. Hoe E, McKay F, Schibeci S, et al. Interleukin 7 receptor alpha chain haplotypes vary in their influence on multiple sclerosis susceptibility and response to interferon Beta. J Interferon Cytokine Res 2010;30(5):291–8.

38. Lee SK, Jeon EK, Kim YJ, et al. A global gene expression analysis of the peripheral blood mononuclear cells reveals the gene expression signature in psoriasis. Ann Dermatol 2009;21(3):237–42.

39. Crawley AM, Faucher S, Angel JB. Soluble IL-7R alpha (sCD127) inhibits IL-7 activity and is increased in HIV infection. J Immunol 2010;184(9):4679–87.

40. Olerup O, Hillert J. HLA class II-associated genetic susceptibility in multiple sclerosis: a critical evaluation. Tissue Antigens 1991;38(1):1–15.

41. Baranzini SE, Wang J, Gibson RA, et al. Genome-wide association analysis of susceptibility and clinical phenotype in multiple sclerosis. Hum Mol Genet 2009;18(4):767–78.

42. Burton PR, Clayton DG, Cardon LR, et al. Association scan of 14,500 nonsynonymous SNPs in four diseases identifies autoimmunity variants. Nat Genet 2007; 39(11):1329–37.

43. Comabella M, Craig DW, Camina-Tato M, et al. Identification of a novel risk locus for multiple sclerosis at 13q31.3 by a pooled genome-wide scan of 500,000 single nucleotide polymorphisms. PLoS One 2008;3(10):e3490.

44. Allen M, Sandberg-Wollheim M, Sjogren K, et al. Association of susceptibility to multiple sclerosis in Sweden with HLA class II DRB1 and DQB1 alleles. Hum Immunol 1994;39(1):41–8.

45. Boon M, Nolte IM, Bruinenberg M, et al. Mapping of a susceptibility gene for multiple sclerosis to the 51 kb interval between G511525 and D6S1666 using a new method of haplotype sharing analysis. Neurogenetics 2001;3(4):221–30.

46. Fernandez O, Fernandez V, Alonso A, et al. DQB1*0602 allele shows a strong association with multiple sclerosis in patients in Malaga, Spain. J Neurol 2004; 251(4):440–4.
47. Spurkland A, Ronningen KS, Vandvik B, et al. HLA-DQA1 and HLA-DQB1 genes may jointly determine susceptibility to develop multiple sclerosis. Hum Immunol 1991;30(1):69–75.
48. Oksenberg JR, Barcellos LF, Cree BA, et al. Mapping multiple sclerosis suscep- tibility to the HLA-DR locus in African Americans. Am J Hum Genet 2004;74(1): 160–7.
49. Caillier SJ, Briggs F, Cree BA, et al. Uncoupling the roles of HLA-DRB1 and HLA-DRB5 genes in multiple sclerosis. J Immunol 2008;181(8):5473–80.
50. Cree BA, Rioux JD, McCauley JL, et al. A major histocompatibility Class I locus contributes to multiple sclerosis susceptibility independently from HLA- DRB1*15:01. PLoS One 2010;5(6):e11296.
51. McElroy JP, Cree BA, Caillier SJ, et al. Refining the association of MHC with multiple sclerosis in African Americans. Hum Mol Genet 2010;19(15):3080–8.
52. Alcina A, Fedetz M, Ndagire D, et al. IL2RA/CD25 gene polymorphisms: uneven association with multiple sclerosis (MS) and type 1 diabetes (T1D). PLoS One 2009;4(1):e4137.
53. Cavanillas ML, Alcina A, Nunez C, et al. Polymorphisms in the IL2, IL2RA and IL2RB genes in multiple sclerosis risk. Eur J Hum Genet 2010;18(7):794–9.
54. Matesanz F, Caro-Maldonado A, Fedetz M, et al. IL2RA/CD25 polymorphisms contribute to multiple sclerosis susceptibility. J Neurol 2007;254(5):682–4.
55. Perera D, Stankovich J, Butzkueven H, et al. Fine mapping of multiple sclerosis susceptibility genes provides evidence of allelic heterogeneity at the IL2RA locus. J Neuroimmunol 2009;211(1/2):105–9.
56. Weber F, Fontaine B, Cournu-Rebeix I, et al. IL2RA and IL7RA genes confer susceptibility for multiple sclerosis in two independent European populations. Genes Immun 2008;9(3):259–63.
57. Dickson SP, Wang K, Krantz I, et al. Rare variants create synthetic genome-wide associations. PLoS Biol 2010;8(1):e1000294.
58. Brand OJ, Lowe CE, Heward JM, et al. Association of the interleukin-2 receptor alpha (IL-2Ralpha)/CD25 gene region with Graves' disease using a multilocus test and tag SNPs. Clin Endocrinol (Oxf) 2007;66(4):508–12.
59. Hinks A, Ke X, Barton A, et al. Association of the IL2RA/CD25 gene with juvenile idiopathic arthritis. Arthritis Rheum 2009;60(1):251–7.
60. Kurreeman FA, Daha NA, Chang M, et al. Association of IL2RA and IL2RB with rheumatoid arthritis: a replication study in a Dutch population. Ann Rheum Dis 2009;68(11):1789–90.
61. Qu HQ, Bradfield JP, Belisle A, et al. The type I diabetes association of the IL2RA locus. Genes Immun 2009;10(Suppl 1):S42–8.
62. Hoffjan S, Akkad DA. The genetics of multiple sclerosis: an update 2010. Mol Cell Probes 2010;24(5):237–43.
63. Baranzini SE. The genetics of autoimmune diseases: a networked perspective. Curr Opin Immunol 2009;21(6):596–605.
64. Swaminathan B, Matesanz F, Cavanillas ML, et al. Validation of the CD6 and TNFRSF1A loci as risk factors for multiple sclerosis in Spain. J Neuroimmunol 2010;223(1/2):100–3.
65. Sarrias MR, Farnos M, Mota R, et al. CD6 binds to pathogen-associated molec- ular patterns and protects from LPS-induced septic shock. Proc Natl Acad Sci U S A 2007;104(28):11724–9.

66. Masson C, Simon V, Hoppe E, et al. Tumor necrosis factor receptor-associated periodic syndrome (TRAPS): definition, semiology, prognosis, pathogenesis, treatment, and place relative to other periodic joint diseases. Joint Bone Spine 2004;71(4):284–90.

67. Cantarini L, Lucherini OM, Baldari CT, et al. Familial clustering of recurrent pericarditis may disclose tumour necrosis factor receptor-associated periodic syndrome. Clin Exp Rheumatol 2010;28(3):405–7.

68. Zoledziewska M, Costa G, Pitzalis M, et al. Variation within the CLEC16A gene shows consistent disease association with both multiple sclerosis and type 1 diabetes in Sardinia. Genes Immun 2009;10(1):15–7.

69. Geijtenbeek TB, van Vliet SJ, Engering A, et al. Self- and nonself-recognition by C-type lectins on dendritic cells. Annu Rev Immunol 2004;22:33–54.

70. Marquez A, Varade J, Robledo G, et al. Specific association of a CLEC16A/KIAA0350 polymorphism with NOD2/CARD15(-) Crohn's disease patients. Eur J Hum Genet 2009;17(10):1304–8.

71. Skinningsrud B, Husebye ES, Pearce SH, et al. Polymorphisms in CLEC16A and CIITA at 16p13 are associated with primary adrenal insufficiency. J Clin Endocrinol Metab 2008;93(9):3310–7.

72. Awata T, Kawasaki E, Tanaka S, et al. Association of type 1 diabetes with two Loci on 12q13 and 16p13 and the influence coexisting thyroid autoimmunity in Japanese. J Clin Endocrinol Metab 2009;94(1):231–5.

73. Skinningsrud B, Lie BA, Husebye ES, et al. A CLEC16A variant confers risk for juvenile idiopathic arthritis and anti-CCP negative rheumatoid arthritis. Ann Rheum Dis 2010;69(8):1471–4.

74. Wang H, Morse HC III. IRF8 regulates myeloid and B lymphoid lineage diversification. Immunol Res 2009;43(1–3):109–17.

75. Giese NA, Gabriele L, Doherty TM, et al. Interferon (IFN) consensus sequence-binding protein, a transcription factor of the IFN regulatory factor family, regulates immune responses in vivo through control of interleukin 12 expression. J Exp Med 1997;186(9):1535–46.

76. Alcina A, Vandenbroeck K, Otaegui D, et al. The autoimmune disease-associated KIF5A, CD226 and SH2B3 gene variants confer susceptibility for multiple sclerosis. Genes Immun 2010;11(5):439–45.

77. Hafler JP, Maier LM, Cooper JD, et al. CD226 Gly307Ser association with multiple autoimmune diseases. Genes Immun 2009;10(1):5–10.

78. International MS. Genetics Consortium. The expanding genetic overlap between multiple sclerosis and type I diabetes. Genes Immun 2009;10(1):11–4.

79. Wieczorek S, Hoffjan S, Chan A, et al. Novel association of the CD226 (DNAM-1) Gly307Ser polymorphism in Wegener's granulomatosis and confirmation for multiple sclerosis in German patients. Genes Immun 2009;10(6):591–5.

80. Xu Z, Jin B. A novel interface consisting of homologous immunoglobulin superfamily members with multiple functions. Cell Mol Immunol 2010;7(1):11–9.

81. Dardalhon V, Schubart AS, Reddy J, et al. CD226 is specifically expressed on the surface of Th1 cells and regulates their expansion and effector functions. J Immunol 2005;175(3):1558–65.

82. Tao D, Shangwu L, Qun W, et al. CD226 expression deficiency causes high sensitivity to apoptosis in NK T cells from patients with systemic lupus erythematosus. J Immunol 2005;174(3):1281–90.

83. Mero IL, Lorentzen AR, Ban M, et al. A rare variant of the TYK2 gene is confirmed to be associated with multiple sclerosis. Eur J Hum Genet 2010; 18(4):502–4.

84. Spach KM, Noubade R, McElvany B, et al. A single nucleotide polymorphism in Tyk2 controls susceptibility to experimental allergic encephalomyelitis. J Immunol 2009;182(12):7776–83.
85. Bieber AJ, Suwansrinon K, Kerkvliet J, et al. Allelic variation in the Tyk2 and EGF genes as potential genetic determinants of CNS repair. Proc Natl Acad Sci U S A 2010;107(2):792–7.
86. International MS. Genetics consortium. Evidence for polygenic susceptibility to multiple sclerosis—the shape of things to come. Am J Hum Genet 2010;86(4): 621–5.
87. Stankiewicz P, Lupski JR. Structural variation in the human genome and its role in disease. Annu Rev Med 2010;61:437–55.
88. Baranzini SE, Mudge J, van Velkinburgh JC, et al. Genome, epigenome and RNA sequences of monozygotic twins discordant for multiple sclerosis. Nature 2010;464(7293):1351–6.
89. Haines JL, Ter-Minassian M, Bazyk A, et al. A complete genomic screen for multiple sclerosis underscores a role for the major histocompatability complex. The multiple sclerosis genetics group. Nat Genet 1996;13(4):469–71.
90. Sawcer S, Jones HB, Feakes R, et al. A genome screen in multiple sclerosis reveals susceptibility loci on chromosome 6p21 and 17q22. Nat Genet 1996; 13(4):464–8.
91. Ebers GC, Kukay K, Bulman DE, et al. A full genome search in multiple sclerosis. Nat Genet 1996;13(4):472–6.
92. Kuokkanen S, Gschwend M, Rioux JD, et al. Genomewide scan of multiple sclerosis in Finnish multiplex families. Am J Hum Genet 1997;61(6):1379–87.
93. International MS Genetics Consortium. A high-density screen for linkage in multiple sclerosis. Am J Hum Genet 2005;77(3):454–67.
94. Reich D, Patterson N, De Jager PL, et al. A whole-genome admixture scan finds a candidate locus for multiple sclerosis susceptibility. Nat Genet 2005;37(10): 1113–8.
95. Alves-Leon SV, Papais-Alvarenga R, Magalhaes M, et al. Ethnicity-dependent association of HLA DRB1-DQA1-DQB1 alleles in Brazilian multiple sclerosis patients. Acta Neurol Scand 2007;115(5):306–11.
96. Barcellos LF, Sawcer S, Ramsay PP, et al. Heterogeneity at the HLA-DRB1 locus and risk for multiple sclerosis. Hum Mol Genet 2006;15(18):2813–24.
97. Benedek G, Paperna T, Avidan N, et al. Opposing effects of the HLA-DRB1*0301-DQB1*0201 haplotype on the risk for multiple sclerosis in diverse Arab populations in Israel. Genes Immun 2010;11(5):423–31.
98. Dyment DA, Herrera BM, Cader MZ, et al. Complex interactions among MHC haplotypes in multiple sclerosis: susceptibility and resistance. Hum Mol Genet 2005;14(14):2019–26.
99. Fernando MM, Stevens CR, Walsh EC, et al. Defining the role of the MHC in autoimmunity: a review and pooled analysis. PLoS Genet 2008;4(4):e1000024.
100. Ligers A, Dyment DA, Willer CJ, et al. Evidence of linkage with HLA-DR in DRB1*15-negative families with multiple sclerosis. Am J Hum Genet 2001; 69(4):900–3.
101. Lincoln MR, Ramagopalan SV, Chao MJ, et al. Epistasis among HLA-DRB1, HLA-DQA1, and HLA-DQB1 loci determines multiple sclerosis susceptibility. Proc Natl Acad Sci U S A 2009;106(18):7542–7.
102. Marrosu MG, Murru R, Murru MR, et al. Dissection of the HLA association with multiple sclerosis in the founder isolated population of Sardinia. Hum Mol Genet 2001;10(25):2907–16.

Individual and Joint Action of Environmental Factors and Risk of MS

I.A.F. van der Mei, PhD[a,b],*, S. Simpson Jr, MPH[a],
J. Stankovich, PhD[a], B.V. Taylor, MD[a]

KEYWORDS

- Multiple sclerosis • Environmental factors
- Gene-environment interaction • Review • Cause

This review discusses the leading environmental and lifestyle factors suspected to play a role in the onset of multiple sclerosis (MS). The authors utilize the framework of the Rothman Causal Pie Model[1] to discuss the joint action, or interaction, of different factors that that may be causally involved in MS. A key feature of many environmental exposures is that the period of life in which exposure occurs and possibly the timing of a sequence of events can affect how they mediate their effects. Evidence on the timing of each environmental factor is discussed.

A CAUSAL PIE MODEL FOR MULTIPLE SCLEROSIS

MS is a complex multifactorial disease wherein a variety of environmental and genetic factors interplay to manifest in the clinical disorder recognized by all neurologists. Rothman's "Causal Pie Model"[1] is a useful framework to understand this interplay of etiological factors, allowing a structure wherein individual components can act together to cause disease. These components may be simplified as "slices of a pie" (**Fig. 1**), with a given causal mechanism requiring the joint action of many slices, or component causes. Each slice (single component cause) is an event or condition that plays a necessary role in the occurrence of disease in some people. To get the disorder a person must complete their pie, though different people or groups of people might have different slices in their pie. **Fig. 1** shows 3 different pies (causal mechanisms) that can lead to the same end point, in this case clinical MS. Factor A may be high Epstein-Barr virus (EBV) antibody titers, factor B may be low ultraviolet radiation (UVR) exposure, factor C may be smoking, and factor D may be *HLA-DR15*1501*

Financial disclosures and/or conflicts of interest: The authors have nothing to disclose.
[a] Menzies Research Institute, University of Tasmania, 17 Liverpool Street, Hobart, Tasmania, Australia 7000
[b] Menzies Research Institute, University of Tasmania, Private Bag 23, Hobart, Tasmania, Australia 7000
* Corresponding author.
E-mail address: Ingrid.vanderMei@utas.edu.au

Neurol Clin 29 (2011) 233–255
doi:10.1016/j.ncl.2010.12.007
0733-8619/11/$ – see front matter © 2011 Elsevier Inc. All rights reserved.

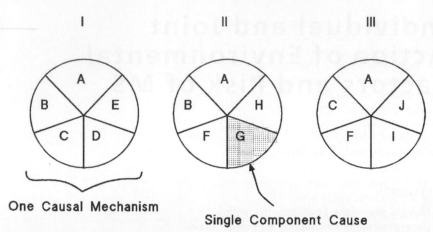

I

II

III

One Causal Mechanism

Single Component Cause

Fig. 1. Three "causal pies" of disease for 3 individuals or groups of people. (*Reproduced from* Rothman KJ. What is causation? In: Rothman KJ. Epidemiology, an introduction. New York: Oxford University Press; 2002. Chapter 2; with permission.)

(HLA-DR15) genotype and so forth, with each slice representing gene regions or environmental exposures (known and unknown) that play a causal role in MS.

It is important to realize that different groups of people have different slices in their pie, and that some slices (single component causes) will act in many different pathways while some may feature in relatively few. Thus, disease is caused by a different combination of component causes in different groups; this explains why some people develop MS even though they, for example, do not have high EBV antibody titers or do not have the high-risk HLA-DR15 genotype. In addition, single component causes need not act at the same time. Such is the case in MS, where different causal factors seem to act in different phases of life (pregnancy, antenatal, early life, adult life).

In epidemiology, a process of "causal inference" is used to decide on how strongly we believe that a factor is *causally* related to a disease. Based on the original criteria from Hill,[2] it includes information on the consistency of findings in different studies, the strength of an association, whether there is evidence of a dose-response relationship, whether there is biologic evidence of the mechanism, whether it has been established that the cause preceded the effect (temporality), and whether there is experimental evidence (randomized controlled trials).[1] These aspects are taken into consideration in the examination of the putative risk factors discussed here.

EPSTEIN-BARR VIRUS

Infections are usual suspects among potential etiological factors in autoimmune disease, thought to act by molecular mimicry, for example, *Campylobacter* and Guillain-Barré syndrome, or by passive changes in immune modulation. EBV is the only viral agent with convincing and consistent evidence for an association with MS onset. EBV is a member of the Herpesviridae group. Whereas primary EBV infection in childhood is normally asymptomatic, infection at or after adolescence often results in clinical symptoms, manifest as infectious mononucleosis (IM), also known as glandular fever. After primary exposure, EBV establishes a latent infection in B cells that persists for life, maintained through expression of a limited set of viral latency genes and low level of viral production in lymphoid tissue.[3] In immunocompetent individuals, EBV infection is largely held in check by the host immune system, although periodic subclinical reactivations occur throughout life.[4]

Over the last two decades, evidence supporting a role for EBV in MS has been steadily accumulating. This evidence is based on several lines of research including epidemiologic studies linking MS occurrence with EBV serology and/or a history of IM, studies on the host immunologic responses to EBV, and neuropathological studies.

Numerous serologic case-control studies have shown that MS is very uncommon in people who are IgG seronegative to EBV antigens, with a meta-analyses yielding a pooled odds ratio (OR) of 0.06 (0.03–0.13).[5] Conversely, people with MS are almost universally seropositive for EBV (99% cases, 90% controls).[6] Further, a history of IM is significantly more common among cases than among controls: an analysis combining 14 studies found a combined relative risk (RR) of 2.3 (1.7–3.0).[7] More recent studies have found similar risk estimates, ranging from 2.06 (1.71–2.48) to 2.50 (1.73–2.86).[8–10] There has been some inconsistency in relation to the timing of IM, however; one study found a higher risk of MS if IM occurred after age 15 years,[11] while another found a higher risk of MS when IM occurred earlier.[9] Regardless of the timing of exposure, the risk is long lasting, with one study finding that the increased risk persisted for more than 30 years after having had IM.[9]

High EBV antibody titers are strongly associated with MS onset. Of importance, prospective studies also observe this association,[12–16] indicating that the high titers develop before the clinical onset of MS rather than being a post-onset phenomenon. The strongest associations have been seen with Epstein-Barr nuclear antigen (EBNA) antibodies, driven by a marked increase of EBNA-1 antibodies, and a less prominent increase in EBNA-2 and viral capsid antigen (VCA).[12,14–16] EBNA-1 is most consistently expressed in infected memory B cells in healthy virus carriers.[17] EBNA is a complex of 6 distinct proteins, one of which (EBNA-1) is primarily recognized in the conventional EBNA complex assay. EBNA-2 antibodies appear in the acute phase of the infection and decline during convalescence, whereas EBNA-1 antibodies become detectable during convalescence and titers remain stable throughout life.

It is unclear as to the significance of having had IM in relation to high EBNA titers. Unfortunately, prospective studies of EBNA titers did not report or have data on IM. In a retrospective case-control study in Tasmania, where 25.7% of the cases and 14.3% of the controls reported a history of IM (OR = 2.10 [1.24–3.55]),[18] mean EBNA IgG titers among EBNA IgG-positive people were higher among those with a history of IM compared with those without, in both cases (312 units vs 295 units) and controls (264 units vs 253 units); however, the difference was similar for cases and controls ($P = .77$ for interaction).

The question is whether the high EBNA titers occur directly after the primary EBV infection or whether there is an increase in titers sometime later, or whether both occur. A longitudinal study suggests that among persons who later develop MS, EBNA IgG titers were similar for cases and controls who were younger than 20 years, whereas titers were 2 to 3 times higher for cases who were 25 to 29 years and those older than 30 years.[15] This result suggests that titers increase sometime between 20 and 30 years of age and then remain elevated.[15] However, the higher EBNA IgG titers may occur earlier in some cases, because EBV seropositivity is also more prevalent among pediatric MS cases than in controls (99% vs 72%, $P = .001$,[19] or 86% vs 64%, $P = .025$[20]), and higher EBNA-1 IgG titers are found in pediatric MS cases than in controls, although the latter might simply be the result of having more EBNA-1 IgG-positive cases.[19]

Enhanced humoral and cellular immune responses to EBV have also been observed in MS patients. For example, increased EBV-specific $CD4^+$ and $CD8^+$ T-cell responses have been detected in the cerebrospinal fluid (CSF) and blood of MS patients, consistent with an abnormal immune activation toward EBV.[21,22]

Furthermore, several reports have shown in MS patients a reactivity of immunoglobulin in CSF to EBV antigens.[21,23] Cepok and colleagues[23] screened CSF IgG with a protein expression array containing 37,000 tagged proteins generated from a human brain cDNA expression library, finding that the 2 most frequent MS-specific reactivities were directed at peptide sequences derived from 2 proteins of EBV, namely EBNA-1 and BRRF2. In addition, T-cell clones, recognizing an immunodominant epitope of myelin basic protein from patients with MS, cross-reacted with EBV-derived proteins as did EBV-reactive T cells isolated from MS patients.[24]

Evidence on the presence of EBV in the brain in postmortem brain tissue is conflicting, however. A comprehensive 2007 study from Serafini and colleagues[25] reported a regular accumulation of EBV-infected B cells/plasma cells in the meninges and perivascular compartment of white matter lesion in MS patients. In addition, viral reactivation appeared restricted to ectopic B-cell follicles and acute lesions.[25] However, 2 recent studies had different findings.[26,27] One study, using multiple methodologies including in situ hybridization, immunohistochemistry, and 2 real-time polymerase chain reaction methodologies, could not detect EBV in white matter lesions and detected low levels of EBV-infected cells in only 2 of 12 MS meningeal specimens.[26] The other study also could not detect latent or productive EBV infection in the MS brain or CSF, and found no specific anti-EBV intrathecal antibody response.[27]

A recent review indicates that there are different hypotheses on how EBV might cause MS: the EBV cross-reactivity hypothesis, the EBV bystander damage hypothesis, the EBV-infected autoreactive B-cell hypothesis, and the alpha B-crystalline (mistaken self) hypothesis.[28] The cross-reactivity hypothesis postulates that T cells primed by exposure to EBV antigens cross-react with central nervous system (CNS) antigens. Under the bystander damage hypothesis, the immune attack on the CNS is primarily directed against EBV reactivation, which results in bystander damage to the CNS. The EBV-infected autoreactive B-cell hypothesis proposes that, in genetically susceptible people, EBV-infected autoreactive B-cells see the target organ where they produce pathogenic autoantibodies, and provide costimulatory survival signals to autoreactive T cells that would otherwise die in the target organ by activation-induced apoptosis. The alpha B-crystalline hypothesis proposes that exposure to infectious agents induces the expression of alpha B-crystalline, a small heat-shock protein, in lymphoid cells that do not normally express this protein in humans. The immune system mistakes self alpha B-crystalline for a microbial antigen and generates a $CD4^+$ T-cell response against it. These T cells then target alpha B-crystalline derived from oligodendrocytes in the CNS, with resultant inflammatory demyelination. A dual role for EBV is also possible where the infection of autoreactive B cells, which seed the CNS and set the stage for chronic disease, is combined with the induction of alpha B-crystalline in B cells that prime $CD4^+$ T cells that target this protein induced in oligodendrocytes in response to EBV infection in the CNS.

Overall, there is convincing epidemiologic evidence that EBV is involved in the etiology of MS. In addition, people with MS seem to have an altered immune response to EBV. However, the evidence on the presence of EBV in the brain is currently inconsistent, and the mechanism by which EBV produces its effect has been difficult to definitively establish.

SUN EXPOSURE/VITAMIN D

It has long been recognized that MS has a distinct geographic variability in its distribution, with the frequency of MS increasing with increasing latitude,[29,30] and this gradient has been borne out in meta-analyses of MS prevalence and incidence.[31,32]

Of interest, a recent study conducted in Australia found a latitudinal gradient in the incidence of first demyelinating events, with the incidence rate increasing by 9.55% per degree increase in latitude.[33] Although differences in allele frequencies of *HLA-DRB1* alleles might explain some of the variance in the European MS prevalence,[34,35] it is probable that the latitudinal gradient also has an environmental component. This finding is demonstrated by the gradient in relatively ethnically homogeneous populations in Australia[36,37] and New Zealand.[38] In addition, the risk associated with latitude alters if people move after birth.[39,40] While it is classically understood that the risk of MS is largely determined before the age of 15 years,[41] migration data from Australia suggest it may operate over a period of many years into adulthood.[40] In 1961 it was observed that MS prevalence was highly correlated with ambient UVR,[42] but it was not until the 1990s that new insights into photoimmunology provided possible mechanisms for this association, prompting further research into this exposure.

There is now substantial epidemiologic evidence that low personal UV exposure or low circulating vitamin D is associated with an increased risk of MS, including case-control studies and prospective cohort studies. A prospective nested case-control study, which measured 25-hydroxyvitamin D (25(OH)D) levels before disease onset, showed that higher 25(OH)D levels were associated with a lower risk of MS (OR = 0.59 [0.36–0.97] per 50-nmol/L increase in 25(OH)D).[43] Of note, even though diet contributes less than 5% of the circulating 25(OH)D, dietary intake of vitamin D was also prospectively associated with MS risk (RR = 0.59 [0.38–0.91], when comparing >400 IU/d vitamin D supplements vs no supplemental vitamin D intake).[44]

Although personal sun exposure has been measured in epidemiologic studies, it has not yet been evaluated in prospective studies. Higher sun exposure in childhood has been found to be associated with a reduced risk of MS in a study of disease-discordant monozygotic twins.[45] The advantage of this study design is that it controls for age, sex, latitude of birth, skin color, socioeconomic status, and family history as well as genotype. In an MS case-control study in Tasmania (41–43°S), it was found that higher sun exposure at 6 to 15 years of age was particularly important in reducing the risk of MS. Further, this study found that winter sun exposure was more important than summer exposure.[46] However, a Norwegian case-control study (66–71°N) found that summer sun exposure at age 16 to 20 years was most important.[47] The fact that winter sun exposure was less important in this study may be explained by the fact that the winter ambient UV levels in Norway are such that no vitamin D is produced for around 4 months of the year, as well as that there is a higher dietary component of vitamin D at these latitudes in Scandinavia.[47,48] Occupational sun exposure has been associated with a reduced MS mortality in 2 studies.[49,50] In a record linkage study, skin cancer was used as a surrogate measure of personal sun exposure, finding that skin cancer was significantly less common in people with MS than in the main comparison cohort (rate ratio 0.49 [0.24–0.91]).[51] Overall, the findings are consistent in identifying associations between different measures of sun exposure or vitamin D and MS onset or mortality.

One important aspect with regard to sun exposure and vitamin D is that it does not seem to be limited to one phase of life. Rather, studies demonstrate effects with MS for sun exposure or vitamin D in different phases of life, ranging from early childhood to adulthood. Whereas some studies show that childhood and adolescence might be particularly important, other studies find that measures of cumulative exposure (eg, skin cancer) or measures of adult life exposure (eg, occupational sun exposure) are important as well.

Whether sun exposure or vitamin D is also important in utero has been indirectly assessed by the season of birth. A large pooled analysis of births in the northern hemisphere found an excess (~10%) of MS among people born in spring (and thus having fetal gestation in winter) and a relative deficit (~10%) among those born in autumn (and thus having fetal gestation in summer).[52] The findings of a recent study in the southern hemisphere were consistent with this (an excess in spring and a deficit in autumn).[53] Moreover, this latter study observed a strong inverse association between ambient UVR in the first trimester and risk of MS. On adjustment for ambient UVR in the first trimester, the association with season of birth was totally abrogated, suggesting that exposure to UVR is the primary mediator of the season of birth effect. Maternal UVR exposure and levels of vitamin D have been found to have a significant role on the brain development of offspring,[54,55] providing a potential biologic mechanism for the observed association. Work in animal models has found that maternal vitamin D deficiency causes abnormal brain development,[55–62] especially during the later stages of development.[60] Vitamin D–deficient mice also have an altered apoptosis[56] and neurogenesis[57] during brain formation, further resulting in altered development of brain structure. Vitamin D–deficient mice have altered or dysregulated expression of several key proteins in the brain, including some related to synapse formation,[58–60] as well as neurotransmitters.[59,60] The expression of these proteins is also altered in MS and other neurologic disorders, but this could be a consequence of the neurologic disorder rather than implying a causal relationship.

From the epidemiologic studies, it is currently unclear whether UVR mediates its effect only via the vitamin D pathway or whether there are additional effects independent of this pathway. There is extensive evidence of immunomodulatory actions of both UVR exposure and the active metabolite of vitamin D, 1,25-dihydroxyvitamin D $(1,25(OH)_2D_3)$.

$1,25(OH)_2D_3$ has been demonstrated to reduce the activity of T_h1 immune cells,[63–66] while simultaneously stimulating activity in T_h2 cells and T_{reg} cells.[65–67] $1,25(OH)_2D_3$ depresses or inhibits the production of T_h1 cytokines including interleukin (IL)-1,[68,69] interferon (IFN)-γ,[70–72] and tumor necrosis factor (TNF)-α,[69,73] as well as the T_h17 cytokine IL-17,[69,71,74] while stimulating the production of T_h2 and T_{reg} cytokines[65,66,70] including IL-10[71,74–76] and transforming growth factor (TGF)-β.[74,77,78] In an animal model of MS, experimental autoimmune encephalitis (EAE), treatment of mice with $1,25(OH)_2D_3$ has been found to significantly affect the development and course of the disease, preventing the onset of EAE when given prior to induction,[79,80] as well as improving the progression of the disease when given after induction.[80–82]

Epidemiologic studies in subjects with MS found that among those with higher serum 25(OH)D, the immune response was weighted toward a T_h2 over T_h1 response, with a concomitant improvement in T_{reg} ability to suppress T_h1 cell proliferation.[83] Other work found that among those with higher $1,25(OH)_2D_3$, the proportion of T_{reg} among immune cells was higher than those with lower levels of $1,25(OH)_2D_3$.[84] Recent work, however, has found that among human subjects with MS, there was no relationship between levels of 25(OH)D or $1,25(OH)_2D_3$ and the number or proportion of T_{reg}, though higher 25(OH)D was still associated with greater T_{reg} function.[85] $1,25(OH)_2D_3$ reduced the proliferation of T_h1 cells in people with MS and reduced the numbers of cells producing IL-6 and IL-17, while at the same time stimulating the development of IL-10–producing cells and T_{reg} cells.[86]

UV also has immunomodulatory effects outside the vitamin D pathway.[87–89] At the most basic level, large-scale apoptosis of immune cells in the epidermis following UV exposure[90] can result in local immunosuppression until these cells can be repopulated. UV modulates the activity of the key immune cells in the skin, the Langerhans cells, impairing normal antigen presentation[91] and inducing their migration to local lymph nodes,[92] where they preferentially activate T_h2 and T_{reg} cells.[93,94] In addition to direct effects on the viability and activation of local immune cells, UV exposure has been demonstrated to affect the local and systemic immunologic milieu via its impact on the production of cytokines and other immunologic agents. UV exposure has been found to induce keratinocytes to directly or indirectly increase levels of several immunomodulatory agents, including IL-4[95] and IL-10.[95–97]

Overall, these data strongly suggest that low vitamin D and/or low UV exposure are important factors in the causation of MS. These factors mediate their effect via the modification of the systemic and local immune status and seem to be important in more than one stage of life. It is possible that the important period for low UV exposure or low vitamin D is different for individuals; it may depend on the occurrence of other factors or change in other factors at a particular point in time (eg, the increase in EBNA IgG titers).

SMOKING

A large number of studies, including prospective studies,[98–101] have found a positive association between smoking and MS. The results have been very consistent in that few have reported a null finding and none an inverse association. The magnitude of effect is modest, with a 2007 meta-analysis of 6 epidemiologic studies finding a pooled estimate for ever smoking versus never smoking of 1.34 (1.17–1.54).[102] Of note, the 3 retrospective studies provided a slightly stronger risk estimate (OR = 1.51 [1.22–1.87]) compared with the 3 prospective studies (1.24 [1.04–1.48]), suggesting that recall bias in retrospective studies might increase the association somewhat. Since then, several studies have found significant risk estimates for ever smoking, ranging from 1.4 to 2.18.[103–107] One recent study found no association in multiplex families[108]; however, by using unaffected siblings as controls they matched, to a certain extent, on both environmental and genetic factors, possibly leading to overmatching on their exposure of interest.

Dose-response relationships have been observed with increasing number of cigarettes,[98,101,105,109] years smoked,[105] or pack-years smoked (pack-years combines the amount and number of years smoked),[104] which increases the confidence that smoking is causally related to MS. For example, in the Nurses' Health Cohorts, compared with never smokers, those who had 1 to 9 pack-years of smoking had an RR of 1.1 (0.8–1.6), those with 10 to 24 pack-years of smoking had an RR of 1.5 (1.2–2.1), and those with 25 or more pack-years of smoking had an RR of 1.7 (1.2–2.4).[98] However, it remains possible that the effect of smoking is driven by another factor. While most studies adjusted (or matched) on some potential confounders such as age, sex, place of residence, or socioeconomic status, few adjusted for established risk factors like ancestry,[98,104,110] latitude of residence,[98] or EBV exposure markers.[107] The latter study, interestingly, which pooled data from 3 studies, found an interaction between smoking and EBNA IgG titers, with the effect of smoking present among those with high EBNA antibody titers (OR = 1.7 [1.1–2.6]) but absent among those with low EBNA titers (OR = 0.97 [0.7–1.3] (test for interaction P = .001).[107] This interaction provides an example of the causal pathways described earlier, with higher EBNA titers allowing an execution of effect by smoking which is absent without it.

In relation to the time period by which smoking might mediate its effect, the demonstrated dose-response relationship with duration of smoking[105] and pack-years smoked[104] seems to suggest a cumulative effect over time. Some studies found an effect for current smoking, but not for past smoking,[99] or a reduced effect for past smoking.[104] An intriguing aspect of the latter study is that it found that the increased risk for MS associated with smoking remained up to 5 years after stopping smoking.[104] Only one study found this relationship inverted, with a greater risk among ex-smokers than current smokers,[103] although this may be due to small numbers in the ex-smoking group. Passive smoking was associated with a doubling in childhood-onset MS (RR = 2.12 [1.43–3.15]),[111] indicating that smoking can already mediate its effect during childhood (<16 years). In addition, the effect was larger among those who were 10 years or older (RR = 2.49 [1.53–4.08]) than in those who were younger (RR = 1.47 [0.73–2.96]), indicating again the importance of duration of exposure.[111] A prospective case-control study found no effect of maternal smoking during pregnancy on MS in offspring.[112] However, this study did not have data on paternal smoking, which is useful when maternal smoking during pregnancy is viewed as a proxy for (maternal) smoking during the early life of the offspring.

The biologic mechanisms by which smoking might mediate these effects are less clear cut, because tobacco contains several proinflammatory and anti-inflammatory components. Tobacco and the resultant smoke from cigarettes contain over 4500 compounds and chemicals, including several known carcinogens and other toxic substances.[113] Among these substances are some with known immunomodulatory effects, most particularly nicotine. The immunomodulatory effects of nicotine have been well studied, having been demonstrated to significantly affect both innate and adaptive immunity. Nicotine has been found to bind to and stimulate the T-cell receptor on T cells which, in the absence of costimulatory molecules, induces a state of anergy in these cells.[114] Long-term exposure to cigarette smoke has been found to have considerable effects on the immune system, including attenuation of the innate immune cells in the respiratory tract, as well as systemic effects such as an increase in number but decrease in function and responsiveness of blood leukocytes, and lower levels and half-lives of circulating antibodies.[113] Cigarette smoke has also been found to up-regulate apoptotic signaling molecules (Fas) on the surface of immune cells, thus increasing the rate of depletion of these cells by apoptosis.[114]

Cigarette smoke has also been found to have an antiestrogenic effect and several proinflammatory immune effects.[114,115] Cigarette smoke contains and induces the production of free radicals,[114,115] which can damage tissue and particularly DNA. Levels of C-reactive protein and IL-6 are increased.[114] In addition, while the levels of circulating antibodies are reduced, cigarette smoke has been found to significantly increase the levels of circulating autoantibodies,[113,115] particularly anti-dsDNA autoantibodies.[115] Nicotine has been found to modulate immune cell activation/differentiation and responsiveness to stimuli, as well as to interfere with the function of activated immune cells, including cell-mediated lysis of target T cells and the production of proinflammatory cytokines, including IL-2, IL-12, IFN-γ, TNF-α, and macrophage inflammatory protein 1α.[116,117] Although nicotine can induce a state of anergy in T cells, low doses of nicotine have been demonstrated to have the opposite effect on dendritic cells, stimulating the expression of costimulatory molecules and increasing the secretion of IL-12, with an overall effect of stimulating T-cell proliferation and production of proinflammatory cytokines.[117,118]

Overall, the findings are consistent with a moderate adverse effect of smoking on MS onset, which increases with an increasing dose or duration of smoking. The increased risk seems to accumulate over time and appears to be reversible after quitting.

INFECTIONS AS A PROTECTIVE FACTOR

Infections might also play a protective role. Bach[119] demonstrated that the increased incidence over time of autoimmune and allergic diseases such as MS, type 1 diabetes,

Crohn disease, and asthma coincided with the decrease in incidence of measles, mumps, rheumatic fever, hepatitis A, and tuberculosis. These observations might be related to infection load during early childhood. In atopic disease, there is evidence for the so-called Hygiene Hypothesis, where increased hygiene and smaller family size over the last decades is thought to be associated with a reduced opportunity for infection in early childhood and an increased risk of atopic disease.[120]

Sibship structure has been used as a marker of infection load. The authors reported in 2005 that having more younger siblings was associated with a reduced risk of MS, and further, having a shorter interval between the index case and siblings reduced risk.[121] The authors combined these 2 aspects by calculating a cumulative exposure to younger infant siblings by the age of 6 years, and this measure was strongly associated with a reduced risk of MS. The replication of this finding has been somewhat inconsistent, however. Whereas a Swedish study found that having 3 or more younger siblings or having 2 or more older siblings was associated with a reduced risk of MS,[122] a Danish study did not find any sibling patterns.[123] A nested case-control study did not report directly on younger siblings but found that among families with 4 or more children, being the first born (equivalent to having 3 or more younger siblings, but no older siblings) was associated with an increased risk (OR = 2.1 [1.2–3.5]), though this was not the case in families with only 2 or 3 children (OR = 0.8 [0.5–1.2]).[11] This study found no effect of birth order and a weak protective effect for the increasing number of older siblings.[11] In general, studies on birth order, which reflects the number of older siblings but not younger siblings, have found no association.[26]

Younger siblings may provide a repeated source of exposure to common early-life microbial infections. Of interest, the authors also found that higher infant sibling exposure was associated with a reduced risk of IM and a lower rate of higher EBV IgG antibody titers among controls.[121] Moreover, higher infant sibling exposure was also associated with higher herpes simplex virus 1 (HSV-1) IgG antibody titers among controls[124] and HSV-1 IgG seropositivity was inversely associated with MS,[124,125] which was also reported in a study of pediatric MS.[125] A possible biologic mechanism is that younger siblings promote repeated exposure to common infant infections in early life, such as HSV-1, that may confer protection against an adverse autoimmune triggering effect of such infectious agents in later life.[121,125] Infant sibling exposure seems to interact with HLA-DR15, as the combined effect of HLA-DR15 positivity and low infant sibling exposure on MS was nearly fourfold higher than expected based on the effects of HLA-DR15 positivity and low infant sibling exposure alone.[18] This interaction was observed irrespective of EBNA IgG titers, indicating that it could not be explained by EBNA IgG titers alone. A similar interaction was observed between HLA-DR15 and being HSV-1 IgG seronegative.[18] These results raise the intriguing possibility that it partly reflects inadequate immune priming for those with the HLA-DR15 haplotype not only to EBV but also to related early-life viruses, as suggested in pediatric MS.[125]

Further studies are required in this area, and although the sibling method has been useful in older populations where the use of childcare was low, childcare needs to be taken into account when examining younger populations.

OTHER FACTORS

Several studies have investigated the relationship between human herpes virus (HHV)-6 and MS, but the results have been mixed. A systematic review of the literature between 1965 and 2001, which included 28 studies of serum, CSF, and/or pathology for the presence and quantity of serologic and/or direct evidence of HHV-6 infection, found no conclusive evidence of a difference in HHV-6 infection between cases and controls and thus, no association between HHV-6 and MS.[126] Subsequent studies have continued along similar veins, comparing MS cases and controls by the presence of HHV-6 infection and/or reactivation. However, no study has used samples obtained prior to onset, as has been done with EBV, so temporality has not been established.

The female predominance in many autoimmune diseases has intrigued many scientists. Significant increases in the female to male sex ratio of MS incidence have been observed in Canada[127] (1.014-fold increase per year over 1931–1980) and Oslo[128] (sex ratio increased from 1.48 to 2.30 over 1910–1980). The authors recently showed that the female to male ratio in first demyelinating events was much higher at a lower latitude, with the ratio being 6.7 in Brisbane (27°S), 3.4 in Newcastle (33°S), and 2.5 in Geelong (37°S) and Tasmania (43°S).[33] It is possible that environmental factors such as sun exposure affect males and females differentially across the latitude range. For example, males are more likely to be outdoors than females,[129] and the differences between males and females are likely to be larger in a high ambient UV environment. Indeed, the reverse latitudinal variation in sex ratio has been found for malignant melanoma incidence in Australia.[130] A recent review nicely outlines an array of differences between males and females that may influence differences in the incidence of autoimmune diseases.[131] These include differences in exposure to environmental factors, biologic response to environmental factors (eg, response of gene expression to vitamin D in mice),[132] general immune system function (eg, T-cell counts, ratios of CD4+ to CD8+), the level of sex hormones and their mediated effects (eg, estrogen, progesterone, androgens, prolactin, and luteinizing hormone releasing hormone), allele frequencies of genes or risk associated with genotypes (eg, HLA-DR15 was more frequent in female MS patients compared with male),[133] and interactions between, for example, sex hormones and genes.[131]

Numerous other environmental factors have been proposed over time. Some deserve more investigation, as there is either insufficient or inconsistent evidence; these include *Chlamydia pneumoniae*, organic solvents, psychological stress, physical trauma, and dietary fat.[5,134] For other factors a substantial number of studies have been conducted, but they do not support an association with MS; these include herpes simplex virus 1, varicella zoster, measles, mumps, and rubella.[5] In 1998, concern was raised in relation to hepatitis B vaccinations.[135] This positive association between hepatitis B vaccination and MS has been found in one other study,[136] but could not be confirmed in several other studies.[27,137–140] Several factors have been proposed to reduce the risk of MS, including vitamin D and juice intake, tetanus toxoid vaccination, use of antibiotics and antihistamines, and increased blood levels of uric acid; however, a role for these factors remains to be elucidated.[134]

THE JOINT ACTION OF RISK FACTORS

Recently, an increasing number of research groups has examined the combined action of 2 or more risk factors. In the most general sense, two risk factors are said to interact with one another if the effect of the first factor on disease risk depends on the level of the second factor, and vice versa. For gene-environment interaction, attention has largely focused on the major genetic risk factor HLA-DR15. Thus, the effect of an environmental exposure on MS might depend on whether a person is HLA-DR15 positive or HLA-DR15 negative, and also, the effect of HLA-DR15 might depend on the level of the environmental factor.

Two different methods have been used to examine and test for interaction, and there has been some debate about which method is preferable. The most common approach is to test for interaction on the multiplicative scale, by adding a product term to an exponential model such as a logistic or log-binomial model, then testing whether the coefficient of the product term is significant. Under this scenario, interaction is present when the increased risk in the presence of both factors is larger than the product of the risk increases conferred by the 2 factors separately. While this test is easy to apply, it has been argued that it is more useful biologically to test for interaction on an additive scale. A positive departure from additivity of effects implies that the total number of cases attributable to the 2 factors is larger than the sum of the number of cases caused by each factor separately (in the absence of the other factor). In the Rothman Causal Pie Model, this means that the 2 factors are present in the same causal mechanism as 2 slices of the same pie, for one or more pies.

The methods to test for interaction on the additive scale are less well developed, but include the use of measures such as the relative excess risk due to interaction (RERI), attributable proportion, or synergy index. Several methods have been proposed to calculate confidence intervals for these measures.[53,141–143] Of importance is that whether interaction is present can depend on whether a multiplicative or additive scale is used. It is therefore proposed to present the data in a 2-by-4 table (**Table 1**) where risk estimates are calculated for having factor 1 but not factor 2 (OR_{F1}), for having factor 2 but not factor 1 (OR_{F2}), and for having both factors together (OR_{both}). The reference group is the group that does not have factors 1 or 2. By presenting the data in this way, interaction can be assessed on both scales.

Interaction Between EBV and HLA-DR15

HLA class II allelic variation may play an important role in how people develop appropriate immune responses. Class II HLA genes produce molecules that participate in the recognition and presentation of antigens to T cells.[144] Class II HLA molecules are expressed on the surfaces of antigen-presenting cells (APCs). These molecules bind to peptides, and the HLA molecule/peptide complex is presented to T-cell receptors (TCRs) on T cells.[144] A T-cell receptor with the ability to bind to certain self-peptides is called a self-reactive T-cell receptor. Genetic differences in class II MHC

Table 1 Example of a presentation of the joint action of two factors for disease in a case-control study				
Factor 1	**Factor 2**		**OR**	**95% CI**
Absent	Absent	Reference	1	
Present	Absent	OR_{F1}	3.7	1.28–6.32
Absent	Present	OR_{F2}	6.9	1.83–31.80
Present	Present	OR_{both}	34.7	7.83–310.0
	Expected OR$_{interaction}$		Departure from expected	
Additive	3.7 + 6.9 – 1 = 9.6		34.7 – 9.6 = 25.07	
Multiplicative	3.7 × 6.9 = 25.7		34.7/25.7 = 1.4	

Factor 1 is oral contraceptive use, factor 2 is the factor V Leiden allele, and disease is venous thromboembolism.
OR_{F1} is the odds ratio for disease among those with factor 1 and without factor 2.
OR_{F2} is the odds ratio for disease among those with factor 2 and without factor 1.
OR_{both} is the odds ratio for disease among those with both factor 1 and factor 2.
Abbreviation: CI, confidence interval.
Data from Vandenbroucke JP, Koster T, Briet E, et al. Increased risk of venous thrombosis in oral-contraceptive users who are carriers of factor V Leiden mutation. Lancet 1994;344(8935):1453–57; *modified from* Botto LD, Khoury MJ. Commentary: facing the challenge of gene-environment interaction: the two-by-four table and beyond. Am J Epidemiol 2001;153(10):1016–20.

genes might result in differences in the affinity and the stimulatory potency of the complex between the class II molecules, the peptide, and the T-cell receptor. It is possible that EBV and HLA-DR15 interact with each other, as the HLA-DR15 haplotype seems to be an important determinant in the type of CD4$^+$ Th-mediated immune response to EBV infections.[145] A study examining processed EBV antigen epitope recognition by HLA-DR–restricted T cells showed that HLA-DR alleles, including DR15, DR4, and DR11, were involved in the presentation of the EBV antigen, EBNA1$_{482}$.[146] HLA class II molecules are important as a coreceptor for EBV entry into B cells,[147] and MHC polymorphisms alter the dynamics of the peptide-MHC landscape, resulting in fine-tuning of T-cell responses between closely related allotypes.[148]

Epidemiologic studies examining the interaction between HLA-DR15 and EBV, however, have provided mixed results. A Danish study indicated an association between EBV VCA IgG titers and *HLA-DRB1* among 517 healthy controls (P = .05).[149] De Jager and colleagues[150] observed that HLA-DR15 and EBNA seemed to operate independently in an additive fashion (nested case-control study in the Nurses' Health Study/Nurses' Health Study II). A pooled study, including data from 3 MS case-control studies (nested case-control study in the Nurses' Health Study/Nurses' Health Study II, the Tasmanian MS Study, and a Swedish MS study) did not observe interaction on a multiplicative scale between HLA-DR15 and EBNA.[107] The effect of increasing EBNA IgG titers on MS was similar for those who were HLA-DR15 positive (OR = 2.2 [1.6–3.0]) compared with those who were HLA-DR15 negative (OR = 2.4 [1.3–4.3]) (P = .95 for interaction).[107] In the Swedish MS study (which was also included in the pooled study), no interaction was observed between HLA-DR15 and EBNA-1. However, when the investigators examined specific epitopes of EBNA-1,[151] they found that the association of a short fragment of EBNA-1 (amino acids 385–420) was a much stronger predictor of MS in HLA-DR15–positive people than in HLA-DR15–negative people.[152]

A Danish study found an interaction between IM and HLA-DR15 and the risk of MS, observing that the association between HLA-DR15 and MS was stronger among those with a history of IM (OR = 7.0 [3.3–15.4]) than in those without a history of IM (OR = 2.4 [2.0–3.0]) (OR for multiplicative interaction 2.9 [1.3–6.5]).[153] Similar findings were observed in the Canadian Collaborative Study on the Genetic Susceptibility of MS, although this data should be interpreted with caution because of the small proportion of patients with a history of IM and possible ascertainment bias.[154]

Interaction Between EBV and Smoking

The only study that directly examined the interaction between EBV and smoking is the pooled study mentioned previously.[107] This study found that the increased risk of MS associated with high EBNA IgG titers was stronger among ever-smokers (OR = 3.9 [2.7–5.7]) than never-smokers (OR = 1.8 [1.4–2.3]) (P = .001 for interaction), or alternatively, the effect of smoking is present among those with high EBNA IgG titers (OR = 1.7 [1.1–2.6]) but absent among those with low EBNA titers (OR = 0.97 [0.7–1.3]).[107] A Danish study observed that EBV VCA IgG titers were higher among smokers in 517 healthy controls[149]; this was also observed in controls of the Tasmanian MS case-control study, though not in the Swedish MS study or the Nurses' Health Study/Nurses' Health Study II.[107]

Although there is limited evidence on the possible biologic mechanisms for this interaction, there are some similarities in relation to the consequences of exposure to nicotine or EBV. For example, EBV activation and nicotine metabolism have been shown to have shared molecular pathways including Jun-c-kinase,[155,156]

MAPK,[157,158] PKC,[157,159] and NF-κB.[160–162] In addition, changes in immune cell profiles may show some similar characteristics that are relevant for MS. There is some support for a role for CD8+ T cells[23] in MS, and EBV infection elicits strong and persistent epitope-specific CD8+ T-cell responses.[163] It has also been reported that smoking, particularly heavy smoking, may increase CD8+ T-cell counts, though this finding has not been consistent.[164]

Interaction Between Infant Sibling Exposure and HLA-DR15

In Tasmania, the authors found that the combined effect of HLA-DR15 positivity and low infant sibling exposure on MS (OR = 7.88 [3.43–18.11]) was nearly fourfold higher than expected based on the effects of HLA-DR15 positivity and low infant sibling exposure alone (P = .019 for interaction) (HLA-DR15 positivity alone, OR = 2.12 [1.00–4.50]; low infant sibling exposure alone, OR = 1.06 [0.56–2.01]). This interaction was observed irrespective of EBNA IgG titers (P = .79 for difference in interactions).[18] The modification of HLA-DR15 and MS risk by infant sibling exposure provides support for the concept that the apparent protective effect of infant sibling exposure is mediated through modulation of the immune system. The findings indicate that the adverse effect of HLA-DR15 on MS is not entirely predestined, but susceptible to modulation in early life. It is hypothesized that the decrease in the adverse HLA-DR15 effect by higher early-life infant sibling exposure could occur because people with the HLA-DR15 haplotype have CD4+ effector cells that particularly benefit from increased opportunities for T-cell receptor affinity refinement afforded by increased infant exposure. Past infection may influence cellular strategies in the thymus[144,165] that reduce the production of T lymphocytes with self-reactive receptors.

Interaction Between EBV and UV Exposure or Vitamin D

There have been no epidemiologic studies that have examined the interaction between EBV and UV exposure or vitamin D, but several mechanisms of interaction have been proposed. Hayes and Donald Acheson[166] proposed that an IL-10–like cytokine produced by EBV might induce dysfunction in IL-10–producing anti-inflammatory lymphocytes, thereby undermining the protective functions of UV exposure, 25(OH) D3, and 1,25(OH)2D3. This virally induced IL-10 could elicit a host immune response capable of neutralizing or depleting IL-10, or could compete with IL-10 for its receptor as an antagonist. Holmøy[167] proposed that vitamin D modulates the immune response to EBV and that detrimental activation of autoreactive T cells leading to MS is more likely if the vitamin D status is suboptimal. Holmøy argues that vitamin D receptors are expressed on EBV infected B cells, APCs, and activated lymphocytes, and that 1,25(OH)2D3 suppresses antibody production and T-cell proliferation and skews T cells toward a less detrimental T_h2 phenotype.

Interaction Between HLA-DR15 and UV Exposure or Vitamin D

A recent study provided functional evidence of an interaction between HLA and vitamin D. Ramagopalan and colleagues[168] identified a vitamin D response element (VDRE) in the proximal *HLA-DRB1* promoter. The VDRE was highly conserved on HLA-DR15 haplotypes (no mutations on more than 600 chromosomes) but not on some other *HLA-DRB1* haplotypes, suggesting a selective pressure to maintain this response element on the HLA-DR15 haplotype. The VDRE was responsive to 1,25 (OH)2D3 and was demonstrated to influence gene expression in B cells that were transiently transfected with the HLA-DR15 promoter. The extent of conservation of the VDRE still needs to be assessed on a wider range of haplotypes, but it raises the interesting possibility that vitamin D responsiveness rather than any antigen specificity determines the increased MS risk of HLA-DR15.

One study examined the interaction between HLA-DR15 and month of birth and MS. In a study of 4834 people with MS and a similar number of controls, people with MS who were born in April were more often HLA-DR15 positive (10.3% of HLA-DR15$^+$ vs 7.8% of HLA-DR15$^-$ were born in April, $P = .004$), whereas if born in November they were less often HLA-DR15 positive (6.0% of HLA-DR15$^+$ vs 7.9% of HLA-DR15$^-$ were born in November, $P = .023$).[169] Although this provides some support for the notion that timing of birth might interact with HLA-DR15 in MS, the investigators do not observe an effect of month of birth on MS risk in the total sample and do not examine the interaction directly.

Other Interactions

The Tasmanian MS case-control study provided some evidence for an interaction between a vitamin D receptor (VDR) polymorphism and sun exposure.[170] Whereas no significant univariate associations between the polymorphisms rs11574010 (Cdx-2A>G), rs10735810 (Fok1T>C), or rs731236 (Taq1C>T) and MS risk were observed, a significant interaction was observed between winter sun exposure during childhood, genotype at rs11574010, and MS risk ($P = .012$), with the "G" allele conferring an increased risk of MS in the low sun exposure group (≤ 2 hours per day). No significant interactions were observed for either rs10735810 or rs731236 following stratification by sun exposure. The same study found an interaction between the melanocortin 1 receptor gene (MC1R) alleles associated with red hair (RHC variant defined as having any Arg151Cys, Arg160Trp, or Asp294His alleles).[171] It was observed that the inverse association between increasing summer sun exposure at ages 6 to 10 years and MS was evident among those with no RHC variant ($P = .005$), but not among those with RHC variant genotype ($P = .18$; difference in effect, $P = .008$), and similar findings were evident for other past sun exposure measures.[171]

Conclusions on the Joint Action of Risk Factors

The number of studies examining interactions is increasing. Given that research on how genes influence susceptibility to MS is rapidly advancing, the area of gene-environment interactions will expand. Epidemiologic interactions will provide additional knowledge on the mechanisms by which different factors might mediate their effect and will, together with other areas of research, slowly unravel this complex disease. In addition, the demonstration of interactions also assists with the process of "causal inference." Given that randomized clinical trials are often unfeasible or unethical to be conducted when examining factors in relation to MS onset, causality needs to be inferred from other types of studies. Studies that can identify interaction are a welcome addition to the repertoire. The studies cited here describe some interesting interactions, but replication is still needed for most of them.

SUMMARY

The etiology of MS is a complex story with multiple factors playing a role at different times during life, interacting with each other to ultimately manifest in MS. Using the Rothman Causal Pie Model helps demonstrate that the way these factors come together to cause disease is somewhat idiosyncratic, with different individuals having different paths to disease; this complicates the task of epidemiologists. Defining causal associations is only a part of the whole equation. Knowing how causal and, for that matter, protective factors interact may provide further answers to the puzzle—teasing out these interactions and associations requires meticulous data collection and often complex analyses. The methodologies for assessing interactions are not as well elaborated as one would like (multiplicative vs additive interactions), thus complicating the area of study. However, these investigations are opening up MS research to a new frontier where we can understand the causal relationships between environmental, personal, and genetic characteristics that influence the risk of developing MS. The increase in knowledge on causal factors, the joint action of these factors, and the underlying mechanisms opens up the real possibility that MS risk could be reduced at the population and individual level by public health measures, including population-wide vitamin D supplementation or EBV vaccination if proven safe.

REFERENCES

1. Rothman KJ, Greenland S. Causation and causal inference in epidemiology. Am J Public Health 2005;95(Suppl 1):S144–50.
2. Hill AB. The environment and disease: association or causation? Proc R Soc Med 1965;58:295–300.
3. Thorley-Lawson DA. Epstein-Barr virus: exploiting the immune system. Nat Rev Immunol 2001;1(1):75–82.
4. Haahr S, Hollsberg P. Multiple sclerosis is linked to Epstein-Barr virus infection. Rev Med Virol 2006;16(5):297–310.
5. Ascherio A, Munger KL. Environmental risk factors for multiple sclerosis. Part I: the role of infection. Ann Neurol 2007;61(4):288–99.
6. Ascherio A, Munch M. Epstein-Barr virus and multiple sclerosis. Epidemiology 2000;11(2):220–4.
7. Thacker EL, Mirzaei F, Ascherio A. Infectious mononucleosis and risk for multiple sclerosis: a meta-analysis. Ann Neurol 2006;59(3):499–503.
8. Zaadstra BM, Chorus AM, van Buuren S, et al. Selective association of multiple sclerosis with infectious mononucleosis. Mult Scler 2008;14(3):307–13.
9. Nielsen TR, Rostgaard K, Nielsen NM, et al. Multiple sclerosis after infectious mononucleosis. Arch Neurol 2007;64(1):72–5.
10. Ramagopalan SV, Valdar W, Dyment DA, et al. Association of infectious mononucleosis with multiple sclerosis. A population-based study. Neuroepidemiology 2009;32(4):257–62.
11. Hernan MA, Zhang SM, Lipworth L, et al. Multiple sclerosis and age at infection with common viruses. Epidemiology 2001;12(3):301–6.
12. Ascherio A, Munger KL, Lennette ET, et al. Epstein-Barr virus antibodies and risk of multiple sclerosis: a prospective study. JAMA 2001;286(24):3083–8.
13. Levin LI, Munger KL, Rubertone MV, et al. Multiple sclerosis and Epstein-Barr virus. JAMA 2003;289(12):1533–6.
14. DeLorenze GN, Munger KL, Lennette ET, et al. Epstein-Barr virus and multiple sclerosis: evidence of association from a prospective study with long-term follow-up. Arch Neurol 2006;63(6):839–44.
15. Levin LI, Munger KL, Rubertone MV, et al. Temporal relationship between elevation of Epstein-Barr virus antibody titers and initial onset of neurological symptoms in multiple sclerosis. JAMA 2005;293(20):2496–500.
16. Sundstrom P, Juto P, Wadell G, et al. An altered immune response to Epstein-Barr virus in multiple sclerosis: a prospective study. Neurology 2004;62(12):2277–82.
17. Hochberg D, Middeldorp JM, Catalina M, et al. Demonstration of the Burkitt's lymphoma Epstein-Barr virus phenotype in dividing latently infected memory cells in vivo. Proc Natl Acad Sci U S A 2004;101(1):239–44.

18. van der Mei IA, Ponsonby AL, Taylor BV, et al. Human leukocyte antigen-DR15, low infant sibling exposure and multiple sclerosis: gene-environment interaction. Ann Neurol 2010;67(2):261–5.

19. Pohl D, Krone B, Rostasy K, et al. High seroprevalence of Epstein-Barr virus in children with multiple sclerosis. Neurology 2006;67(11):2063–5.

20. Banwell B, Krupp L, Kennedy J, et al. Clinical features and viral serologies in children with multiple sclerosis: a multinational observational study. Lancet Neurol 2007;6(9):773–81.

21. Hollsberg P, Hansen HJ, Haahr S. Altered CD8+ T cell responses to selected Epstein-Barr virus immunodominant epitopes in patients with multiple sclerosis. Clin Exp Immunol 2003;132(1):137–43.

22. Lunemann JD, Edwards N, Muraro PA, et al. Increased frequency and broadened specificity of latent EBV nuclear antigen-1-specific T cells in multiple sclerosis. Brain 2006;129(Pt 6):1493–506.

23. Cepok S, Zhou D, Srivastava R, et al. Identification of Epstein-Barr virus proteins as putative targets of the immune response in multiple sclerosis. J Clin Invest 2005;115(5):1352–60.

24. Lunemann JD, Jelcic I, Roberts S, et al. EBNA1-specific T cells from patients with multiple sclerosis cross react with myelin antigens and co-produce IFN-gamma and IL-2. J Exp Med 2008;205(8):1763–73.

25. Serafini B, Rosicarelli B, Franciotta D, et al. Dysregulated Epstein-Barr virus infection in the multiple sclerosis brain. J Exp Med 2007;204(12):2899–912.

26. Willis SN, Stadelmann C, Rodig SJ, et al. Epstein-Barr virus infection is not a characteristic feature of multiple sclerosis brain. Brain 2009;132(Pt 12):3318–28.

27. Sargsyan SA, Shearer AJ, Ritchie AM, et al. Absence of Epstein-Barr virus in the brain and CSF of patients with multiple sclerosis. Neurology 2010;74(14):1127–35.

28. Pender MP. Preventing and curing multiple sclerosis by controlling Epstein-Barr virus infection. Autoimmun Rev 2009;8(7):563–8.

29. McLeod JG, Hammond SR, Hallpike JF. Epidemiology of multiple sclerosis in Australia. With NSW and SA survey results. Med J Aust 1994;160(3):117–22.

30. Kurtzke JF. Geography in multiple sclerosis. J Neurol 1977;215(1):1–26.

31. Zivadinov R, Iona L, Monti-Bragadin L, et al. The use of standardized incidence and prevalence rates in epidemiological studies on multiple sclerosis. A meta-analysis study. Neuroepidemiology 2003;22(1):65–74.

32. Alonso A, Hernan MA. Temporal trends in the incidence of multiple sclerosis: a systematic review. Neurology 2008;71(2):129–35.

33. Taylor BV, Lucas RM, Dear K, et al. Latitudinal variation in incidence and type of first central nervous system demyelinating events. Mult Scler 2010;16(4):398–405.

34. McGuigan C, Dunne C, Crowley J, et al. Population frequency of HLA haplotypes contributes to the prevalence difference of multiple sclerosis in Ireland. J Neurol 2005;252(10):1245–8.

35. Handel AE, Handunnetthi L, Giovannoni G, et al. Genetic and environmental factors and the distribution of multiple sclerosis in Europe. Eur J Neurol 2010;17(9):1210–4.

36. McCall MG, Brereton TL, Dawson A, et al. Frequency of multiple sclerosis in three Australian cities—Perth, Newcastle, and Hobart. J Neurol Neurosurg Psychiatry 1968;31(1):1–9.

37. Hammond SR, McLeod JG, Millingen KS, et al. The epidemiology of multiple sclerosis in three Australian cities: Perth, Newcastle and Hobart. Brain 1988;111(Pt 1):1–25.

38. Skegg DC, Corwin PA, Craven RS, et al. Occurrence of multiple sclerosis in the north and south of New Zealand. J Neurol Neurosurg Psychiatry 1987;50(2): 134–9.
39. Alter M, Leibowitz U, Speer J. Risk of multiple sclerosis related to age at immigration to Israel. Arch Neurol 1966;15(3):234–7.
40. Hammond SR, English DR, McLeod JG. The age-range of risk of developing multiple sclerosis: evidence from a migrant population in Australia. Brain 2000;123(Pt 5):968–74.
41. Dean G, Elian M. Age at immigration to England of Asian and Caribbean immigrants and the risk of developing multiple sclerosis. J Neurol Neurosurg Psychiatry 1997;63(5):565–8.
42. Acheson ED, Bachrach CA, Wright FM. Some comments on the relationship of the distribution of multiple sclerosis to latitude, solar radiation, and other variables. Acta Psychiatr Scand Suppl 1960;35(147):132–47.
43. Munger KL, Levin LI, Hollis BW, et al. Serum 25-hydroxyvitamin D levels and risk of multiple sclerosis. JAMA 2006;296(23):2832–8.
44. Munger KL, Zhang SM, O'Reilly E, et al. Vitamin D intake and incidence of multiple sclerosis. Neurology 2004;62(1):60–5.
45. Islam T, Gauderman WJ, Cozen W, et al. Childhood sun exposure influences risk of multiple sclerosis in monozygotic twins. Neurology 2007;69(4):381–8.
46. van der Mei IA, Ponsonby AL, Dwyer T, et al. Past exposure to sun, skin phenotype, and risk of multiple sclerosis: case-control study. BMJ 2003;327(7410): 316.
47. Kampman MT, Wilsgaard T, Mellgren SI. Outdoor activities and diet in childhood and adolescence relate to MS risk above the Arctic Circle. J Neurol 2007; 254(4):471–7.
48. Brustad M, Alsaker E, Engelsen O, et al. Vitamin D status of middle-aged women at 65-71 degrees N in relation to dietary intake and exposure to ultraviolet radiation. Public Health Nutr 2004;7(2):327–35.
49. Freedman DM, Dosemeci M, Alavanja MC. Mortality from multiple sclerosis and exposure to residential and occupational solar radiation: a case-control study based on death certificates. Occup Environ Med 2000;57(6):418–21.
50. Westberg M, Feychting M, Jonsson F, et al. Occupational exposure to UV light and mortality from multiple sclerosis. Am J Ind Med 2009;52(5):353–7.
51. Goldacre MJ, Seagroatt V, Yeates D, et al. Skin cancer in people with multiple sclerosis: a record linkage study. J Epidemiol Community Health 2004;58(2): 142–4.
52. Willer CJ, Dyment DA, Sadovnick AD, et al. Timing of birth and risk of multiple sclerosis: population based study. BMJ 2005;330(7483):120.
53. Staples J, Ponsonby AL, Lim L, et al. Low maternal exposure to ultraviolet radiation in pregnancy, month of birth, and risk of multiple sclerosis in offspring: longitudinal analysis. BMJ 2010;340:c1640.
54. Levenson CW, Figueiroa SM. Gestational vitamin D deficiency: long-term effects on the brain. Nutr Rev 2008;66(12):726–9.
55. Handel AE, Giovannoni G, Ebers GC, et al. Environmental factors and their timing in adult-onset multiple sclerosis. Nat Rev Neurol 2010;6(3):156–66.
56. Ko P, Burkert R, McGrath J, et al. Maternal vitamin D3 deprivation and the regulation of apoptosis and cell cycle during rat brain development. Brain Res Dev Brain Res 2004;153(1):61–8.
57. Cui X, McGrath JJ, Burne TH, et al. Maternal vitamin D depletion alters neurogenesis in the developing rat brain. Int J Dev Neurosci 2007;25(4):227–32.

58. Eyles D, Brown J, Mackay-Sim A, et al. Vitamin D3 and brain development. Neuroscience 2003;118(3):641–53.
59. Feron F, Burne TH, Brown J, et al. Developmental vitamin D3 deficiency alters the adult rat brain. Brain Res Bull 2005;65(2):141–8.
60. Almeras L, Eyles D, Benech P, et al. Developmental vitamin D deficiency alters brain protein expression in the adult rat: implications for neuropsychiatric disorders. Proteomics 2007;7(5):769–80.
61. Eyles DW, Feron F, Cui X, et al. Developmental vitamin D deficiency causes abnormal brain development. Psychoneuroendocrinology 2009;34(Suppl 1): S247–57.
62. O'Loan J, Eyles DW, Kesby J, et al. Vitamin D deficiency during various stages of pregnancy in the rat; its impact on development and behaviour in adult offspring. Psychoneuroendocrinology 2007;32(3):227–34.
63. Tsoukas CD, Provvedini DM, Manolagas SC. 1,25-Dihydroxyvitamin D3: a novel immunoregulatory hormone. Science 1984;224(4656):1438–40.
64. Bhalla AK, Amento EP, Krane SM. Differential effects of 1,25-dihydroxyvitamin D3 on human lymphocytes and monocyte/macrophages: inhibition of interleukin-2 and augmentation of interleukin-1 production. Cell Immunol 1986;98(2):311–22.
65. Lemire J. 1,25-Dihydroxyvitamin D3—a hormone with immunomodulatory properties. Z Rheumatol 2000;59(Suppl 1):24–7.
66. Lemire JM. Immunomodulatory actions of 1,25-dihydroxyvitamin D3. J Steroid Biochem Mol Biol 1995;53(1–6):599–602.
67. Meehan MA, Kerman RH, Lemire JM. 1,25-Dihydroxyvitamin D3 enhances the generation of nonspecific suppressor cells while inhibiting the induction of cytotoxic cells in a human MLR. Cell Immunol 1992;140(2):400–9.
68. Tsoukas CD, Watry D, Escobar SS, et al. Inhibition of interleukin-1 production by 1,25-dihydroxyvitamin D3. J Clin Endocrinol Metab 1989;69(1):127–33.
69. Tang J, Zhou R, Luger D, et al. Calcitriol suppresses antiretinal autoimmunity through inhibitory effects on the Th17 effector response. J Immunol 2009; 182(8):4624–32.
70. Boonstra A, Barrat FJ, Crain C, et al. 1alpha,25-Dihydroxyvitamin D3 has a direct effect on naive CD4(+) T cells to enhance the development of Th2 cells. J Immunol 2001;167(9):4974–80.
71. Jeffery LE, Burke F, Mura M, et al. 1,25-Dihydroxyvitamin D3 and IL-2 combine to inhibit T cell production of inflammatory cytokines and promote development of regulatory T cells expressing CTLA-4 and FoxP3. J Immunol 2009;183(9):5458–67.
72. Baeke F, Korf H, Overbergh L, et al. Human T lymphocytes are direct targets of 1,25-dihydroxyvitamin D(3) in the immune system. J Steroid Biochem Mol Biol 2010;121(1/2):221–7.
73. Giulietti A, van Etten E, Overbergh L, et al. Monocytes from type 2 diabetic patients have a pro-inflammatory profile. 1,25-Dihydroxyvitamin D(3) works as anti-inflammatory. Diabetes Res Clin Pract 2007;77(1):47–57.
74. Daniel C, Sartory NA, Zahn N, et al. Immune modulatory treatment of trinitrobenzene sulfonic acid colitis with calcitriol is associated with a change of a T helper (Th) 1/Th17 to a Th2 and regulatory T cell profile. J Pharmacol Exp Ther 2008; 324(1):23–33.
75. Penna G, Adorini L. 1 Alpha,25-dihydroxyvitamin D3 inhibits differentiation, maturation, activation, and survival of dendritic cells leading to impaired alloreactive T cell activation. J Immunol 2000;164(5):2405–11.
76. Heine G, Niesner U, Chang HD, et al. 1,25-Dihydroxyvitamin D(3) promotes IL-10 production in human B cells. Eur J Immunol 2008;38(8):2210–8.

77. Cantorna MT, Woodward WD, Hayes CE, et al. 1,25-Dihydroxyvitamin D3 is a positive regulator for the two anti-encephalitogenic cytokines TGF-beta 1 and IL-4. J Immunol 1998;160(11):5314–9.
78. Garcion E, Sindji L, Nataf S, et al. Treatment of experimental autoimmune encephalomyelitis in rat by 1,25-dihydroxyvitamin D3 leads to early effects within the central nervous system. Acta Neuropathol 2003;105(5):438–48.
79. Lemire JM, Archer DC. 1,25-Dihydroxyvitamin D3 prevents the in vivo induction of murine experimental autoimmune encephalomyelitis. J Clin Invest 1991;87(3): 1103–7.
80. Cantorna MT, Hayes CE, DeLuca HF. 1,25-Dihydroxyvitamin D3 reversibly blocks the progression of relapsing encephalomyelitis, a model of multiple sclerosis. Proc Natl Acad Sci U S A 1996;93(15):7861–4.
81. Garcion E, Nataf S, Berod A, et al. 1,25-Dihydroxyvitamin D3 inhibits the expression of inducible nitric oxide synthase in rat central nervous system during experimental allergic encephalomyelitis. Brain Res Mol Brain Res 1997;45(2): 255–67.
82. Pedersen LB, Nashold FE, Spach KM, et al. 1,25-Dihydroxyvitamin D3 reverses experimental autoimmune encephalomyelitis by inhibiting chemokine synthesis and monocyte trafficking. J Neurosci Res 2007;85(11):2480–90.
83. Smolders J, Thewissen M, Peelen E, et al. Vitamin D status is positively correlated with regulatory T cell function in patients with multiple sclerosis. PLoS One 2009;4(8):e6635.
84. Royal W 3rd, Mia Y, Li H, et al. Peripheral blood regulatory T cell measurements correlate with serum vitamin D levels in patients with multiple sclerosis. J Neuroimmunol 2009;213(1/2):135–41.
85. Smolders J, Menheere P, Thewissen M, et al. Regulatory T cell function correlates with serum 25-hydroxyvitamin D, but not with 1,25-dihydroxyvitamin D, parathyroid hormone and calcium levels in patients with relapsing remitting multiple sclerosis. J Steroid Biochem Mol Biol 2010;121(1/2):243–6.
86. Correale J, Ysrraelit MC, Gaitan MI. Immunomodulatory effects of Vitamin D in multiple sclerosis. Brain 2009;132(Pt 5):1146–60.
87. Garssen J, van Loveren H. Effects of ultraviolet exposure on the immune system. Crit Rev Immunol 2001;21(4):359–97.
88. Murphy GM. Ultraviolet radiation and immunosuppression. Br J Dermatol 2009; 161(Suppl 3):90–5.
89. Schwarz T. Mechanisms of UV-induced immunosuppression. Keio J Med 2005; 54(4):165–71.
90. Kulms D, Zeise E, Poppelmann B, et al. DNA damage, death receptor activation and reactive oxygen species contribute to ultraviolet radiation-induced apoptosis in an essential and independent way. Oncogene 2002;21(38):5844–51.
91. Weiss JM, Renkl AC, Denfeld RW, et al. Low-dose UVB radiation perturbs the functional expression of B7.1 and B7.2 co-stimulatory molecules on human Langerhans cells. Eur J Immunol 1995;25(10):2858–62.
92. Dandie GW, Clydesdale GJ, Jacobs I, et al. Effects of UV on the migration and function of epidermal antigen presenting cells. Mutat Res 1998;422(1):147–54.
93. Simon JC, Cruz PD Jr, Bergstresser PR, et al. Low dose ultraviolet B-irradiated Langerhans cells preferentially activate CD4+ cells of the T helper 2 subset. J Immunol 1990;145(7):2087–91.
94. Simon JC, Hara H, Denfeld RW, et al. UVB-irradiated dendritic cells induce nonproliferating, regulatory type T cells. Skin Pharmacol Appl Skin Physiol 2002; 15(5):330–4.

95. Shreedhar V, Giese T, Sung VW, et al. A cytokine cascade including prosta-glandin E2, IL-4, and IL-10 is responsible for UV-induced systemic immune suppression. J Immunol 1998;160(8):3783–9.

96. Nishigori C, Yarosh DB, Ullrich SE, et al. Evidence that DNA damage triggers interleukin 10 cytokine production in UV-irradiated murine keratinocytes. Proc Natl Acad Sci U S A 1996;93(19):10354–9.

97. Rivas JM, Ullrich SE. Systemic suppression of delayed-type hypersensitivity by supernatants from UV-irradiated keratinocytes. An essential role for keratinocyte-derived IL-10. J Immunol 1992;149(12):3865–71.

98. Hernan MA, Oleky MJ, Ascherio A. Cigarette smoking and incidence of multiple sclerosis. Am J Epidemiol 2001;154(1):69–74.

99. Hernan MA, Jick SS, Logroscino G, et al. Cigarette smoking and the progression of multiple sclerosis. Brain 2005;128(Pt 6):1461–5.

100. Thorogood M, Hannaford PC. The influence of oral contraceptives on the risk of multiple sclerosis. Br J Obstet Gynaecol 1998;105(12):1296–9.

101. Villard-Mackintosh L, Vessey MP. Oral contraceptives and reproductive factors in multiple sclerosis incidence. Contraception 1993;47(2):161–8.

102. Hawkes CH. Smoking is a risk factor for multiple sclerosis: a metanalysis. Mult Scler 2007;13(5):610–5.

103. Rodriguez Regal A, del Campo Amigo M, Paz-Esquete J, et al. A case-control study of the influence of the smoking behaviour in multiple sclerosis. Neurologia 2009;24(3):177–80 [in Spanish].

104. Hedstrom AK, Baarnhielm M, Olsson T, et al. Tobacco smoking, but not Swedish snuff use, increases the risk of multiple sclerosis. Neurology 2009;73(9):696–701.

105. Pekmezovic T, Drulovic J, Milenkovic M, et al. Lifestyle factors and multiple scle-rosis: a case-control study in Belgrade. Neuroepidemiology 2006;27(4):212–6.

106. Silva KR, Alvarenga RM, Fernandez YFO, et al. Potential risk factors for multiple sclerosis in Rio de Janeiro: a case-control study. Arq Neuropsiquiatr 2009; 67(2A):229–34.

107. Simon KC, van der Mei IA, Munger KL, et al. Combined effects of smoking, anti-EBNA antibodies, and HLA-DRB1*1501 on multiple sclerosis risk. Neurology 2010;74(17):1365–71.

108. Jafari N, Hoppenbrouwers IA, Hop WC, et al. Cigarette smoking and risk of MS in multiplex families. Mult Scler 2009;15(11):1363–7.

109. Piao WH, Campagnolo D, Dayao C, et al. Nicotine and inflammatory neurolog-ical disorders. Acta Pharmacol Sin 2009;30(6):715–22.

110. Warren SA, Warren KG, Greenhill S, et al. How multiple sclerosis is related to animal illness, stress and diabetes. Can Med Assoc J 1982;126(4):377–82, 385.

111. Mikaeloff Y, Caridade G, Tardieu M, et al. Parental smoking at home and the risk of childhood-onset multiple sclerosis in children. Brain 2007;130(Pt 10):2589–95.

112. Montgomery SM, Bahmanyar S, Hillert J, et al. Maternal smoking during preg-nancy and multiple sclerosis amongst offspring. Eur J Neurol 2008;15(12):1395–9.

113. Sopori M. Effects of cigarette smoke on the immune system. Nat Rev Immunol 2002;2(5):372–7.

114. Piao WH, Campagnolo D, Dayao C, et al. Nicotine and inflammatory neurolog-ical disorders. Acta Pharmacol Sin 2009;30(6):715–22.

115. Costenbader KH, Karlson EW. Cigarette smoking and autoimmune disease: what can we learn from epidemiology? Lupus 2006;15(11):737–45.

116. Harel-Meir M, Sherer Y, Shoenfeld Y. Tobacco smoking and autoimmune rheu-matic diseases. Nat Clin Pract Rheumatol 2007;3(12):707–15.

117. Gahring LC, Rogers SW. Neuronal nicotinic acetylcholine receptor expression and function on nonneuronal cells. AAPS J 2005;7(4):E885–94.

118. Aicher A, Heeschen C, Mohaupt M, et al. Nicotine strongly activates dendritic cell-mediated adaptive immunity: potential role for progression of atherosclerotic lesions. Circulation 2003;107(4):604–11.

119. Bach JF. The effect of infections on susceptibility to autoimmune and allergic diseases. N Engl J Med 2002;347(12):911–20.

120. Leeder SR, Corkhill R, Irwig LM, et al. Influence of family factors on the incidence of lower respiratory illness during the first year of life. Br J Prev Soc Med 1976;30(4):203–12.

121. Ponsonby AL, van der Mei I, Dwyer T, et al. Exposure to infant siblings during early life and risk of multiple sclerosis. JAMA 2005;293(4):463–9.

122. Montgomery SM, Lambe M, Olsson T, et al. Parental age, family size, and risk of multiple sclerosis. Epidemiology 2004;15(6):717–23.

123. Bager P, Nielsen NM, Bihrmann K, et al. Sibship characteristics and risk of multiple sclerosis: a nationwide cohort study in Denmark. Am J Epidemiol 2006;163(12):1112–7.

124. Ponsonby AL, Dwyer T, van der Mei I, et al. Asthma onset prior to multiple sclerosis and the contribution of sibling exposure in early life. Clin Exp Immunol 2006;146(3):463–70.

125. Alotaibi S, Kennedy J, Tellier R, et al. Epstein-Barr virus in pediatric multiple sclerosis. JAMA 2004;291(15):1875–9.

126. Moore FG, Wolfson C. Human herpes virus 6 and multiple sclerosis. Acta Neurol Scand 2002;106(2):63–83.

127. Orton SM, Herrera BM, Yee IM, et al. Sex ratio of multiple sclerosis in Canada: a longitudinal study. Lancet Neurol 2006;5(11):932–6.

128. Celius EG, Smestad C. Change in sex ratio, disease course and age at diagnosis in Oslo MS patients through seven decades. Acta Neurol Scand Suppl 2009;189:27–9.

129. Fritschi L, Green A, Solomon PJ. Sun exposure in Australian adolescents. J Am Acad Dermatol 1992;27(1):25–8.

130. Jones ME, Shugg D, Dwyer T, et al. Interstate differences in incidence and mortality from melanoma. A re-examination of the latitudinal gradient. Med J Aust 1992;157(6):373–8.

131. McCombe PA, Greer JM, Mackay IR. Sexual dimorphism in autoimmune disease. Curr Mol Med 2009;9(9):1058–79.

132. Song Y, Fleet JC. 1,25 Dihydroxycholecalciferol-mediated calcium absorption and gene expression are higher in female than in male mice. J Nutr 2004; 134(8):1857–61.

133. Celius EG, Harbo HF, Egeland T, et al. Sex and age at diagnosis are correlated with the HLA-DR2, DQ6 haplotype in multiple sclerosis. J Neurol Sci 2000;178(2):132–5.

134. Ascherio A, Munger KL. Environmental risk factors for multiple sclerosis. Part II: Noninfectious factors. Ann Neurol 2007;61(6):504–13.

135. Marshall E. A shadow falls on hepatitis B vaccination effort. Science 1998; 281(5377):630–1.

136. Hernan MA, Jick SS, Olek MJ, et al. Recombinant hepatitis B vaccine and the risk of multiple sclerosis: a prospective study. Neurology 2004;63(5): 838–42.

137. Touze E, Fourrier A, Rue-Fenouche C, et al. Hepatitis B vaccination and first central nervous system demyelinating event: a case-control study. Neuroepidemiology 2002;21(4):180–6.

138. Zipp F, Weil JG, Einhaupl KM. No increase in demyelinating diseases after hepatitis B vaccination. Nat Med 1999;5(9):964–5.
139. DeStefano F, Verstraeten T, Jackson LA, et al. Vaccinations and risk of central nervous system demyelinating diseases in adults. Arch Neurol 2003;60(4):504–9.
140. Sadovnick AD, Scheifele DW. School-based hepatitis B vaccination programme and adolescent multiple sclerosis. Lancet 2000;355(9203):549–50.
141. Hosmer DW, Lemeshow S. Confidence interval estimation of interaction. Epidemiology 1992;3(5):452–6.
142. Zou GY. On the estimation of additive interaction by use of the four-by-two table and beyond. Am J Epidemiol 2008;168(2):212–24.
143. Richardson DB, Kaufman JS. Estimation of the relative excess risk due to interaction and associated confidence bounds. Am J Epidemiol 2009;169(6):756–60.
144. Klein J, Sato A. The HLA system. First of two parts. N Engl J Med 2000;343(10): 702–9.
145. Lunemann JD, Kamradt T, Martin R, et al. Epstein-Barr virus: environmental trigger of multiple sclerosis? J Virol 2007;81(13):6777–84.
146. Kruger S, Schroers R, Rooney CM, et al. Identification of a naturally processed HLA-DR-restricted T-helper epitope in Epstein-Barr virus nuclear antigen type 1. J Immunother 2003;26(3):212–21.
147. Haan KM, Longnecker R. Coreceptor restriction within the HLA-DQ locus for Epstein-Barr virus infection. Proc Natl Acad Sci U S A 2000;97(16):9252–7.
148. Archbold JK, Macdonald WA, Gras S, et al. Natural micropolymorphism in human leukocyte antigens provides a basis for genetic control of antigen recognition. J Exp Med 2009;206(1):209–19.
149. Nielsen TR, Pedersen M, Rostgaard K, et al. Correlations between Epstein-Barr virus antibody levels and risk factors for multiple sclerosis in healthy individuals. Mult Scler 2007;13(3):420–3.
150. De Jager PL, Simon KC, Munger KL, et al. Integrating risk factors: HLA-DRB1*1501 and Epstein-Barr virus in multiple sclerosis. Neurology 2008; 70(13 Pt 2):1113–8.
151. Sundstrom P, Nystrom L, Jidell E, et al. EBNA-1 reactivity and HLA DRB1*1501 as statistically independent risk factors for multiple sclerosis: a case-control study. Mult Scler 2008;14(8):1120–2.
152. Sundstrom P, Nystrom M, Ruuth K, et al. Antibodies to specific EBNA-1 domains and HLA DRB1*1501 interact as risk factors for multiple sclerosis. J Neuroimmunol 2009;215(1/2):102–7.
153. Nielsen T, Rostgaard K, Askling J, et al. Effects of infectious mononucleosis and HLA-DRB1*15 in multiple sclerosis. Mult Scler 2009;15(4):431–6.
154. Ramagopalan SV, Sadovnick AD, Ebers GC, et al. Effects of infectious mononucleosis and HLA-DRB1*15 in multiple sclerosis. Mult Scler 2010;16(1):127–8.
155. Eliopoulos AG, Young LS. Activation of the cJun N-terminal kinase (JNK) pathway by the Epstein-Barr virus-encoded latent membrane protein 1 (LMP1). Oncogene 1998;16(13):1731–42.
156. Hoshino S, Yoshida M, Inoue K, et al. Cigarette smoke extract induces endothelial cell injury via JNK pathway. Biochem Biophys Res Commun 2005;329(1):58–63.
157. Heusch WL, Maneckjee R. Signalling pathways involved in nicotine regulation of apoptosis of human lung cancer cells. Carcinogenesis 1998;19(4):551–6.
158. Satoh T, Hoshikawa Y, Satoh Y, et al. The interaction of mitogen-activated protein kinases to Epstein-Barr virus activation in Akata cells. Virus Genes 1999;18(1): 57–64.

159. Baumann M, Mischak H, Dammeier S, et al. Activation of the Epstein-Barr virus transcription factor BZLF1 by 12-O-tetradecanoylphorbol-13-acetate-induced phosphorylation. J Virol 1998;72(10):8105–14.
160. Shen Y, Rattan V, Sultana C, et al. Cigarette smoke condensate-induced adhesion molecule expression and transendothelial migration of monocytes. Am J Physiol 1996;270(5 Pt 2):H1624–33.
161. Zhang S, Day I, Ye S. Nicotine induced changes in gene expression by human coronary artery endothelial cells. Atherosclerosis 2001;154(2):277–83.
162. Adamson AL, Kenney S. The Epstein-Barr virus BZLF1 protein interacts physically and functionally with the histone acetylase CREB-binding protein. J Virol 1999;73(8):6551–8.
163. Rickinson AB, Kieff E. Epstein-Barr virus. In: Knipe DM, Howley PM, Griffin DE, et al, editors. Fields virology, vol. 2. 5th edition. Philadelphia: Wolters Kluwer Health/Lippincott Williams & Wilkins; 2007. p. 2655–700.
164. Arcavi L, Benowitz NL. Cigarette smoking and infection. Arch Intern Med 2004; 164(20):2206–16.
165. Goodnow CC, Sprent J, Fazekas de St Groth B, et al. Cellular and genetic mechanisms of self tolerance and autoimmunity. Nature 2005;435(7042):590–7.
166. Hayes CE, Donald Acheson E. A unifying multiple sclerosis etiology linking virus infection, sunlight, and vitamin D, through viral interleukin-10. Med Hypotheses 2008;71(1):85–90.
167. Holmøy T. Vitamin D status modulates the immune response to Epstein Barr virus: synergistic effect of risk factors in multiple sclerosis. Med Hypotheses 2008;70(1):66–9.
168. Ramagopalan SV, Maugeri NJ, Handunnetthi L, et al. Expression of the multiple sclerosis-associated MHC class II allele HLA-DRB1*1501 is regulated by vitamin D. PLoS Genet 2009;5(2):e1000369.
169. Ramagopalan SV, Link J, Byrnes JK, et al. HLA-DRB1 and month of birth in multiple sclerosis. Neurology 2009;73(24):2107–11.
170. Dickinson JL, Perera DI, van der Mei AF, et al. Past environmental sun exposure and risk of multiple sclerosis: a role for the Cdx-2 Vitamin D receptor variant in this interaction. Mult Scler 2009;15(5):563–70.
171. Dwyer T, van der Mei I, Ponsonby AL, et al. Melanocortin 1 receptor genotype, past environmental sun exposure, and risk of multiple sclerosis. Neurology 2008;71(8):583–9.

The Immunopathophysiology of Multiple Sclerosis

Gregory F. Wu, MD, PhD*, Enrique Alvarez, MD, PhD

KEYWORDS

- Multiple sclerosis • Neuroimmunology • Demyelination
- Pathogenesis

OVERVIEW

The cause of multiple sclerosis (MS) is elusive. However, clues to the pathogenesis of this condition have traditionally been derived from the basic pathologic characterization of the central nervous system (CNS) tissues of patients with MS. Although ongoing debate lingers over the autoimmune nature of MS, it is well established that the immune system directly participates in the destruction of myelin and nerve cells. Understanding the mechanisms of immune-mediated destruction of the CNS components in MS not only promises to promote the effective design of MS therapeutics but also provides a broader understanding of immune-mediated diseases affecting the CNS.

This review explores the principle features of the immunopathology of MS, in particular of relapsing-remitting MS (RR-MS). It highlights the emerging concepts in the pathogenesis of MS in the context of known features of pathology, including the characterization of cytokine networks promoting inflammatory damage of the CNS, B-cell involvement, and inflammatory damage of axons and neurons. This article preferentially focuses on MS rather than animal models of the disease, such as experimental autoimmune encephalomyelitis (EAE). For a more comprehensive examination of data derived from studies on animal models, the readers are referred to other reviews.[1,2] From human studies alone it is clear that the past 5 to 10 years have been highly productive in advancing the understanding of the pathogenesis of MS. For both the general neurologist and the MS specialist, the fundamental appreciation of the immunopathology of MS should lead to a broader understanding of the disease course and the emerging MS therapeutics that are now more-than-ever tailored to the intricacies of the immune system.

PATHOLOGIC CHARACTERIZATION OF MS LESIONS

Plaques of inflammatory demyelination within the CNS are the pathologic hallmark of MS.[3–5] Myelin destruction is an essential element of the plaque. Yet the MS plaque is

Division of Multiple Sclerosis, Department of Neurology, Washington University, Box 8111, 660 South Euclid Avenue, St Louis, MO 63110, USA
* Corresponding author.
E-mail address: wug@neuro.wustl.edu

Neurol Clin 29 (2011) 257–278
doi:10.1016/j.ncl.2010.12.009   **neurologic.theclinics.com**

not simply a static entity of myelin loss in isolation; rather, the lesions are composed of a wide variety of immunologic and pathologic features. These features have been categorized in an effort to understand the neural-immune mechanisms underlying MS. Constructing a framework around which myelin loss and neuronal/axonal injury occur entails a close examination of the cellular and molecular constituents, timing of damage, and repair processes. Thus, the various features of plaques provide a platform on which hypotheses regarding pathogenic mechanisms underlying MS have been formulated for over a century.

Traditionally, MS plaque classification has been based on temporal progression, or stages, of inflammatory destruction. Accordingly, acute, chronic active, and chronic silent lesions are thought to occur along a continuous timeline, eventually producing the scarred and hardened areas within the CNS that can be appreciated grossly (**Fig. 1**). The acute MS plaque represents the earliest stage of lesion formation. This plaque is typified by robust inflammatory infiltration combined with demyelination distributed throughout the lesion (see **Fig. 1**).[5–7] Typical features of the acute plaque include ill-defined margins of myelin loss, infiltration of immune cells, and parenchymal edema.[5] The constituents of immune cell influx around vessels (termed perivascular cuffing) include lymphocytes (predominantly T cells), monocytes, and macrophages. A portion of class II major histocompatibility complex (MHC)-expressing cells, distributed evenly throughout the lesion, is loaded with lipids (foamy macrophages, see **Fig. 1**) and participates in active stripping of myelin from axons. Although oligodendrocyte apoptosis has been observed,[8] the degree of oligodendrocyte loss within active lesions can be variable.[6] In spite of the relative degree of axonal sparing, axonal injury

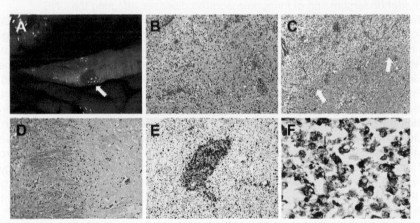

Fig. 1. Gross and histologic features of MS plaques. (A) Gross examination of the brain at autopsy of a 79-year-old patient with RR-MS. A dorsal view of the corpus callosum after separation of the cerebral hemispheres reveals a hardened discolored area within the body of the corpus callosum (*arrow*). (B) Acute MS plaque revealing hypercellularity caused by the perivascular and parenchymal infiltration of leukocytes (hematoxylin-eosin). (C) Section of a plaque margin reveals a blurred but discrete edge (*arrows*) (Luxol fast blue periodic acid–Schiff [LFB-PAS]). (D) Inactive plaque demonstrating borders that are distinct and devoid of inflammation (hematoxylin-eosin). (E) CD3+ lymphocytes clustering in a perivascular cuff within an active lesion area (immunohistochemistochemical stain for CD3+). (F) Foamy macrophages characterized by fragments of myelin (*arrow*) engulfed by macrophages at a plaque margin (LFB-PAS). (*Courtesy of* Dr Robert Schmidt, Washington University, St Louis, MO [A]. *From* Perry A, Brat DJ. Practical surgical neuropathology: a diagnostic approach. Philadelphia: Churchill Livingstone/Elsevier. p. 489, 490, 492, copyright Elsevier 2010; with permission [B–F].)

can be extensive in acute lesions (see section later).[9] There is glial reactivity throughout the lesion, particularly in hypertrophic astrocytes. However, dense glial scarring is not typical of the acute plaque.

The chronic plaque is characterized by a region of hypocellularity with loss of myelin and glial scarring. On gross examination of postmortem tissue, the hardened and discolored appearance of chronic plaques is often appreciable in frequently targeted areas of the CNS (eg, the corpus callosum, see **Fig. 1**). Histologically, the lesion borders of chronic plaques are more distinct than those of acute plaques (see **Fig. 1**). The chronic plaques are divided into 2 forms to signify temporal evolution from active destruction at the edge of the lesion (chronic active plaque) to an entirely "burned-out" lesion devoid of active inflammatory destruction (chronic silent plaque). In chronic active lesions, inflammation continues along the outer border, with the histologic appearance comparable to acute lesions.[6] Thus, borders of the chronic active plaques are populated with activated microglia and macrophages, vessels demonstrating perivascular cuffing, and reactive astrocytes. The presence of antibody and complement is more prominent in chronic active lesions. Areas of remyelination are often observed on the edge of lesions but can encompass the entire lesion.[10] However, the core of the chronic plaque is typically hypocellular and often contains thickened vessels with enlarged perivascular spaces. Chronic silent lesions are characterized by loss of the inflammatory traits along the border of chronic active lesions. Remyelination and the presence of oligodendrocyte progenitors are uncommon.[11] Essentially, the chronic silent plaque is burned out, containing minimal inflammation and lacking the active inflammatory border. This feature is accompanied by a complete loss of oligodendrocytes and a variable, but demonstrable, reduction in axonal density (see **Fig. 1**). Overall, the gross and histologic features of the MS plaque imply a complex progression of inflammatory damage culminating in a scarred region of demyelination.

There is extensive variability across MS plaques, including different degrees of inflammation, demyelination, remyelination, and axonal injury. There is controversy regarding how lesions are grouped, possibly in part as a result of studying a combination of autopsy and biopsied tissues at different stages of the disease. A recent attempt was made to redefine the process of categorizing MS lesions by proposing a system for classification based on suspected pathologic mechanisms. Alongside a temporally based system, Lucchinetti and colleagues[12] described various types of lesions based on the pattern of leukocyte markers, myelin proteins, immunoglobulins, and complements within the lesions. From 83 pathologic specimens obtained at autopsy or that were biopsied, 4 distinct patterns of immunologic and pathologic features of actively demyelinating lesions were discerned, patterns II and III being the most common. Pattern I is characterized by the predominance of T cells and inflammatory macrophages; pattern II, by T cell and macrophage infiltration, along with accentuated immunoglobulin deposition and myelin degradation products within macrophages; pattern III, by pronounced oligodendrocyte loss at the active edge of the lesion and preferential loss of myelin-associated glycoprotein; and pattern IV, by oligodendrocyte dystrophy and the absence of remyelination or shadow plaques. Importantly, these distinct patterns were consistently observed within samples from the same patient but varied between patients. The investigators, based on the results from one open-label clinical trial in patients who had brain biopsies, hypothesized that deficit recovery after plasma exchange indicated the individual pattern of MS pathology. Plasma exchange was effective in patients with biopsy-proven pattern II lesion (with prominent antibody and complement involvement) but not in patients with pattern I or III lesions.[13] Overall, the categorization of MS lesions based on immunopathologic mechanisms has added to the complexity of paradigms for lesion classification.

While the thought that distinct pathologic processes underlie a singular clinical entity referred to as MS is attractive, this concept has recently been disputed. In particular, challenges have emerged to the idea that there is a clear delineation between the different patterns of pathology.[14] Barnett and Prineas[15] have reported acute lesions from the same patient consisting of features from several of the 4 pathologic patterns. Furthermore, in a recent study, 131 tissue specimens from 39 patients with MS had lesions with little interindividual variation in pathologic features. Indeed, lesions from this study exhibited traits consistent with inclusion into pattern II (ie, deposition of complement and antibodies in proximity to macrophages and absence of oligodendrocyte apoptosis).[16] Therefore, the various pathologic patterns of disease may more precisely refer to the stage of lesion; the relevance of the classification system based on 4 individual subtypes of plaques remains to be confirmed.

The timing of lesion evaluation may be a critical factor in reconciling the conflicting data described earlier. One hypothesis proposed regarding initial events during plaque genesis is that early intrinsic oligodendrocyte injury leads to the inflammatory damage historically associated with the pathologic features of MS plaques. Thus, toxic insults directly affecting the oligodendrocyte could serve as a trigger for a common immunopathologic pathway associated with evolution into later stages of the plaque. That 30 of 39 cases examined by Breij and colleagues[16] were from patients who were in the progressive phase of disease would suggest that early heterogeneity of lesions could have been missed. Further support of this hypothesis comes from a study in which 26 active lesions were examined from 15 patients at autopsy, 11 of whom were early in the course of their disease.[8] In this study, tissue immediately adjacent to lesion borders showed microscopic evidence of cellular injury without the presence of immune infiltration. Prineas and colleagues[8] speculate that there are possibly toxic factors that diffuse to the edge of the lesion resulting in oligodendrocyte fragility, and they refer to these areas of initial injury as prephagocytic. Therefore, a critical question remaining in neuropathology is whether differences exist between borders of acute and chronic active lesions. Further work is required in order to more clearly identify white matter within the CNS that is undergoing early changes or at risk for doing so and how this relates to features described in more established MS plaques.

NORMAL-APPEARING WHITE MATTER

There has been a long-standing interest in early white matter changes in MS, with some of the earliest studies on myelin examining tissue outside plaque regions that seem grossly unaffected.[17,18] More recently, normal-appearing white matter (NAWM) defined on conventional magnetic resonance imaging (MRI) sequences has been explored extensively using a variety of novel neuroimaging techniques that show abnormalities in these areas suggestive of decreased myelin integrity and diminished axonal density within nonlesional regions.[19–21]

The histopathologic examination of NAWM in patients with MS also supports the concept that areas outside plaques have immunopathologic changes. Microglial activation, T-cell infiltration, and perivascular cuffing have been reported in NAWM.[22,23] However, these features were found more diffusely in cases of progressive MS. As a transition zone, dirty-appearing white matter, defined by MRI as having intermediate signal intensity between NAWM and type II lesions, showed diffuse loss of myelin histologically.[24] Thus, the greater involvement of NAWM in MS, associated with the progression of disease, may be related to the extent to which inflammation extends beyond the focal lesions.[23] Overall, the extent of white matter abnormalities and the immunopathologic features of NAWM have yet to be precisely defined.

GRAY MATTER PLAQUES

MS plaques are not confined to the white matter. Gray matter lesions are detected by MRI and by examination of pathologic specimens.[25] Almost all gray matter nuclei within the CNS can be affected, as observed in a cohort of patients mostly with progressive forms of MS,[26] but of the several regions of the CNS, including motor cortex, the spinal cord and cerebellum are particularly vulnerable, resulting in demyelination in up to 28.8% of the gray matter on average. As might be expected, inflammatory lesions within the gray matter are associated with neuronal loss and transected axons, which are more common in active lesions.[27] Although gray matter lesions seem to be more common in patients with progressive forms of MS,[23] they can develop early in the disease process and possibly account for some of the disability seen in patients with MS that cannot be explained by white matter lesions. For example, lesions located within the gray matter correlate better with cognitive disability than white matter lesions.[28]

There are several unique features of pathology associated with gray matter lesions. Histologically, gray matter lesions are less inflammatory, with fewer infiltrating T lymphocytes and microglia/macrophages.[27] Purely cortical gray matter lesions have also been described as lacking complement deposition[29] and blood-brain barrier (BBB) breakdown.[30] Whether gray matter plaques arise from distinct immunologic mechanisms is unclear at this time. In an attempt to more carefully evaluate the processes involved, cortical lesions have been categorized based on the depth of penetration from the surface into the brain (**Fig. 2**). Type I lesions include discernable injury to both white and gray matters, type II lesions have perivascular areas of demyelination only in the cortex, and type III lesions demonstrate cortical demyelination below the pial surface, which often cover several gyri and stop at cortical layers 3 or 4.[27] Others have proposed a fourth category, type IV, to describe lesions that affect all cortical layers without extending into the white matter (see **Fig. 2**).[31,32] Type III and IV lesions are the most extensive and difficult to visualize. Although scarce inflammatory cells are found within these lesions, the meninges overlying them contain inflammatory cells that collect in structures resembling ectopic B-cell follicles.[23,33] In support of a role for lymphoid neogenesis in the pathogenesis of these lesions is the fact that patients with ectopic B-cell follicles (41% of patients with secondary progressive MS [SPMS]) had a more rapid disease progression.[33] More solid determination of the role for ectopic B-cell follicle formation in MS will depend on the reliable detection of cortical lesions by MRI and identification of the immunopathologic mechanisms leading to lymphoid neogenesis within the CNS.

THE ROLE OF T LYMPHOCYTES IN MS

The lymphocytic presence within plaques and bordering areas suggests that inflammatory destruction in MS is driven by antigen-specific targeting of myelin and other CNS components. In particular, adaptive immune responses by T lymphocytes are thought to mediate injury to myelin and nerves within the CNS during MS. The determination that EAE can be mediated by CD4 T cells has promoted intense investigation into the potential CD4 T-cell targets in MS. The relevance of antigen-specific CD4 T-cell responses in MS was highlighted by the results of trials using an altered peptide ligand of myelin basic protein (MBP) designed for therapeutic suppression of CD4 T-cell responses, which resulted in disease exacerbations in multiple patients.[34] T cells from patients with MS can recognize a variety of myelin protein targets, including MBP,[35,36] proteolipid protein (PLP),[37] myelin oligodendrocyte glycoprotein (MOG),[38] and myelin-associated oligodendrocyte basic protein[39] among others.

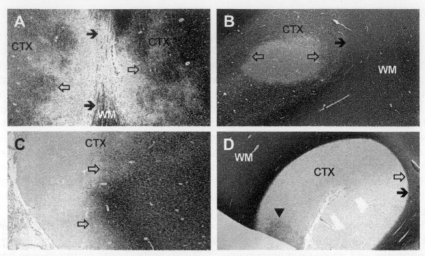

Fig. 2. Cortical lesions in MS revealed by sections immunohistochemically labeled for myelin basic protein. (*A*) Type I cortical lesions encompass both white and gray matters. Solid arrows indicate the cortex (CTX)/white matter (WM) border, whereas the lesion border is delineated by open arrows. (*B*) Type II lesions are contained entirely within the CTX and do not extend to the subcortical WM (*solid arrow*) or pial surface. The border of this type II lesion is indicated by the open arrows. (*C*) Type III cortical lesions represent cortical demyelination below the pial surface that often cover several gyri and stop at cortical layers 3 or 4. Open arrows indicate the lesion border. (*D*) Type IV lesions (border represented by *filled arrow*) span the entirety of the CTX without involvement of WM (*solid arrow*). The arrowhead indicates a small area likely undergoing remyelination. (*From* Bo L, Vedeler CA, Nyland HI, et al. Subpial demyelination in the cerebral cortex of multiple sclerosis patients. J Neuropathol Exp Neurol 62:723, copyright Wolters Kluwer Health 2003; with permission.)

Nonmyelin T-cell antigens have also been described, including αB crystalline[40] and neuronal proteins such as contactin-2.[41] Further, autoreactive CD8 T cells are also observed.[42] Although autoreactive T cells are found in similar frequencies in patients with MS and healthy subjects,[42,43] the myelin-specific T-cell avidity[44] and activation profiles[38] seem to be elevated in patients with MS.

Newer technologies such as arrays of protein,[45] lipid,[46] and gene expression[47] have allowed fresh insight into targets that were heretofore unknown. For example, highly expressed genes in MS plaques compared with nonlesional CNS tissue include osteopontin[48]; however, elevated gene expression does not necessarily imply targeting by the adaptive immune response in MS. Genes encoding myelin proteins actually display reduced expression.[47] Thus, although several of these targets have been validated in EAE,[48,49] their involvement in MS has yet to be fully demonstrated. Again, it is likely that multiple CNS antigens exist for T cells during the inflammatory targeting in MS; results from array experiments highlight how diverse and extensive these targets may be.

How these T cells become abnormally activated toward CNS antigens remains unclear. A popular concept invoked to explain how T cells become pathogenic in patients with MS is molecular mimicry.[50,51] Several infectious agents have been postulated to serve as activation triggers for autoreactive T cells. The most consistently reported one is Epstein-Barr virus (EBV).[52] Other infectious agents may also serve to trigger cross-reactivity with myelin components.[53,54] One advantage of the adaptive immune response in MS lies in the ability to harness the specificity of

T-cell responses.[55] As such, discrete immunologic targets of therapy may be available for treating MS, including vaccines[56] and antigen-presenting cell (APC)-mediated delivery of antigens[57] designed to induce antigen-specific tolerance. Clearly, antigen-specific therapeutics for MS must address the potentially wide array of T-cell targets as well as HLA-specific presentation of antigens intrinsic to the genetic heterogeneity of individuals with MS.

THE ROLE OF Th17 CELLS IN MS

Since the identification of interleukin (IL) 17 as a novel cytokine in 1993, there has been an intense inquiry into the role of IL-17 in EAE and MS. Two members of the IL-17 gene family, IL-17A and IL-17F, are expressed by CD4 T cells.[58] Cua and colleagues[59] identified IL-23, and not IL-12, as a critical cytokine regulator of EAE. This identification quickly led to a new pathway for investigation into the immunologic basis for MS after the discovery that IL-23 regulates IL-17 production by CD4 T cells.[59–61] Subsequently, IL-17–secreting CD4 T cells have emerged as a distinct lineage of T-helper cells, termed Th17 cells. In EAE, Th17 cells participate in early infiltration of the CNS[62] and alone induce a unique neutrophil-predominant pathologic condition.[63] However, unlike IL-23, the neutralization or genetic deletion of IL-17 in EAE does not result in complete absence of the disease.[64] Hence, the direct contribution of Th17 cells during autoimmune demyelination remains unclear.

Human studies have emerged to bolster the relevance of IL-17 to the pathogenesis of MS. A greater proportion of IL-17–secreting cells, but not interferon (IFN) γ^+ CD4 T cells, is found in the cerebrospinal fluid (CSF) of patients with MS compared with those with noninflammatory neurologic diseases.[65] The percentage of IL-17–producing memory CD4 T cells is elevated in peripheral blood from patients with MS experiencing relapses,[66] suggesting a prominent role for Th17 cells in MS. Further, IL-17 gene expression is upregulated in lesions of patients with MS,[47] and Th17 cells are found in perivascular cuffs and borders of active lesions,[67] indicating that Th17 cells are home to areas of inflammatory demyelination (**Fig. 3**). These studies clearly highlight the association between Th17 cells and MS immune pathology.

How might Th17 cells contribute to the pathogenesis of MS? In vitro mobilization studies suggest that Th17 cells cross the BBB more efficiently than other T cells. IL-17–secreting CD4 T cells are capable of eliciting damage to the BBB,[68] which would promote greater influx of other inflammatory cells. Once present in the CNS parenchyma, Th17 cells are capable of mediating injury via recruitment of polymorphonuclear neutrophils[63] and monocytes, along with coproduction of other cytokines, such as IL-22 and IL-21.[69] In addition, Th17 cells are more adept at killing human neurons in vitro than unactivated T cells, providing data to suggest that Th17 cells are potential mediators of axonal and neuronal damage in MS lesions.[68] These initial studies support the idea that Th17 cells may be critical mediators of immune destruction of myelin and axons during MS.

Recent data highlight the potential for targeting Th17 cells in MS. CD4 T cells from healthy individuals skewed to produce IL-17 are more responsive to one current form of treatment of MS, IFN-β, than those from patients with MS.[66] Further, IFN-β can inhibit the differentiation of naive CD4 T cells into Th17 cells.[70] Patient responses to IFN-β may be related to the level of IL-17 before the onset of therapy.[71] This result reemphasizes the complexity and heterogeneity of the disease; in particular, the response to current therapies may signify differences in the pathogenesis of MS between patients.[72] The Th17 pathway offers a new therapeutic target, including the molecular pathways that regulate IL-17.[73] However, consistent with the

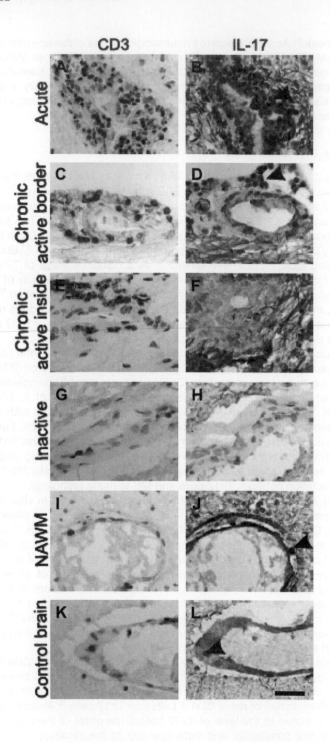

complexity of cytokine networks and regulation, a singular stance that IL-17 is purely pathogenic is likely to be an oversimplification. In particular, IL-17 may participate in limiting tissue destruction during an inflammatory response.[74] Overall, evidence is mounting to suggest that Th17 cells are present during the inflammatory destruction of tissues in MS, but questions remain about the direct contribution of this newly identified lineage of CD4 T cells. At this point, it is reasonable to include Th17 cells in the pathogenesis of MS (**Fig. 4**), but their degree of involvement remains to be shown.

B CELL–MEDIATED CNS DAMAGE IN MS

Evidence gathered from examination of CNS tissue implicates the role of antibodies during the pathogenesis of MS. As noted, the presence of plasma cells, immunoglobulins, and complements is a typical feature of the MS plaque.[5,12] Naturally, this observation has prompted consideration over whether immunoglobulin present within plaques specifically targets myelin antigens. Molecular features of B cells found within MS plaques demonstrate that B-cell receptor genes are modified in a specific way that indicates their evolving response toward specific targets.[75,76] Further specificity of immunoglobulin from MS tissue has been described. MBP-reactive[77,78] and MOG-reactive[79] immunoglobulins have been isolated from CNS tissue of patients with MS. In addition, the in situ deposition of MOG-specific antibodies has been detected in MS lesions, along with MOG- and MBP-specific immunoglobulin complexed with myelin within macrophages.[80] In contrast, immunoglobulins seemed to be nonspecifically dispersed throughout cellular constituents of plaques and NAWM, without significant differences when compared with control tissues, suggesting that immunoglobulin presence may be secondary to white matter injury rather than antigen-specific B-cell activation unique to MS.[81] Thus, while controversy persists regarding the antigen-specific nature of B-cell involvement in MS, the presence of plasma cells and immunoglobulins continues to fuel investigation into their involvement during MS plaque development.

As a representation of B-cell involvement in parenchymal damage of CNS of patients with MS, CSF analysis has afforded several clues on the role of immunoglobulins in the pathogenesis of MS. The localized intrathecal production of immunoglobulins, referred to as oligoclonal bands (OCBs), is detected in more than 90% of patients with RR-MS,[82] and their absence is associated with reduced severity of the disease.[83] While OCBs are thought to be a product of clonally expanded B cells within the CSF compartment, their potential targets remain elusive. Plasma cells from the CSF of patients with inflammatory demyelinating disease produce antibodies that are capable of binding myelin[84] and recognizing MBP.[85] However, a more recent study of the CSF of patients with MS failed to detect IgG from clonally expanded B cells in CSF that bound to MBP, PLP, or MOG.[86] Analysis of OCBs has also included

Fig. 3. Involvement of IL-17 in MS lesions. Immunohistochemical identification of CD3 (*left column*) and IL-17 (*right column*) in consecutive sections. Abundant IL-17 staining (*arrowheads*) is observed in perivascular cells in both acute (*A, B*) and chronic active (*C, D*) lesions. (*E, F*) Whereas CD3+ cells do not colocalize with IL-17 staining within the internal region of a chronic lesion, the fibrillary pattern of IL-17 immunoreactivity is representative of its possible astrocyte production. Minimal staining is observed in tissue from an inactive lesion (*G, H*). Sparse Th17 cells are observed in NAWM in MS or within control tissue (*I–L*) (*arrowheads, I, L*). Scale bar = 30 μm. (*From* Tzartos JS, Friese MA, Craner MJ, et al. Interleukin-17 production in central nervous system-infiltrating T cells and glial cells is associated with active disease in multiple sclerosis. Am J Pathol 2008;172:146; with permission from the American Society for Investigative Pathology.)

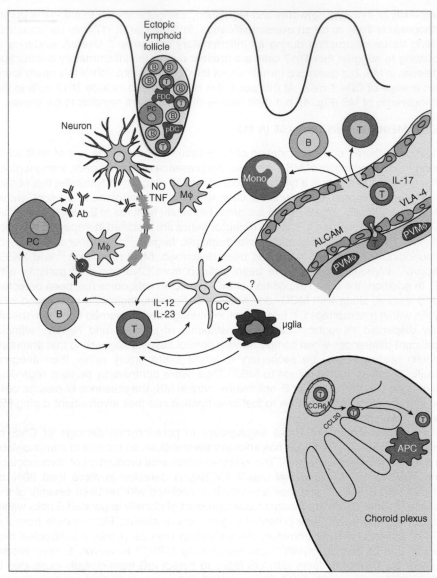

Fig. 4. Cellular and molecular factors involved in the immunopathogenesis of MS. Rather than representing an all-inclusive summary of the immunopathologic features of MS, this diagram highlights recent advances in the understanding of the neural-immune interactions in MS, including factors involved in leukocyte trafficking, axonal injury, and antigen presentation. μglia, microglia; Ab, antibody; B, B lymphocyte; FDC, follicular dendritic cell; Mφ, macrophage; Mono, monocyte; PC, plasma cell; pDC, plasmacytoid dendritic cell; PVMφ, perivascular macrophage; T, T lymphocyte; TNF, tumor necrosis factor; VLA-4, very late activating antigen 4.

investigation of IgM, which is found in a subset of patients with MS.[87] CSF-restricted IgM isolated from patients with MS has been found to target a variety of lipid antigens, predominantly phosphatidylcholine.[87] These persistent lipid-specific IgM OCBs are associated with more aggressive disease[87,88] and might be associated with a poor response to interferon therapy.[89] Taken as a whole, a multitude of potential targets, including those from myelin as well as other CNS antigens,[90] have been proposed and investigated in patients with MS.[91]

Modulation of T-cell function may be an equally important function of B cells in the immune dysregulation in patients with MS. As noted, anti-CD20 monoclonal antibody–targeted depletion of B cells is efficacious for the treatment of RR-MS.[92] This efficacy seems to be independent of antibody effects because anti-CD20 treatment does not directly target immunoglobulin-secreting plasma cells,[82] results in early efficacy in relapse reduction and inflammatory MRI lesions,[92] and does not alter CSF immunoglobulin levels.[93] B cells may promote neuroinflammation in MS via direct and indirect effects on T cells, such as the secretion of the proinflammatory cytokines. For example, B cells from patients with MS produce more tumor necrosis factor (TNF)-α and lymphotoxin in the presence of the T cell–derived proinflammatory cytokine IFN-γ compared with healthy controls.[94] After anti-CD20–mediated B-cell depletion in patients with RR-MS, T cells produced less IFN-γ and were less proliferative in response to T cell antigen receptor engagement.[94] Conversely, B cells are also likely to have immune-suppressive traits that are important in the immunopathogenesis of MS. For example, IL-10 secretion by B cells can serve to limit proinflammatory autoreactive CD4 T-cell responses.[95]

Finally, recent evidence suggests a role for B cells in the generation of ectopic follicles in MS. Building on the observations of Prineas,[96] Aloisi and colleagues[97] have described the presence of B-cell follicles within the meninges in patients with SPMS. These follicles are characterized by features of germinal centers, including the presence of B cells, follicular dendritic cells (DCs), and CXCL13 (a chemokine involved in the genesis of lymphoid organs). These follicles, found in approximately 40% of autopsy specimens only from patients with SPMS,[33] were purported to be a maker for cortical lesions immediately adjacent to the ectopic follicle within the meninges. This finding has been disputed in subsequent work that failed to detect meningeal follicles in 12 patients with SPMS.[98] There may be an association between the presence of EBV infectious material and secondary lymphoid follicles observed in patients with MS.[99] This finding implies that latent infection of B cells with EBV drives the expansion and maturation of B cells along with ectopic follicle generation within the CNS, promoting intrathecal immunoglobulin production and the targeted destruction of underlying myelin in this region.[82] Although only observed in patients with SPMS, it is possible that the generation of these lymphoid organ–like structures begins during the relapsing-remitting phase and evolves over time. Whether these structures are inhibited by B cell–depleting therapy in MS remains to be investigated.

MECHANISMS OF LEUKOCYTE ENTRY DURING MS

Immune access to the CNS is generally considered restricted. In practice, the traditional view of the CNS as an immune-privileged site has been replaced with the more appropriate characterization of the CNS as an immune-specialized organ.[100] Thus, one key element to immune-mediated damage within the CNS during MS is the process by which immune cells are able to gain access to this specialized compartment. Within the context of universal processes governing immune cell trafficking, there are features that are relatively specific for leukocyte migration to, and within, the brain and spinal cord in health and disease. The molecular components, location, and timing of migration are all important factors during the immunopathogenesis of MS.

The BBB serves to actively restrict cellular and macromolecular movement between the blood and CNS tissue. Adequate function of the BBB depends on several unique anatomic and cellular features, including tight junctions between endothelial cells, specialized expression of molecular transporters, and placement of immune cells within the CNS relative to the vasculature.[101] Only by engaging in a critically timed sequence of events are autoreactive lymphocytes able to enter the CNS compartment. Initially, leukocytes engage in rolling, activation, and arrest of the endothelium of the BBB. This initial step is greatly facilitated by upregulation of adhesion molecules by the vasculature, including intercellular adhesion molecule 1 (ICAM-1) and vascular cell adhesion molecule (VCAM-1).[102] Although a trigger for vascular change remains unclear in MS, hypothetically, changes in the vascular endothelium could result from proinflammatory mediators circulating within the vasculature, including TNF and/or lipopolysaccharide. Subsequently, migration of cells through and between endothelial cells takes place.[103] Eventually, concentrated extravasation of immune cells in perivascular cuffs within the CNS parenchyma culminates in a breach of the BBB, which is an essential component to the process of inflammatory destruction of the white matter in MS.[6]

The complex set of molecules that leukocytes depend on for entry into CNS tissues are integrins. Integrins are heterodimeric cell surface molecules that mediate adhesion between cells. Among a panel of leukocyte adhesion receptors, the $\alpha4$ subunit of very late activating antigen (VLA)-4 was identified as a crucial factor for encephalitogenic T-cell binding to CNS endothelium. Blockade of $\alpha4\beta1$ engagement with one of its binding partners, VCAM-1, successfully abrogated disease in an animal model of MS.[104] Clinical trials of a humanized monoclonal antibody targeting the $\alpha4$ subunit of VLA-4, called natalizumab, also demonstrated efficacy in the treatment of MS.[105,106] Hence, selective inhibition of specific adhesion molecules is effective in reducing leukocyte entry into the CNS. Of note, natalizumab reduces the influx of a wide range of leukocytes, including T cells and DCs.[107] In addition to VLA-4, other trafficking molecules impart specificity of migration into the CNS. Recently, ALCAM-1 was shown to be localized to the BBB and upregulated in active MS lesions.[108] In experimental animal systems, blockade of ALCAM-1 delayed disease.[108] In addition, osteopontin also serves as a binding partner for VLA-4 and potentially serves as a separate target for reducing leukocyte migration into the CNS of patients with MS.[109] Hence, a multitude of adhesion molecules participate in effective leukocyte trafficking to and within the CNS and serve as potential targets for therapies in MS.

Chemokines, a broad class of cytokines mediating chemotaxis, also contribute to leukocyte migration to the CNS. Several chemokines and their receptors have been implicated in leukocyte influx to the CNS in MS.[103] For example, CXCL12, constitutively expressed in the CNS, is typically localized to the basolateral aspect of the CNS microvasculature and functions to retain leukocytes within the perivascular space. Redistribution of CXCL12 to the luminal aspect of vessels was observed in autopsy specimens from patients with MS, which would allow for the dissemination of lymphocytes into the CNS parenchyma.[110] Other chemokines are thought to participate in the recruitment of lymphocytes into the CNS in MS. Recent work in the EAE system has demonstrated that the initial wave of T-cell infiltration into the CNS before disease onset is CCR6 dependent.[62] Furthermore, in EAE, the initial wave of inflammatory CD4 T cells expresses IL-17 and is potentially recruited specifically via CCR6 into the CNS via the choroid plexus that expresses the CCR6 ligand, CCL20. These results have yet to be convincingly replicated in humans. Several other chemokines and chemokine receptors expressed by various cell types in MS show dysregulation, including CCR7, CCL19 and CCL21, and CCR5.[111,112] Thus, there may be a unique chemokine signature at different phases of disease and in different regions of the CNS in order for various leukocytes to localize to the CNS during MS.

THE ROLE OF APCS IN MS

APCs process and present antigens to T cells, and in the context of MHC, costimulatory signals and cytokine secretion drive adaptive immune responses.[113] Experimental evidence based on animal models has shown that antigen-specific encounters within the CNS between T cells and APCs is crucial to the unfolding of MS. In EAE, without newly generated myelin antigens from the CNS by APCs, inflammatory demyelination does not proceed, even in the presence of myelin-reactive CD4 T cells.[114,115] Thus, CD4 T cell–mediated disease is thought to be a multistage process, involving the initial activation of autoreactive CD4 T cells as well as reactivation within the CNS immune compartment. DCs are thought to be the major APCs during the secondary phase of cognate interactions with CD4 T cells within the CNS.[116,117] Perivascular spaces within areas bordering edges of active lesions immunostain for CD209, a marker for a subset of DCs, suggesting that antigen presentation by DCs at the interface of the BBB contributes to the earliest inflammatory processes promoting lesion formation.[8] Visualization of APC interactions with encephalitogenic CD4 T cells using intravital microscopy in a murine model of MS suggests that primed CD4 T cells actively engage with these perivascular APCs en route to entry within the CNS.[118]

In addition to DCs, other APCs likely play an important role in antigen presentation during the pathogenesis of MS. Microglia are hematogenously derived resident APCs within the CNS. Upon activation, these cells express greater amounts of class II MHC's and costimulatory molecules,[119] signifying a greater capacity to promote proinflammatory T-cell responses within the CNS. Activated microglia are localized to active plaques.[120] Experimentally, impeding microglial function attenuates EAE.[121] However, relative to other professional APCs, microglia are not as potent in inducing autoreactive T-cell responses[122] and may even downregulate CD4 T-cell functions.[123] Thus, as resident APCs within the CNS, microglia are capable of performing APC functions, but likely are not the lynchpin for driving autoimmunity of the CNS in MS. Another APC potentially involved in driving myelin-reactive CD4 T cells in MS is the B cell. As already mentioned, recent work suggests that B cells play a prominent role in the pathogenesis of MS[82,92] and potentially play important roles in antigen presentation to T cells. In addition to the effects on T cells, class II MHC–dependent interactions with B cells promote immunoglobulin class switching from IgM to IgG. Thus, antigen-specific interactions between B cells and T cells represent a critical step in the generation of immunoglobulin responses in MS. It is important to acknowledge that not all interactions between APCs and T cells promote inflammation. In addition to the effects of regulatory B cells mentioned earlier, APCs can also engender antiinflammatory responses.[124] For example, suppressor myeloid cells are generated after EAE induction and are capable of suppressing T-cell function.[125] In MS, the process of myeloid suppression is thought to be regulated in part by TREM-2, a transmembrane signaling protein expressed by microglial cells, macrophages, monocytes, and DCs.[126] This mechanism may be dysregulated by secretion of soluble TREM-2, which could act as a decoy receptor and prevent inhibitory function of transmembrane TREM-2.[126]

AXONAL AND NEURONAL DAMAGE IN MS

Inflammatory CNS injury in MS has increasingly been associated with axonal damage. Although MS has classically been described as a disease marked by the loss of myelin in greater proportion to the loss of axons, axonal damage was noted in the earliest pathological descriptions of MS lesions.[3] Modern techniques have allowed for precise demonstrations of axonal damage. Antibodies directed at amyloid precursor protein show damaged axons in active areas of MS lesions.[127] Representing a major advance in MS pathology, Trapp and colleagues[9] were able to directly view and quantify transected axons using confocal microscopy by counting axonal ovoids at the ends of transected axons. The active areas of MS lesions were found to contain more transected axons than inactive areas in more chronic lesions. Of note, comparisons of biopsy and autopsy samples from patients with RR-MS, SPMS, and primary progressive MS suggest that axonal pathology is greatest within the first year of disease onset, particularly in patients with RR-MS.[128] These studies propose that axonal pathology occurs in areas of active inflammatory demyelination and early during the course of disease.

In addition, a slower rate of axonal damage is also thought to occur and contribute to the clinical decline observed in patients with MS. Trapp and colleagues[9] and Kornek and colleagues[129] showed that axonal ovoids are more common in inactive demyelinated lesions and in NAWM than in the white matter of control patients. However, remyelinated inactive lesions, or shadow plaques, have the same number of abnormal axons as control tissue.[129] Patients with higher levels of motor disability have fewer surviving corticospinal axons traveling through their spinal cord, demonstrating a direct correlation of axonal damage and disease progression.[130]

The mechanisms involved in axonal damage in MS are under intense investigation. CD8$^+$ T lymphocytes can cause axonal damage via the release of cytotoxic granules, induction of apoptosis through activation of surface receptors such as Fas, the release of cytokines such as TNF-α, or direct transection of axons.[131,132] Macrophages/microglia are also found in close proximity to damaged neurons. Release of toxic molecules by these cells, such as proteases and reactive nitrogen species, can cause oligodendrocyte injury, demyelination, and axonal degeneration; disrupt the BBB; and contribute to the loss of axonal conduction.[133] Axonal damage also occurs by activation of other components of the innate immune response such as toll-like receptors.[134] Toll-like receptor 2 is overexpressed by oligodendrocytes in MS lesions, in which it inhibits remyelination.[135] Antibody-mediated injury to axonal components, such as neurofascin, can result in axonal and neuronal dysfunction.[90] As a consequence of immune injury to myelin, higher energy demands on demyelinated axons and glutamate-mediated excitotoxicity may further impart unsustainable damage.[136,137] Overall, axonal injury in MS is likely mediated by multiple mechanisms in both active and chronic lesions.

Neuronal loss in MS can be severe and occurs throughout the brain. Neuronal loss in the range of 18% to 35% has been reported in the cortex, hippocampus, thalamus, and spinal cord.[31] Damage to axons and neurons has been evaluated in vivo using MRI techniques such as quantitative proton magnetic resonance spectroscopy. In patients presenting with their first clinical attack of MS, the amount of N-acetylaspartate in the whole brain is already decreased, indicating early neuronal damage.[138] This reduction is still present 1 year later and is independent of whether or not the patients progress to develop MS. Other MRI techniques, such as measurement of brain volume or diffusion tensor imaging, have provided more variable results in evaluating axonal and neuronal damage, especially in short-term studies, because factors such as demyelination and edema can confound the results. However, examination of neuronal integrity using optical coherence tomography shows a loss of macular volume in patients with progressive forms of MS, which correlates with poor visual acuity, especially in patients with a history of optic neuritis.[139] Similar to axonal injury, the processes resulting in neuronal loss in MS are likely several-fold. Direct immune injury to the gray matter can result in the loss of neurons, because, within gray matter lesions, a significant increase in apoptotic neurons was observed primarily in large pyramidal cortical neurons.[27] However, in layer II of primary motor cortex from NAWM, paralbumin interneurons were more affected than other neurons that are relatively spared in patients with MS.[140] This differential susceptibility of neurons exposed to the same insult is part of a key consideration in how clinical deterioration, particularly with secondary progression, is related to repeated accumulation of axonal or neuronal damage to various neuronal populations. Further, axonal and neuronal survival may be directly tied to the trophic support provided by myelin, which may be particularly relevant during a high metabolic demand state of neurons exposed to inflammatory stressors.[141]

SUMMARY

Several new features of cellular and molecular immunity have added to the understanding of the pathology of MS. These features include the role of B cells, including antibody-dependent and antibody-independent mechanisms; the extent of axonal and neuronal injury; the contribution of a new lineage of CD4 T cells identified by the production of IL-17; leukocyte trafficking mechanisms to the CNS; and new lymphocyte targets during disease. These features stand out among many other recent developments that due to space limitations are beyond the realms of this review. Topics involving resolution of inflammation in MS lesions, suppressor cells (regulatory T cells, CD8 T cells), and remyelination are bound to be important in driving toward a more comprehensive understanding of the pathogenesis of MS. Overall, an attempt has been made not to detail every mechanism involved in the pathology of MS, but rather highlight the features of disease that are under current study (see **Fig. 4**).

REFERENCES

1. Gold R, Linington C, Lassmann H. Understanding pathogenesis and therapy of multiple sclerosis via animal models: 70 years of merits and culprits in experimental autoimmune encephalomyelitis research. Brain 1953;129:2006.
2. Goverman J. Autoimmune T cell responses in the central nervous system. Nat Rev Immunol 2009;9:393.
3. Charcot JM. Lecons sur les maladies du systeme nerveux faites a la salpetriere. Paris: A. Delahaye; 1872.
4. Compston A, McDonald IR, Noseworthy J, et al. McAlpine's multiple sclerosis. Philadelphia: Churchill Livingstone; 2006.
5. Frohman EM, Racke MK, Raine CS. Multiple sclerosis–the plaque and its pathogenesis. N Engl J Med 2006;354:942.
6. Greenfield JG, Love S, Louis DN, et al. Greenfield's neuropathology. 8th edition. London: Hodder Arnold; 2008.
7. Perry A, Brat DJ. Practical surgical neuropathology: a diagnostic approach. Philadelphia: Churchill Livingstone/Elsevier; 2010.
8. Henderson AP, Barnett MH, Parratt JD, et al. Multiple sclerosis: distribution of inflammatory cells in newly forming lesions. Ann Neurol 2009;66:739.
9. Trapp BD, Peterson J, Ransohoff RM, et al. Axonal transection in the lesions of multiple sclerosis. N Engl J Med 1998;338:278.
10. Lassmann H, Bruck W, Lucchinetti C, et al. Remyelination in multiple sclerosis. Mult Scler 1997;3:133.
11. Wilson HC, Scolding NJ, Raine CS. Co-expression of PDGF alpha receptor and NG2 by oligodendrocyte precursors in human CNS and multiple sclerosis lesions. J Neuroimmunol 2006;176:162.

12. Lucchinetti CF, Bruck W, Lassmann H. Evidence for pathogenic heterogeneity in multiple sclerosis. Ann Neurol 2004;56:308.
13. Keegan M, Konig F, McClelland R, et al. Relation between humoral pathological changes in multiple sclerosis and response to therapeutic plasma exchange. Lancet 2005;366:579.
14. Raine CS. Multiple sclerosis: classification revisited reveals homogeneity and recapitulation. Ann Neurol 2008;63:1.
15. Barnett MH, Prineas JW. Relapsing and remitting multiple sclerosis: pathology of the newly forming lesion. Ann Neurol 2004;55:458.
16. Breij EC, Brink BP, Veerhuis R, et al. Homogeneity of active demyelinating lesions in established multiple sclerosis. Ann Neurol 2008;63:16.
17. Baker RW, Thompson RH, Zilkha KJ. Fatty-acid composition of brain lecithins in multiple sclerosis. Lancet 1963;1:26.
18. Suzuki K, Kamoshita S, Eto Y, et al. Myelin in multiple sclerosis. Composition of myelin from normal-appearing white matter. Arch Neurol 1973;28:293.
19. Ceccarelli A, Rocca MA, Falini A, et al. Normal-appearing white and grey matter damage in MS. A volumetric and diffusion tensor MRI study at 3.0 Tesla. J Neurol 2007;254:513.
20. Filippi M, Campi A, Dousset V, et al. A magnetization transfer imaging study of normal-appearing white matter in multiple sclerosis. Neurology 1995;45:478.
21. Zivadinov R, Stosic M, Cox JL, et al. The place of conventional MRI and newly emerging MRI techniques in monitoring different aspects of treatment outcome. J Neurol 2008;255(Suppl 1):61.
22. Allen IV, McQuaid S, Mirakhur M, et al. Pathological abnormalities in the normal-appearing white matter in multiple sclerosis. Neurol Sci 2001;22:141.
23. Kutzelnigg A, Lucchinetti CF, Stadelmann C, et al. Cortical demyelination and diffuse white matter injury in multiple sclerosis. Brain 2005;128:2705.
24. Moore GR, Laule C, Mackay A, et al. Dirty-appearing white matter in multiple sclerosis: preliminary observations of myelin phospholipid and axonal loss. J Neurol 1802;255:2008.
25. Geurts JJ, Pouwels PJ, Uitdehaag BM, et al. Intracortical lesions in multiple sclerosis: improved detection with 3D double inversion-recovery MR imaging. Radiology 2005;236:254.
26. Gilmore CP, Donaldson I, Bo L, et al. Regional variations in the extent and pattern of grey matter demyelination in multiple sclerosis: a comparison between the cerebral cortex, cerebellar cortex, deep grey matter nuclei and the spinal cord. J Neurol Neurosurg Psychiatry 2009;80:182.
27. Peterson JW, Bo L, Mork S, et al. Transected neurites, apoptotic neurons, and reduced inflammation in cortical multiple sclerosis lesions. Ann Neurol 2001;50:389.
28. Amato MP, Portaccio E, Goretti B, et al. Association of neocortical volume changes with cognitive deterioration in relapsing-remitting multiple sclerosis. Arch Neurol 2007;64:1157.
29. Brink BP, Veerhuis R, Breij EC, et al. The pathology of multiple sclerosis is location-dependent: no significant complement activation is detected in purely cortical lesions. J Neuropathol Exp Neurol 2005;64:147.
30. van Horssen J, Brink BP, de Vries HE, et al. The blood-brain barrier in cortical multiple sclerosis lesions. J Neuropathol Exp Neurol 2007;66:321.
31. Bo L. The histopathology of grey matter demyelination in multiple sclerosis. Acta Neurol Scand Suppl 2009;189:51.

32. Bo L, Vedeler CA, Nyland HI, et al. Subpial demyelination in the cerebral cortex of multiple sclerosis patients. J Neuropathol Exp Neurol 2003;62:723.
33. Magliozzi R, Howell O, Vora A, et al. Meningeal B-cell follicles in secondary progressive multiple sclerosis associate with early onset of disease and severe cortical pathology. Brain 2007;130:1089.
34. Bielekova B, Goodwin B, Richert N, et al. Encephalitogenic potential of the myelin basic protein peptide (amino acids 83-99) in multiple sclerosis: results of a phase II clinical trial with an altered peptide ligand. Nat Med 2000;6:1167.
35. Pette M, Fujita K, Wilkinson D, et al. Myelin autoreactivity in multiple sclerosis: recognition of myelin basic protein in the context of HLA-DR2 products by T lymphocytes of multiple-sclerosis patients and healthy donors. Proc Natl Acad Sci U S A 1990;87:7968.
36. Valli A, Sette A, Kappos L, et al. Binding of myelin basic protein peptides to human histocompatibility leukocyte antigen class II molecules and their recognition by T cells from multiple sclerosis patients. J Clin Invest 1993;91:616.
37. Greer JM, Csurhes PA, Cameron KD, et al. Increased immunoreactivity to two overlapping peptides of myelin proteolipid protein in multiple sclerosis. Brain 1997;120(Pt 8):1447.
38. Zhang J, Markovic-Plese S, Lacet B, et al. Increased frequency of interleukin 2-responsive T cells specific for myelin basic protein and proteolipid protein in peripheral blood and cerebrospinal fluid of patients with multiple sclerosis. J Exp Med 1994;179:973.
39. de Rosbo NK, Kaye JF, Eisenstein M, et al. The myelin-associated oligodendrocytic basic protein region MOBP15-36 encompasses the immunodominant major encephalitogenic epitope(s) for SJL/J mice and predicted epitope(s) for multiple sclerosis-associated HLA-DRB1*1501. J Immunol 2004;173:1426.
40. Bajramovic JJ, Plomp AC, Goes A, et al. Presentation of alpha B-crystallin to T cells in active multiple sclerosis lesions: an early event following inflammatory demyelination. J Immunol 2000;164:4359.
41. Derfuss T, Parikh K, Velhin S, et al. Contactin-2/TAG-1-directed autoimmunity is identified in multiple sclerosis patients and mediates gray matter pathology in animals. Proc Natl Acad Sci U S A 2009;106:8302.
42. Berthelot L, Laplaud DA, Pettre S, et al. Blood CD8+ T cell responses against myelin determinants in multiple sclerosis and healthy individuals. Eur J Immunol 2008;38:1889.
43. Hellings N, Baree M, Verhoeven C, et al. T-cell reactivity to multiple myelin antigens in multiple sclerosis patients and healthy controls. J Neurosci Res 2001; 63:290.
44. Bielekova B, Sung MH, Kadom N, et al. Expansion and functional relevance of high-avidity myelin-specific CD4+ T cells in multiple sclerosis. J Immunol 2004; 172:3893.
45. Han MH, Hwang SI, Roy DB, et al. Proteomic analysis of active multiple sclerosis lesions reveals therapeutic targets. Nature 2008;451:1076.
46. Kanter JL, Narayana S, Ho PP, et al. Lipid microarrays identify key mediators of autoimmune brain inflammation. Nat Med 2006;12:138.
47. Lock C, Hermans G, Pedotti R, et al. Gene-microarray analysis of multiple sclerosis lesions yields new targets validated in autoimmune encephalomyelitis. Nat Med 2002;8:500.
48. Chabas D, Baranzini SE, Mitchell D, et al. The influence of the proinflammatory cytokine, osteopontin, on autoimmune demyelinating disease. Science 2001; 294:1731.

49. Lanz TV, Ding Z, Ho PP, et al. Angiotensin II sustains brain inflammation in mice via TGF-beta. J Clin Invest 2010;120:2782.
50. Munz C, Lunemann JD, Getts MT, et al. Antiviral immune responses: triggers of or triggered by autoimmunity? Nat Rev Immunol 2009;9:246.
51. Sospedra M, Martin R. Immunology of multiple sclerosis. Annu Rev Immunol 2005;23:683.
52. Salvetti M, Giovannoni G, Aloisi F. Epstein-Barr virus and multiple sclerosis. Curr Opin Neurol 2009;22:201.
53. Talbot PJ, Paquette JS, Ciurli C, et al. Myelin basic protein and human corona-virus 229E cross-reactive T cells in multiple sclerosis. Ann Neurol 1996;39:233.
54. Tejada-Simon MV, Zang YC, Hong J, et al. Cross-reactivity with myelin basic protein and human herpesvirus-6 in multiple sclerosis. Ann Neurol 2003;53:189.
55. Steinman L. Antigen-specific therapy of multiple sclerosis: the long-sought magic bullet. Neurotherapeutics 2007;4:661.
56. Bar-Or A, Vollmer T, Antel J, et al. Induction of antigen-specific tolerance in multiple sclerosis after immunization with DNA encoding myelin basic protein in a randomized, placebo-controlled phase 1/2 trial. Arch Neurol 2007;64:1407.
57. Dolgin E. The inverse of immunity. Nat Med 2010;16:740.
58. Miossec P, Korn T, Kuchroo VK. Interleukin-17 and type 17 helper T cells. N Engl J Med 2009;361:888.
59. Cua DJ, Sherlock J, Chen Y, et al. Interleukin-23 rather than interleukin-12 is the critical cytokine for autoimmune inflammation of the brain. Nature 2003;421:744.
60. Langrish CL, Chen Y, Blumenschein WM, et al. IL-23 drives a pathogenic T cell population that induces autoimmune inflammation. J Exp Med 2005;201:233.
61. Mangan PR, Harrington LE, O'Quinn DB, et al. Transforming growth factor-beta induces development of the T(H)17 lineage. Nature 2006;441:231.
62. Reboldi A, Coisne C, Baumjohann D, et al. C-C chemokine receptor 6-regulated entry of TH-17 cells into the CNS through the choroid plexus is required for the initiation of EAE. Nat Immunol 2009;10:514.
63. Kroenke MA, Carlson TJ, Andjelkovic AV, et al. IL-12- and IL-23-modulated T cells induce distinct types of EAE based on histology, CNS chemokine profile, and response to cytokine inhibition. J Exp Med 2008;205:1535.
64. Haak S, Croxford AL, Kreymborg K, et al. IL-17A and IL-17F do not contribute vitally to autoimmune neuro-inflammation in mice. J Clin Invest 2009;119:61.
65. Brucklacher-Waldert V, Stuerner K, Kolster M, et al. Phenotypical and functional characterization of T helper 17 cells in multiple sclerosis. Brain 2009;132:3329.
66. Durelli L, Conti L, Clerico M, et al. T-helper 17 cells expand in multiple sclerosis and are inhibited by interferon-beta. Ann Neurol 2009;65:499.
67. Tzartos JS, Friese MA, Craner MJ, et al. Interleukin-17 production in central nervous system-infiltrating T cells and glial cells is associated with active disease in multiple sclerosis. Am J Pathol 2008;172:146.
68. Kebir H, Kreymborg K, Ifergan I, et al. Human TH17 lymphocytes promote blood-brain barrier disruption and central nervous system inflammation. Nat Med 2007;13:1173.
69. Spolski R, Leonard WJ. Cytokine mediators of Th17 function. Eur J Immunol 2009;39:658.
70. Ramgolam VS, Sha Y, Jin J, et al. IFN-beta inhibits human Th17 cell differentia-tion. J Immunol 2009;183:5418.
71. Axtell RC, de Jong BA, Boniface K, et al. T helper type 1 and 17 cells determine efficacy of interferon-beta in multiple sclerosis and experimental encephalomy-elitis. Nat Med 2010;16:406.

72. Koike F, Satoh J, Miyake S, et al. Microarray analysis identifies interferon beta-regulated genes in multiple sclerosis. J Neuroimmunol 2003;139:109.
73. Du C, Liu C, Kang J, et al. MicroRNA miR-326 regulates TH-17 differentiation and is associated with the pathogenesis of multiple sclerosis. Nat Immunol 2009;10:1252.
74. O'Connor W Jr, Zenewicz LA, Flavell RA. The dual nature of T(H)17 cells: shifting the focus to function. Nat Immunol 2010;11:471.
75. Baranzini SE, Jeong MC, Butunoi C, et al. B cell repertoire diversity and clonal expansion in multiple sclerosis brain lesions. J Immunol 1999;163:5133.
76. Owens GP, Burgoon MP, Anthony J, et al. The immunoglobulin G heavy chain repertoire in multiple sclerosis plaques is distinct from the heavy chain repertoire in peripheral blood lymphocytes. Clin Immunol 2001;98:258.
77. Warren KG, Catz I. Autoantibodies to myelin basic protein within multiple sclerosis central nervous system tissue. J Neurol Sci 1993;115:169.
78. Wucherpfennig KW, Catz I, Hausmann S, et al. Recognition of the immunodominant myelin basic protein peptide by autoantibodies and HLA-DR2-restricted T cell clones from multiple sclerosis patients. Identity of key contact residues in the B-cell and T-cell epitopes. J Clin Invest 1997;100:1114.
79. O'Connor KC, Appel H, Bregoli L, et al. Antibodies from inflamed central nervous system tissue recognize myelin oligodendrocyte glycoprotein. J Immunol 1974;175:2005.
80. Genain CP, Cannella B, Hauser SL, et al. Identification of autoantibodies associated with myelin damage in multiple sclerosis. Nat Med 1999;5:170.
81. Barnett MH, Parratt JD, Cho ES, et al. Immunoglobulins and complement in postmortem multiple sclerosis tissue. Ann Neurol 2009;65:32.
82. Franciotta D, Salvetti M, Lolli F, et al. B cells and multiple sclerosis. Lancet Neurol 2008;7:852.
83. Avasarala JR, Cross AH, Trotter JL. Oligoclonal band number as a marker for prognosis in multiple sclerosis. Arch Neurol 2001;58:2044.
84. von Budingen HC, Harrer MD, Kuenzle S, et al. Clonally expanded plasma cells in the cerebrospinal fluid of MS patients produce myelin-specific antibodies. Eur J Immunol 2008;38:2014.
85. Lambracht-Washington D, O'Connor KC, Cameron EM, et al. Antigen specificity of clonally expanded and receptor edited cerebrospinal fluid B cells from patients with relapsing remitting MS. J Neuroimmunol 2007;186:164.
86. Owens GP, Bennett JL, Lassmann H, et al. Antibodies produced by clonally expanded plasma cells in multiple sclerosis cerebrospinal fluid. Ann Neurol 2009;65:639.
87. Villar LM, Sadaba MC, Roldan E, et al. Intrathecal synthesis of oligoclonal IgM against myelin lipids predicts an aggressive disease course in MS. J Clin Invest 2005;115:187.
88. Bosca I, Magraner MJ, Coret F, et al. The risk of relapse after a clinically isolated syndrome is related to the pattern of oligoclonal bands. J Neuroimmunol 2010;226:143.
89. Bosca I, Villar LM, Coret F, et al. Response to interferon in multiple sclerosis is related to lipid-specific oligoclonal IgM bands. Mult Scler 2010;16:810.
90. Mathey EK, Derfuss T, Storch MK, et al. Neurofascin as a novel target for autoantibody-mediated axonal injury. J Exp Med 2007;204:2363.
91. Reindl M, Khalil M, Berger T. Antibodies as biological markers for pathophysiological processes in MS. J Neuroimmunol 2006;180:50.
92. Hauser SL, Waubant E, Arnold DL, et al. B-cell depletion with rituximab in relapsing-remitting multiple sclerosis. N Engl J Med 2008;358:676.

93. Cross AH, Stark JL, Lauber J, et al. Rituximab reduces B cells and T cells in cerebrospinal fluid of multiple sclerosis patients. J Neuroimmunol 2006;180:63.

94. Bar-Or A, Fawaz L, Fan B, et al. Abnormal B-cell cytokine responses a trigger of T-cell-mediated disease in MS? Ann Neurol 2010;67:452.

95. Fillatreau S, Sweenie CH, McGeachy MJ, et al. B cells regulate autoimmunity by provision of IL-10. Nat Immunol 2002;3:944.

96. Prineas JW. Multiple sclerosis: presence of lymphatic capillaries and lymphoid tissue in the brain and spinal cord. Science 1979;203:1123.

97. Serafini B, Rosicarelli B, Magliozzi R, et al. Detection of ectopic B-cell follicles with germinal centers in the meninges of patients with secondary progressive multiple sclerosis. Brain Pathol 2004;14:164.

98. Kooi EJ, Geurts JJ, van Horssen J, et al. Meningeal inflammation is not associated with cortical demyelination in chronic multiple sclerosis. J Neuropathol Exp Neurol 2009;68:1021.

99. Serafini B, Rosicarelli B, Franciotta D, et al. Dysregulated Epstein-Barr virus infection in the multiple sclerosis brain. J Exp Med 2007;204:2899.

100. Ransohoff RM, Kivisakk P, Kidd G. Three or more routes for leukocyte migration into the central nervous system. Nat Rev Immunol 2003;3:569.

101. Daneman R, Rescigno M. The gut immune barrier and the blood-brain barrier: are they so different? Immunity 2009;31:722.

102. Piccio L, Rossi B, Scarpini E, et al. Molecular mechanisms involved in lymphocyte recruitment in inflamed brain microvessels: critical roles for P-selectin glycoprotein ligand-1 and heterotrimeric G(i)-linked receptors. J Immunol 1940; 168:2002.

103. Holman DW, Klein RS, Ransohoff RM. The blood-brain barrier, chemokines and multiple sclerosis. Biochim Biophys Acta 2011;1812(2):220–30.

104. Yednock TA, Cannon C, Fritz LC, et al. Prevention of experimental autoimmune encephalomyelitis by antibodies against alpha 4 beta 1 integrin. Nature 1992; 356:63.

105. Polman CH, O'Connor PW, Havrdova E, et al. A randomized, placebo-controlled trial of natalizumab for relapsing multiple sclerosis. N Engl J Med 2006;354:899.

106. Rudick RA, Stuart WH, Calabresi PA, et al. Natalizumab plus interferon beta-1a for relapsing multiple sclerosis. N Engl J Med 2006;354:911.

107. del Pilar Martin M, Cravens PD, Winger R, et al. Decrease in the numbers of dendritic cells and CD4+ T cells in cerebral perivascular spaces due to natalizumab. Arch Neurol 2008;65:1596.

108. Cayrol R, Wosik K, Berard JL, et al. Activated leukocyte cell adhesion molecule promotes leukocyte trafficking into the central nervous system. Nat Immunol 2008;9:137.

109. Steinman L. A molecular trio in relapse and remission in multiple sclerosis. Nat Rev Immunol 2009;9:440.

110. McCandless EE, Piccio L, Woerner BM, et al. Pathological expression of CXCL12 at the blood-brain barrier correlates with severity of multiple sclerosis. Am J Pathol 2008;172:799.

111. Pashenkov M, Teleshova N, Kouwenhoven M, et al. Elevated expression of CCR5 by myeloid (CD11c+) blood dendritic cells in multiple sclerosis and acute optic neuritis. Clin Exp Immunol 2002;127:519.

112. Teleshova N, Pashenkov M, Huang YM, et al. Multiple sclerosis and optic neuritis: CCR5 and CXCR3 expressing T cells are augmented in blood and cerebrospinal fluid. J Neurol 2002;249:723.

113. Chastain EM, Duncan DS, Rodgers JM, et al. The role of antigen presenting cells in multiple sclerosis. Biochim Biophys Acta 2011;1812(2):265–74.
114. Slavin AJ, Soos JM, Stuve O, et al. Requirement for endocytic antigen processing and influence of invariant chain and H-2M deficiencies in CNS autoimmunity. J Clin Invest 2001;108:1133.
115. Tompkins SM, Padilla J, Dal Canto MC, et al. De novo central nervous system processing of myelin antigen is required for the initiation of experimental autoimmune encephalomyelitis. J Immunol 2002;168:4173.
116. Becher B, Bechmann I, Greter M. Antigen presentation in autoimmunity and CNS inflammation: how T lymphocytes recognize the brain. J Mol Med 2006; 84:532.
117. Greter M, Heppner FL, Lemos MP, et al. Dendritic cells permit immune invasion of the CNS in an animal model of multiple sclerosis. Nat Med 2005;11:328.
118. Bartholomaus I, Kawakami N, Odoardi F, et al. Effector T cell interactions with meningeal vascular structures in nascent autoimmune CNS lesions. Nature 2009;462:94.
119. Aloisi F, Ria F, Adorini L. Regulation of T-cell responses by CNS antigen-presenting cells: different roles for microglia and astrocytes. Immunol Today 2000;21:141.
120. Lassmann H, Bruck W, Lucchinetti C. Heterogeneity of multiple sclerosis pathogenesis: implications for diagnosis and therapy. Trends Mol Med 2001;7:115.
121. Heppner FL, Greter M, Marino D, et al. Experimental autoimmune encephalomyelitis repressed by microglial paralysis. Nat Med 2005;11:146.
122. McMahon EJ, Bailey SL, Castenada CV, et al. Epitope spreading initiates in the CNS in two mouse models of multiple sclerosis. Nat Med 2005;11:335.
123. Ortler S, Lodor C, Mittelbronn M, et al. B7-H1 restricts neuroantigen-specific T cell responses and confines inflammatory CNS damage: implications for the lesion pathogenesis of multiple sclerosis. Eur J Immunol 2008;38:1734.
124. Gabrilovich DI, Nagaraj S. Myeloid-derived suppressor cells as regulators of the immune system. Nat Rev Immunol 2009;9:162.
125. Zhu B, Bando Y, Xiao S, et al. CD11b+Ly-6C(hi) suppressive monocytes in experimental autoimmune encephalomyelitis. J Immunol 2007;179:5228.
126. Piccio L, Buonsanti C, Cella M, et al. Identification of soluble TREM-2 in the cerebrospinal fluid and its association with multiple sclerosis and CNS inflammation. Brain 2008;131:3081.
127. Ferguson B, Matyszak MK, Esiri MM, et al. Axonal damage in acute multiple sclerosis lesions. Brain 1997;120(Pt 3):393.
128. Kuhlmann T, Lingfeld G, Bitsch A, et al. Acute axonal damage in multiple sclerosis is most extensive in early disease stages and decreases over time. Brain 2002;125:2202.
129. Kornek B, Storch MK, Weissert R, et al. Multiple sclerosis and chronic autoimmune encephalomyelitis: a comparative quantitative study of axonal injury in active, inactive, and remyelinated lesions. Am J Pathol 2000;157:267.
130. Tallantyre EC, Bo L, Al-Rawashdeh O, et al. Clinico-pathological evidence that axonal loss underlies disability in progressive multiple sclerosis. Mult Scler 2010;16:406.
131. Medana I, Martinic MA, Wekerle H, et al. Transection of major histocompatibility complex class I-induced neurites by cytotoxic T lymphocytes. Am J Pathol 2001;159:809.
132. Neumann H, Medana IM, Bauer J, et al. Cytotoxic T lymphocytes in autoimmune and degenerative CNS diseases. Trends Neurosci 2002;25:313.

133. Smith KJ, Lassmann H. The role of nitric oxide in multiple sclerosis. Lancet Neurol 2002;1:232.

134. Fernandez M, Montalban X, Comabella M. Orchestrating innate immune responses in multiple sclerosis: molecular players. J Neuroimmunol 2010; 225(1–2):5–12.

135. Sloane JA, Batt C, Ma Y, et al. Hyaluronan blocks oligodendrocyte progenitor maturation and remyelination through TLR2. Proc Natl Acad Sci U S A 2010; 107:11555.

136. Mahad DJ, Ziabreva I, Campbell G, et al. Mitochondrial changes within axons in multiple sclerosis. Brain 2009;132:1161.

137. Pitt D, Werner P, Raine CS. Glutamate excitotoxicity in a model of multiple sclerosis. Nat Med 2000;6:67.

138. Rovaris M, Gambini A, Gallo A, et al. Axonal injury in early multiple sclerosis is irreversible and independent of the short-term disease evolution. Neurology 2005;65:1626.

139. Burkholder BM, Osborne B, Loguidice MJ, et al. Macular volume determined by optical coherence tomography as a measure of neuronal loss in multiple sclerosis. Arch Neurol 2009;66:1366.

140. Clements RJ, McDonough J, Freeman EJ. Distribution of parvalbumin and calretinin immunoreactive interneurons in motor cortex from multiple sclerosis post-mortem tissue. Exp Brain Res 2008;187:459.

141. Nave KA, Trapp BD. Axon-glial signaling and the glial support of axon function. Annu Rev Neurosci 2008;31:535.

Natural History of Multiple Sclerosis: Early Prognostic Factors

Ellen M. Mowry, MD, MCR

KEYWORDS

• Prognostic factors • Natural history • Multiple sclerosis
• Relapses • Disability • Severity

Although a small number of patients have slowly progressive neurologic deficits from the onset of the disease (primary progressive multiple sclerosis [PPMS]), most (85%) experience intermittent, subacute attacks of neurologic dysfunction, otherwise known as relapses or exacerbations, without clinical worsening between attacks (relapsing-remitting [RRMS]). There are also individuals who have a first multiple sclerosis (MS) attack who may or may not develop further symptoms thereof (clinically isolated syndrome [CIS]) and still others who have subclinical evidence of MS discovered incidentally on brain imaging (radiologically isolated syndrome [RIS]). The outcomes associated with each of these diagnoses are variable, but the short-term prognostic factors that have been assessed are discussed in the following sections.

RADIOLOGICALLY ISOLATED SYNDROME

It has long been established that there are individuals who have demyelinating lesions in the brain typical of MS at autopsy who never reported symptoms thereof during life.[1,2] The advent and increasing use of brain magnetic resonance imaging (MRI) have led to an increase in the identification of lesions typical of MS in asymptomatic individuals. The term "RIS" was coined to describe patients who have had no clinical symptoms suggestive of MS and have a normal neurologic examination but, on brain MRI, have ovoid, well-circumscribed lesions of at least 3 mm that fulfill the Barkhof MRI criteria for dissemination in space.[3,4]

In a retrospective study, 23 of 30 patients with RIS (77%) developed further lesions on follow-up brain MRI; 11 (37%) developed clinical symptoms consistent with MS (mean time to symptoms 2.3 years after initial MRI).[5] In another study of 44 patients

This work was supported by a National MS Society Lawry Fellowship Award.
Multiple Sclerosis Center, University of California, San Francisco, 350 Parnassus Avenue, Suite 908, San Francisco, CA 94117, USA
E-mail address: ellen.mowry@ucsf.edu

Neurol Clin 29 (2011) 279–292
doi:10.1016/j.ncl.2011.01.001
0733-8619/11/$ – see front matter © 2011 Elsevier Inc. All rights reserved.

neurologic.theclinics.com

with RIS, 24 (59%) developed further lesions on brain MRI, whereas 10 (23%) developed clinical symptoms consistent with a CIS.[3] Age, ethnicity, gender, and cerebrospinal fluid (CSF) anomalies did not seem to be meaningfully associated with the risk of conversion to CIS. The presence of a contrast-enhancing lesion on the RIS-defining brain MRI was associated with an increased risk of subsequent radiological progression (dissemination in time; hazard ratio [HR], 3.4; 95% CI, 1.3–8.7). In a follow-up study, 71 patients with RIS (some of whom were included in the initial study) who had undergone cervical spinal cord imaging before the development of clinical symptoms (either CIS/RRMS or PPMS) were also assessed (Okuda and colleagues, unpublished data, 2010).[3] The presence of a cervical spine lesion was associated with a large increase in the odds of subsequently developing MS, although the estimate was imprecise because of the small sample size (odds ratio [OR], 128.0; 95% CI, 13.0–1256.5). Younger age and the presence of a posterior fossa lesion were also associated with increased odds of developing clinical symptoms consistent with CIS/RRMS or PPMS. These studies were all retrospective and may have been biased by indications for, timing of, and differential techniques for scanning as well as loss to follow-up.

A prospective study of 70 patients with RIS in France demonstrated that 64 (91%) patients had dissemination in time on brain MRI scans performed after the RIS-defining scan, whereas 23 (33%) developed clinical symptoms consistent with CIS (mean time to symptoms 2.3 years).[6] In univariate models, the presence of gadolinium-enhancing lesions on MRI, abnormal visual evoked potentials, and the presence of a CSF anomaly (oligoclonal bands or elevated IgG index) in combination with 9 or more T2 hyperintense lesions on initial brain MRI (compared with neither) were associated with an increased risk of developing CIS. The study was limited by the lack of use of multivariate models and because it appeared that some (n = 14) patients did not actually meet the Barkhof MRI criteria for MS, although such patients were said to have been excluded.

The study of patients with RIS is of interest, particularly because evaluating why some individuals with MS pathology remain clinically asymptomatic may help develop new therapeutic strategies for people with MS.

CLINICALLY ISOLATED SYNDROME

CIS is considered a first clinical demyelinating event that is consistent with MS. Because many of the disease-modifying therapies approved for MS have been shown to reduce the risk of a second attack,[7–10] many experts recommend initiating disease-modifying therapy for MS at the time of the CIS.[11] However, not all patients with CIS subsequently develop new symptoms or brain MRI lesions consistent with MS. Therefore, understanding prognostic factors for MS after a CIS may help identify patients at highest risk for early disease activity.

A few studies have assessed clinical and demographic prognostic factors in patients with CIS. In a prospective study of 163 patients with CIS (who were required to have 3 or more brain MRI lesions 3 mm or larger compatible with MS, with at least one 6 mm or larger and in the brainstem or periventricular region), 94 (58%) had a second attack within a year and an additional 42 (26%) developed a second episode in the remaining period of follow-up, largely within the first 3 years.[12] In univariate models, patients who had optic neuritis were more likely to remain relapse-free than those who had onset in other regions (P = .02). Among those who did experience a second attack, the presence of motor symptoms at the time of the initial attack, a higher Expanded Disability Status Scale (EDSS) score, and polysymptomatic onset were associated with an increased risk of a second attack within the first year. However, some of these characteristics have overlapping features, and their relative contribution to the risk of early attack is unknown. In another study, 186 patients with CIS, of nonwhite race (HR, 2.47; 95% CI, 1.42–4.29), with age less than 30 years at onset (HR, 1.43; 95% CI, 0.86–2.39), and with a lower number of functional systems involved (HR, 1.39; 95% CI, 1.01–1.92) were associated in multivariate models with an increased risk of a second attack within a year of the CIS.[13] In a larger study (n = 330) at the same center that incorporated some of the same patients as the study by West and colleagues, the association of nonwhite race, younger age, and a lower number of functional systems with an increased risk of early second attack was confirmed. There was a tendency for incomplete recovery to be associated with a lower risk of early second attack.[14]

The initial brain MRI can also help to predict which individuals with CIS are at greatest risk of developing further disease activity. The Barkhof criteria for dissemination in space require 3 of the following: at least 1 gadolinium-enhancing lesion, at least 3 periventricular lesions, at least 1 juxtacortical lesion, or at least 1 infratentorial lesion.[4] These criteria were modified such that 9 T2 lesions can replace the gadolinium-enhancing lesion.[15] In a prospective study of 52 individuals with CIS, the modified Barkhof criteria were associated with a positive predictive value of 93% and a negative predictive value of 63%, with a sensitivity of 74% and a specificity of 88%.[16] In another prospective study of 415 patients with CIS, the investigators assessed the effect of the number of Barkhof criteria on the risk of subsequent attacks during a mean follow-up of 50 months.[17] Adjusted for age, gender, time on MS therapy, and the presence of oligoclonal bands, meeting 1 or 2 Barkhof criteria on baseline brain MRI was associated with an HR for conversion to clinically definite MS of 3.8 (95% CI, 2.0–7.2); meeting 3 or 4 Barkhof criteria was associated with an HR for MS of 8.9 (95% CI, 4.8–16.4). Several others studies have shown an association of a greater number of or fully meeting Barkhof criteria and increased risk of converting to MS over short periods.[18–22] Among the Barkhof criteria, the presence of a greater number of lesions[18,21,23] or the presence of gadolinium-enhancing lesions[18,20,24] has been most consistently associated with MS risk; the presence of an infratentorial lesion[23] or of 3 or more periventricular lesions[18,21] was also predictive of MS in some studies.

The development of new lesions on follow-up MRI scan is predictive of increased risk of another clinical attack.[18,24] Thus, more recent diagnostic criteria for MS (which incorporate further revised Barkhof criteria for dissemination in space to incorporate spinal cord lesions) have suggested that after a CIS, a patient can be diagnosed with MS based solely on the development of new lesions on follow-up brain MRI (dissemination in time).[25,26]

More contemporary studies have suggested that fewer lesions than required by the Barkhof dissemination in space criteria can be used to predict conversion to clinically definite MS. These criteria required that at least 1 or more lesions be present in at least 2 of the following locations: spinal cord, infratentorial region, periventricular region, or juxtacortical region.[27,28] When combined with the Swanton dissemination in time requirement (new T2 lesion on follow-up MRI, regardless of when the initial MRI was performed), these criteria were shown to have similar sensitivity and specificity as the 2001 and 2005 McDonald criteria[25,26] for the development of clinically definite MS. An even more recent study has shown that a single brain MRI scan can be used to fulfill criteria for dissemination in space and time[29]; further revisions to the diagnostic criteria have recently been updated.[30]

Characteristics of the MRI at the time of a CIS may also predict risk of early or intermediate disability. In models adjusted for age of onset, gender, location of first attack, and use of disease-modifying therapies for MS in a longitudinal cohort study of 175 patients with CIS, the presence of 3 or 4 Barkhof criteria at baseline was associated with a HR of 3.9 (95% CI, 1.1–13.6) for developing an EDSS score of 3 or more, which occurred at a mean of more than 8 years[19]; another study showed that meeting 3 or 4 Barkhof criteria conferred an HR of 35.8 for an EDSS score of 3 or more (95% CI, 4.4–294.6).[31] In a study of patients with CIS who had a follow-up brain MRI at the time of onset and 1 year later, an increased odds of developing an EDSS score of 6 over the next 6 years was associated with the presence of gadolinium-enhancing lesions on baseline MRI (OR for each standard deviation greater gadolinium-enhancing lesion number, 1.73; 95% CI, 1.05–2.84) or an increase in T2 lesion load over the first year (OR for each SD greater increase T2 lesion burden, 2.21; 95% CI, 1.23–3.97).[23]

CSF and other paraclinical data may also help predict which patients with CIS will have subsequent clinical symptoms consistent with RRMS. In the study by Masjuan and colleagues,[16] the presence of oligoclonal bands in the CSF had a positive predictive value for developing MS of 97%, with a negative predictive value of 84% (sensitivity 91%, specificity 94%). In the study by Tintore and colleagues[17] of 415 patients with CIS, those who had oligoclonal bands, regardless of age, gender, time on MS therapy, or number of Barkhof criteria on brain MRI, had nearly twice the risk of having a second clinical attack of MS (HR, 1.7; 95% CI, 1.1–2.7).[17] Visual, somatosensory, or brainstem auditory evoked potentials may be helpful as well. The HR for developing clinically definite MS if all 3 evoked potentials were abnormal at the time of CIS was 1.6 (95% CI, 0.8–3.2].[31] Similarly, if all 3 tests were abnormal, the risk of developing an EDSS score of 3 or more was substantially increased (HR, 7.0; 95% CI, 1.4–34.9).

Although only investigational at this time, several CSF and genetic biomarkers have been associated with the conversion from CIS to MS.[32–35] For example, among patients with brain lesions at the time of a CIS, those who were *HLA-DRB1*1501*-positive were more likely to develop MS within 5 years of CIS than those who were *DRB1*1501*-negative ($P<.025$).[35] As such, it is plausible that such biomarkers may be validated and incorporated into clinical use in the future.

In terms of environmental factors, one study assessed whether cigarette smoking, a risk factor for developing MS, also influences the likelihood of conversion from CIS to RRMS. In multivariate models, patients with CIS who smoked were at an increased risk of converting to RRMS (HR, 1.8; 95% CI, 1.2–2.8).[36] Titers of antibodies to Epstein-Barr virus antigens may also predict conversion to MS. Among patients with CIS, each unit increase in Epstein-Barr virus–encoded nuclear antigen 1 titer was associated with a tendency for increased conversion to MS (defined by McDonald criteria; HR, 1.6; 95% CI, 0.9–3.0).[37] However, there did not seem to be an increased risk of converting when only clinical conversion (ie, a second relapse) was the outcome. Thus, the relation between such titers and clinical disease activity remains uncertain.

Four first-line therapies initially approved for RRMS have also been shown to reduce the likelihood of converting from CIS to RRMS,[7–10] thus altering the natural history of the disease. The use of disease-modifying therapies in CIS is discussed in an article elsewhere in this issue.

RELAPSING-REMITTING MS
Clinical and Demographic Predictors of Early Attack Features

In a cohort study of 330 adult patients with RRMS or CIS seen within a year of onset, predictors of early attack severity and recovery were assessed.[38] Younger age at onset was associated with a small increase in the severity of the onset attack in adults (OR for greater severity associated with 10-year lower age, 1.3; 95% CI, 1.0–1.6). Further, older age seemed to be associated with worse recovery from the first (OR per 10-year greater age, 1.2; 95% CI, 1.0–1.5,) and second (OR, 1.4; 95% CI, 1.0–2.0) attacks. In a study of the predictors of attack severity and recovery in children with MS, those who were younger were also at an increased risk of a more severe onset attack (OR for greater severity associated with 1 year older, 0.9; 95% CI, 0.8–1.0); the same was true for the second, but not the third, attack (Fay and colleagues, unpublished data, 2011). Older children were at an increased risk of incomplete recovery from the first attack (OR per year greater age, 1.1; 95% CI, 1.0–1.3).

Race and ethnicity may also be important to attack features. In a retrospective study of 375 African Americans and 427 white individuals with all subtypes of MS, African Americans more frequently had multifocal onset and complete (vs partial) transverse myelitis during the course of the disease as well as more opticospinal MS compared with whites.[39] The results were reportedly similar when those with progressive onset were excluded. In a study of predictors of second and third attack locations in patients who had had at least 2 attacks, African American race was associated with an increased odds of having brainstem/cerebellar involvement in the second, but not the third, attack.[40] In the 330-person cohort study described earlier, patients of nonwhite race had a greater risk of a more severe first (HR, 1.6; 95% CI, 0.9–3.0) or second (HR, 2.1; 95% CI, 0.9–4.6) attack than white non-Hispanic individuals[38]; a similar association between nonwhite race and event severity was reported in a pediatric cohort with MS (Fay and colleagues, unpublished data, 2011). Hispanic ethnicity seemed to be associated with an increased relapse rate in a cohort of patients with early pediatric-onset MS/CIS.[41]

There seem to be aspects of MS attacks that remain stereotyped within an individual, at least early in the disease. In multivariate models, a more severe first attack was associated with a greater severity of the second event (OR, 4.7; 95% CI, 1.8–12.6); a more severe second event was also associated with a more severe third event.[38] Similarly, poor recovery from the first attack was associated with greater odds of worse recovery from the second attack (OR, 4.9; 95% CI, 1.7–14.4); second event recovery was associated with third event recovery. This tendency was also described in patients with pediatric MS, particularly for recovery (Fay and colleagues, unpublished data, 2011). Furthermore, in a study of patients with RRMS seen within a year of onset, the location of the first attack was associated with the location of the second attack, particularly if onset was in the spinal cord or optic nerve.[40] If the first 2 events occurred in the same location, the third event was also likely to occur in that location (OR for spinal cord, 2.2 [95% CI, 0.5–9.2]; OR for optic nerve, 4.7 [95% CI, 1.0–22.3]; OR for brainstem/cerebellum, 5.8 [95% CI, 1.3–26.8]). It is unknown if these conserved attack features are caused by underlying genetics alone or by the interplay of genetics and biologic processes.

Clinical and Demographic Predictors of Early and Intermediate-Term Disability

The number of attacks in the first few years after MS onset may influence short- and intermediate-term disability. In a heterogeneous cohort of 2477 patients with RRMS, those who had an attack within the first 5 years were at an increased risk of reaching an EDSS score of 6 within 5 years (HR, 1.5; 95% CI, 1.4–1.6) or 5 to 10 years after onset (HR, 1.3; 95% CI, 1.2–1.3).[42] A similar association was found when the outcome was defined as the development of secondary progressive MS (SPMS). In a pediatric MS cohort of 197 patients who already had 2 attacks, factors influencing the development of an outcome of either a third attack or an EDSS score of 4 or more, female gender, early time to second attack, meeting MRI criteria for pediatric MS, and lack of mental status change were all associated with an increased risk of a third attack or of reaching an EDSS of 4 in multivariate models.[43] The study included some patients with a progressive course, which was independently associated with an increased risk of reaching the endpoint. Further, some patients seemed to reach an EDSS score of 4 before the second attack; it is unclear if they were removed from the analysis because the study focus was to assess whether features of the first and second attacks, as well as demographics, were predictive of a subsequent attack or disability.

Runmarker and Andersen[44] studied a heterogeneous group of patients with MS. Among the 202 patients with "bout-onset" [RR] MS, favorable prognostic factors (for maintaining an EDSS score <6 or not converting to a progressive course) at 5 years included female gender, younger age, afferent (sensory or optic neuritis) symptoms as the first attack, monoregional onset, and full recovery from the first attack. These factors were all assessed as univariate correlates, so it is unclear if they are truly independent prognostic factors. In a prospective study that included 190 patients with RRMS (disease duration less than 3 years at study entry) who were followed for an average of 10 years, several univariate features of the initial attack were associated with an increased risk of reaching SPMS, including a greater number of functional systems involved; a higher visual, sphincteric, cerebellar, or pyramidal functional system score; and poor recovery from the attack.[45] A shorter time to second attack was also associated with an increased risk of disability in the intermediate term. Notably, many of these variables are likely related, so the relative contribution of each is unclear. In a cohort of 1609 patients with relapsing-onset MS, female gender, older age, the number of attacks that occurred in the 2 years after onset, and the presence of residual deficits after the first attack were all associated with being assigned an irreversible EDSS score of 3, which occurred after a median of 7.4 years (95% CI, 6.9–7.9).[46]

Nonwhite race has been implicated as a predictor of disability in MS, even in the short- to intermediate- term. In a retrospective study of patients with RRMS and PPMS, disability was greater in African American patients than in white patients at diagnosis and at a 4- to 6-year follow-up.[47] However, the analyses did not account for the fact that more African Americans had PPMS than whites, which is important because patients with PPMS acquire disability more rapidly than those with RRMS.[44]

MRI as a Predictor of the Early and Intermediate Course of RRMS

MRI has been studied less rigorously as a predictor of short-term outcomes in established RRMS than as a predictor of conversion from CIS to RRMS or as a predictor of long-term disability. In a convenience sample of 46 patients with RRMS (median disease duration 3 years) who had a gadolinium-enhanced brain MRI monthly for at least 9 months, baseline T2 lesion load correlated with an increase in disability over the study period (correlation coefficient [r] = 0.44, $P = .002$), and the number of gadolinium-enhancing lesions at baseline weakly correlated with relapse rate in the period of follow-up (r = 0.35, $P = .02$).[48] An association between gadolinium-enhancing lesions and subsequent relapse rate was also noted in a study that assessed patients with RRMS or SPMS of varied disease duration with monthly brain MRI scans in natural history studies or clinical trials.[49] In 63 patients who had been followed since their CIS, an increase in T2 lesion volume from baseline to the fifth year was correlated with an increase in EDSS score over the intermediate to late term (r = 0.6; 95% CI, 0.4–0.7; $P<.001$).[50] In a 48-patient subset of individuals from a prospective study on optic neuritis CIS who developed definite MS within the next 6 years, there seemed to be no association between baseline brain MRI metrics and the EDSS score after 5 years, although spinal cord lesions were associated with a higher EDSS score at 5 years.[51]

Environmental, Biologic, and Genetic Predictors in Early and Intermediate RRMS

Several environmental factors have been shown to be associated with an increased risk of developing MS, including vitamin D deficiency, cigarette smoking, and Epstein-Barr virus infection. Some studies have begun to assess whether these factors influence the course of established MS. In a 110-subject study of pediatric-onset MS/CIS (median disease duration at entry 1 year), vitamin D status, adjusted for date of blood draw, was assessed for its association with subsequent relapse rate. In multivariate models, each 10 ng/mL higher serum 25-hydroxyvitamin D_3 level was associated with a 34% decrease in the rate of subsequent attacks (incidence rate ratio, 0.66; 95% CI, 0.46–0.95).[41] A similar magnitude of association was found in a study of 145 adults with a longer MS duration (mean 11 years). Each 10-nmol/L (4 ng/mL) increase of 25-hydroxyvitamin D_3 level was associated with a lower risk of relapse over the following 6 months (HR, 0.91; 95% CI, 0.85–0.97).[52] It is still unknown if vitamin D supplementation is associated with a reduction in relapses. Cigarette smoking was assessed as a risk factor for conversion to SPMS in a subgroup analysis of 179 patients with RRMS in a larger nested case-control study assessing smoking as a risk factor for SPMS.[53] The disease duration was not reported, although the MS diagnosis had occurred within 7 years. Smokers were at increased risk of developing SPMS (HR, 3.6; 95% CI, 1.3–9.9). The lack of adjustment for disease duration is a potential concern.

Physical trauma and psychological stress have been proposed as risk factors for exacerbations. A systematic review by the American Academy of Neurology Therapeutics and the Technology Assessment Subcommittee concluded that physical trauma is unlikely to influence MS exacerbation risk, whereas the association between stress and MS attacks is still uncertain based on the evidence available.[54] Pregnancy seems to influence the risk of MS relapse. In a prospective study of 254 women with RRMS (who had a total of 269 pregnancies), the relapse rate during and after the pregnancy was compared with the relapse rate before pregnancy.[55] The relapse rate decreased during pregnancy and was lowest in the third trimester. There was a higher risk of relapse immediately after delivery, which persisted for the first 3 months postpartum; subsequently, the relapse rate returned to what it had been prepregnancy. The influence of pregnancy on the course of MS is reviewed more thoroughly in an article elsewhere in this issue.

Infections and some vaccinations have also been assessed for their association with increased risk of relapse. In 142 patients with RRMS with a mean disease duration of 11 years, there was a trend for upper respiratory infections to be concurrently associated with relapses.[56] Among 41 patients with RRMS or SPMS (median disease duration 6 years), symptomatic upper respiratory tract infection was associated with a relative risk for relapse of 2 (95% CI, 1.3–3.2, P = .004).[57] A similar magnitude of association was found in a prospective study of the association of clinical infections with attacks in 73 patients with RRMS (mean disease duration 5 years).[58] Vaccinations have also been considered as putative triggers of MS relapse. In a randomized, double-blind, placebo-controlled study of 104 patients with RRMS, influenza vaccination was not associated with an increased risk of relapse in the following 6 months.[59] A case-crossover study of 643 patients with relapsing MS assessed whether recent vaccination was associated with an increased risk of relapse and did not find an

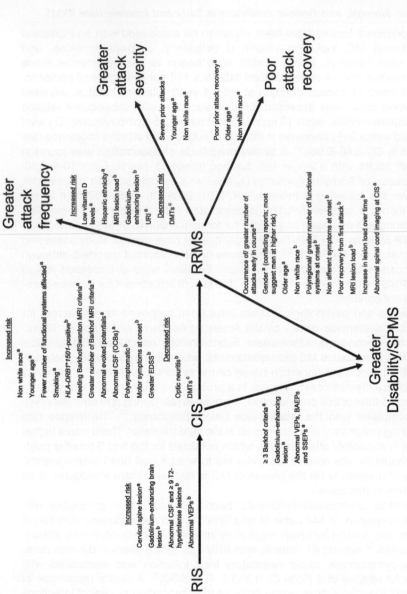

Fig. 1. Predictors of conversion from RIS to CIS and from CIS to RRMS are demonstrated. In addition, factors associated with relapse frequency, severity, and recovery in patients with RRMS are provided, as are predictors of disability (or the development of SPMS) after CIS or RRMS. VEPs, visual evoked potentials; BAEPs, brainstem auditory evoked potentials; SSEPs, somatosensory evoked potentials; OCBs, oligoclonal bands; DMTs, disease-modifying therapies; URI, upper respiratory tract infection. [a] Univariate analysis. [b] Multivariate analysis. [c] Randomized controlled trials.

Predictors of the Early and Intermediate Course of MS

Greater attack frequency

Increased risk
Low vitamin D levels[a]
Hispanic ethnicity[a]
MRI lesion load[b]
Gadolinium-enhancing lesion[b]
URI[a]

Decreased risk
DMTs[c]

Greater attack severity

Severe prior attacks[a]
Younger age[a]
Non white race[a]

Poor attack recovery

Poor prior attack recovery[a]
Older age[a]
Non white race[a]

RRMS

Occurrence of/ greater number of attacks early in course[a]
Gender[a] (conflicting reports, most suggest men at higher risk)
Older age[a]
Non white race[b]
Polyregional/ greater number of functional systems at onset[b]
Non afferent symptoms at onset[b]
Poor recovery from first attack[b]
MRI lesion load[b]
Increase in lesion load over time[b]
Abnormal spinal cord imaging at CIS[a]

Greater Disability/SPMS

CIS

Increased risk
Non white race[a]
Younger age[a]
Fewer number of functional systems affected[a]
Smoking[a]
HLA-DRB1*1501-positive[b]
Meeting Barkhof/Swanton MRI criteria[a]
Greater number of Barkhof MRI criteria[a]
Abnormal evoked potentials[a]
Abnormal CSF (OCBs)[a]
Polysymptomatic[b]
Motor symptoms at onset[b]
Greater EDSS[b]

Decreased risk
Optic neuritis[c]
DMTs[c]

≥ 3 Barkhof criteria[a]
Gadolinium-enhancing lesion[a]
Abnormal VEPs, BAEPs and SSEPs[a]

RIS

Increased risk
Cervical spine lesion[a]
Gadolinium-enhancing brain lesion[b]
Abnormal CSF and ≥ 9 T2-hyperintense lesions[b]
Abnormal VEPs[b]

association.[60] Tetanus, hepatitis B, and influenza vaccinations were evaluated separately, and none seemed to be associated with an increased risk of relapse.

HLA-DRB1*1501, the gene conferring the largest susceptibility to MS, has also been evaluated as a prognostic factor. Although there may be an association of DRB1 status and disease severity, studies thus far have included heterogeneous patient populations, were cross-sectional, and have included patients of longer disease duration.[61,62] There have been conflicting reports about the association of apolipoprotein E epsilon 4 alleles with disease progression.[63,64] Polymorphisms in genes for several cytokines, chemokines, cell surface proteins or receptors, and enzymes have been assessed for their association with disease progression, relapse rate, and other measures of disease severity; these studies are reviewed extensively elsewhere.[65] Most studies have used heterogeneous cohorts with varied endpoints, and the results remain unclear for most.

Altering the Course of RRMS: Disease-Modifying Therapies

Several disease-modifying therapies have been approved for RRMS, including interferon beta-1b, 2 forms of interferon beta-1a, glatiramer acetate, natalizumab, and mitoxantrone.[66-71] These medications have been shown to decrease the relapse rate, reduce the number of new or gadolinium-enhancing lesion on MRI, and/or reduce the accumulation of disability. Disease-modifying therapies are discussed extensively in an article elsewhere in this issue.

Early Course of RRMS as a Predictor of Longer-Term Prognosis

The course of MS within the first few years of onset may be associated with long-term prognosis. Several studies have demonstrated an association between the number of relapses early in the course and a worse long-term prognosis.[72-76] Poor recovery from the first attack, a longer time to the second attack, early irreversible disability, and sphincter involvement also seem to be important predictors of long-term disability.[77] Long-term prognostic factors are discussed in detail in the following section.

PRIMARY PROGRESSIVE MS

Defined by its relentless progression from onset, prognostic factors for PPMS are more poorly characterized than for relapsing forms of the disease. It is difficult to measure predictors of short-term progression because it takes several years for worsening to occur. Further, because early symptoms are often insidious, defining the exact onset time can be difficult. Some baseline features have been associated with an increased risk of intermediate-term worsening. In a retrospective study of 552 patients with prevalent PPMS (median disease duration at entry 7 years), those with sensory symptoms at onset or who were younger at onset had a longer time to use of a cane (EDSS score of 6).[78] Despite a longer time to EDSS score 6, younger age at onset was associated with a younger age of reaching that end point. Other studies published enrolled patients with a very long disease duration, thus possibly introducing bias. More thorough prospective studies of prognostic factors for PPMS outcomes are needed.

SUMMARY

MS is a heterogeneous disease, and predicting the short- and intermediate-term course is difficult. Clinical and demographic features at disease onset and early in the disease course, along with MRI, CSF, and evoked potential abnormalities, can be used to predict risk of relapses, relapse severity and recovery, or disability (Fig. 1). These predictors may help clinicians determine when to initiate first-line disease-modifying therapies. Limitations of several published studies include retrospective design, the use of heterogeneous groups of patients with varied disease durations and MS subtypes, the lack of uniform follow-up, and the sole use of univariate models. A better understanding of the factors influencing prognosis and their respective importance allows for a more individualized approach to the treatment of MS.

REFERENCES

1. Gilbert JJ, Sadler M. Unsuspected multiple sclerosis. Arch Neurol 1983;40: 533–6.
2. Phadke JG, Best PV. Atypical and clinically silent multiple sclerosis: a report of 12 cases discovered unexpectedly at autopsy. J Neurol Neurosurg Psychiatry 1983; 46:414–20.
3. Okuda DT, Mowry EM, Beheshtian A, et al. Incidental MRI anomalies suggestive of multiple sclerosis: the radiologically isolated syndrome. Neurology 2009;72: 800–5.
4. Barkhof F, Filippi M, Miller DH, et al. Comparison of MRI criteria at first presentation to predict conversion to clinically definite multiple sclerosis. Brain 1997;120: 2059–69.
5. Lebrun C, Bensa C, Debouverie M, et al. Unexpected multiple sclerosis: follow-up of 30 patients with magnetic resonance imaging and clinical conversion profile. J Neurol Neurosurg Psychiatry 2008;79:195–8.
6. Lebrun C, Bensa C, Debouverie M, et al. Association between clinical conversion to multiple sclerosis in radiologically isolated syndrome and magnetic resonance imaging, cerebrospinal fluid, and visual evoked potential: follow-up of 70 patients. Arch Neurol 2009;66:841–6.
7. Kappos L, Polman CH, Freedman MS, et al. Treatment with interferon beta-1b delays conversion to clinically definite and McDonald MS in patients with clinically isolated syndromes. Neurology 2006;67:1242–9.
8. Jacobs LD, Beck RW, Simon JH, et al. Intramuscular interferon beta-1a therapy initiated during a first demyelinating event in multiple sclerosis. N Engl J Med 2000;343:898–904.
9. Comi G, Filippi M, Barkhof F, et al. Effect of early interferon treatment on conversion to definite multiple sclerosis: a randomised study. Lancet 2001;357: 1576–82.
10. Comi G, Martinelli V, Rodegher M, et al. Effect of glatiramer acetate on conversion to clinically definite multiple sclerosis in patients with clinically isolated syndrome (PreCISe study): a randomized, double-blind, placebo-controlled trial. Lancet 2009;374:1503–11.
11. Frohman E, Havrdova E, Lublin F, et al. Most patients with multiple sclerosis or clinically isolated demyelinating syndrome should be treated at the time of diagnosis. Arch Neurol 2006;63:614–9.
12. Achiron A, Borak Y. Multiple sclerosis—from probable to definite diagnosis. Arch Neurol 2000;57:974–9.
13. West T, Wyatt M, High A, et al. Are initial demyelinating event recovery and time to second event under differential control? Neurology 2006;67:809–13.
14. Mowry EM, Pesic M, Grimes B, et al. Clinical predictors of early second event in patients with clinically isolated syndrome. J Neurol 2009;256:1061–6.
15. Tintore M, Rovira A, Martinez MJ, et al. Isolated demyelinating syndromes: comparison of different MR imaging criteria to predict conversion to clinically definite multiple sclerosis. AJNR Am J Neuroradiol 2000;21:702–6.

16. Masjuan J, Alvarez-Cermeno JC, Garcia-Barragan N, et al. Clinically isolated syndromes: a new oligoclonal band test accurately predicts conversion to MS. Neurology 2006;28:576–8.
17. Tintore M, Rovira A, Rio J, et al. Do oligoclonal bands add information to MRI in first attacks of multiple sclerosis? Neurology 2008;70:1079–83.
18. Moraal B, Pohl C, Uitdehaag MB, et al. Magnetic resonance imaging predictors of conversion to multiple sclerosis in the BENEFIT study. Arch Neurol 2009;66: 1345–52.
19. Tintore M, Rovira A, Rio J. Baseline MRI predicts future attacks and disability in clinically isolated syndromes. Neurology 2006;67:968–72.
20. CHAMPS Study Group. MRI predictors of early conversion to clinically definite MS in the CHAMPS placebo group. Neurology 2002;59:998–1005.
21. Barkhof F, Rocca M, Francis G, et al. Validation of diagnostic magnetic resonance imaging criteria for multiple sclerosis and response to interferon β1a. Ann Neurol 2003;53:718–24.
22. Korteweg T, Tintore M, Uitdehaag B, et al. MRI criteria for dissemination in space in patients with clinically isolated syndromes: a multicentre follow-up study. Lancet Neurol 2006;5:221–7.
23. DiFilippo M, Andersonn VM, Altmann DR, et al. Brain atrophy and lesion load measures over 1 year relate to clinical status after 6 years in patients with clinically isolated syndromes. J Neurol Neurosurg Psychiatry 2010;81:204–8.
24. Brex PA, O'Riordan JI, Miszkiel KA, et al. Multisequence MRI in clinically isolated syndromes and the early development of MS. Neurology 1999;53:1184–90.
25. McDonald WI, Compston A, Edan G, et al. Recommended diagnostic criteria for multiple sclerosis: guidelines from the International Panel on the diagnosis of multiple sclerosis. Ann Neurol 2001;50:121–7.
26. Polman CH, Reingold SC, Edan G, et al. Diagnostic revisions for multiple sclerosis: 2005 revisions to the "McDonald Criteria." Ann Neurol 2005;58: 840–6.
27. Swanton JK, Rovira A, Tintore M, et al. MRI criteria for multiple sclerosis in patients presenting with clinically isolated syndromes: a multicentre retrospective study. Lancet Neurol 2007;6:677–86.
28. Swanton JK, Fernando KT, Dalton CM, et al. Modification of MRI criteria for multiple sclerosis in patients with clinically isolated syndromes. J Neurol Neurosurg Psychiatry 2006;77:830–3.
29. Rovira A, Swanton J, Tintore M, et al. A single, early magnetic resonance imaging study in the diagnosis of multiple sclerosis. Arch Neurol 2009;66:587–92.
30. Polman CH, Reingold SC, Banwell B, et al. Diagnostic criteria for multiple sclerosis: 2010 revisions to the "McDonald criteria". Ann Neurol 2011. DOI: 10.1002/ana.22366.
31. Pelayo R, Montalban X, Minoves T, et al. Do multimodal evoked potentials add information to MRI in clinically isolated syndrome? Mult Scler 2010;16:55–61.
32. Brettschneider J, Petzold A, Junker A, et al. Axonal damage markers in the cerebrospinal fluid of patients with clinically isolated syndrome improve predicting conversion to definite multiple sclerosis. Mult Scler 2006;12:143–8.
33. Comabella M, Fernandez M, Martin R, et al. Cerebrospinal fluid chitinase 3-like levels are associated with conversion to multiple sclerosis. Brain 2010;133: 1082–93.
34. Corvol JC, Pelletier D, Henry RG, et al. Abrogation of T cell quiescence characterizes patients at high risk for multiple sclerosis after the initial neurological event. Proc Natl Acad Sci U S A 2008;105:11839–44.

35. Kelly MA, Cavan DA, Penny MA, et al. The influence of HLA-DR and –DQ alleles on progression to multiple sclerosis following a clinically isolated syndrome. Hum Immunol 1993;37:187–91.

36. DiPauli F, Reindl M, Ehling R, et al. Smoking is a risk factor for early conversion to clinically definite multiple sclerosis. Mult Scler 2008;14:1026–30.

37. Lunemann JD, Tintore M, Messmer B, et al. Elevated Epstein-Barr virus-encoded nuclear antigen-1 immune responses predict conversion to multiple sclerosis. Ann Neurol 2010;67:159–69.

38. Mowry EM, Pesic M, Grimes B, et al. Demyelinating events in early multiple sclerosis have inherent severity and recovery. Neurology 2009;72:602–8.

39. Cree BA, Khan O, Bourdette D, et al. Clinical characteristics of African Americans vs Caucasian Americans with multiple sclerosis. Neurology 2004;63:2039–45.

40. Mowry EM, Deen S, Malikova I, et al. The onset location of multiple sclerosis predicts the location of subsequent relapses. J Neurol Neurosurg Psychiatry 2009;80:400–3.

41. Mowry EM, Krupp LB, Milazzo M, et al. Vitamin D status is associated with relapse rate in pediatric-onset multiple sclerosis. Ann Neurol 2010;67:618–24.

42. Tremlett H, Yousefi M, Devonshire V, et al. Impact of multiple sclerosis relapses on progression diminishes with time. Neurology 2009;73:1616–23.

43. Mikaeloff Y, Caridade G, Assi S, et al. Prognostic factors for early severity in a childhood multiple sclerosis cohort. Pediatrics 2006;118:1133–9.

44. Runmarker B, Andersen O. Prognostic factors in a multiple sclerosis incidence cohort with twenty-five years of follow-up. Brain 1993;116:117–34.

45. Amato MP, Ponziani G. A prospective study on the prognosis of multiple sclerosis. Neurol Sci 2000;21:S831–8.

46. Leray E, Yaouanq J, LePage E, et al. Evidence for a two-stage disability progression in multiple sclerosis. Brain 2010;133(Pt 7):1900–13.

47. Naismith RT, Trinkaus K, Cross AK. Phenotype and prognosis in African-Americans with multiple sclerosis: a retrospective chart review. Mult Scler 2006;12:775–81.

48. Molyneux PD, Filippi M, Barkhof F, et al. Correlations between monthly enhanced MRI lesion rate and changes in T2 lesion volume in multiple sclerosis. Ann Neurol 1998;43:332–9.

49. Kappos L, Moeri D, Radue EW, et al. Predictive value of gadolinium-enhanced magnetic resonance imaging for relapse rate and changes in disability or impairment in multiple sclerosis: a meta-analysis. Gadolinium MRI Meta-analysis Group. Lancet 1999;353:964–9.

50. Brex PA, Ciccarelli O, O'Riordan JI, et al. A longitudinal study of abnormalities on MRI and disability from multiple sclerosis. N Engl J Med 2002;346:158–64.

51. Swanton JK, Fernando KT, Miszkiel KA, et al. Early MRI in optic neuritis. Neurology 2009;72:542–50.

52. Simpson S, Taylor B, Blizzard L, et al. Higher 25-hydroxyvitamin D is associated with lower relapse risk in MS. Ann Neurol 2010;68:193–203.

53. Hernan M, Jick SS, Logroscino G, et al. Cigarette smoking and the progression of multiple sclerosis. Brain 2005;128:1461–5.

54. Goodin DS, Ebers GC, Johnson KP, et al. The relationship of MS to physical trauma and psychological stress. Neurology 1999;52:1737–45.

55. Confavreux C, Hutchinson M, Hours MM, et al. Rate of pregnancy-related relapse in multiple sclerosis. N Engl J Med 1998;339:285–91.

56. Tremlett H, van der Mai IA, Pittas F, et al. Monthly ambient sunlight, infections and relapse rates in multiple sclerosis. Neuroepidemiology 2008;31:271–9.

57. Edwards S, Zvartau M, Clarke H, et al. Clinical relapses and disease activity on magnetic resonance imaging associated with viral upper respiratory tract infections in multiple sclerosis. J Neurol Neurosurg Psychiatry 1998;64:736–41.

58. Buljevac D, Flach HZ, Hop WC, et al. Prospective study on the relationship between infections and multiple sclerosis exacerbations. Brain 2002;125: 952–60.

59. Miller AE, Morgante LA, Buchwald LY, et al. A multicenter, randomized, double-blind, placebo-controlled trial of influenza immunization in multiple sclerosis. Neurology 1997;48:312–4.

60. Confavreux C, Suissa S, Saddier P, et al. Vaccinations and the risk of relapse in multiple sclerosis. N Engl J Med 2001;344:319–26.

61. Okuda DT, Srinivasan R, Oksenberg JR, et al. Genotype-phenotype correlations in multiple sclerosis: HLA genes influence disease severity inferred by 1HMR spectroscopy and MRI measures. Brain 2009;132:250–9.

62. Barcellos LF, Oksenberg JR, Begovich AB, et al. HLA-DR2 dose effect on susceptibility to multiple sclerosis and influence on disease course. Am J Hum Genet 2003;72:710–6.

63. Sedano MJ, Calmarza P, Perez L, et al. No association of apolipoprotein E E4 genotype with faster progression or less recovery of relapses in a Spanish cohort of multiple sclerosis. Mult Scler 2006;12:13–8.

64. Chapman J, Sylantiev C, Nisipeanu P, et al. Preliminary observations on APOE epsilon4 allele and progression of disability in multiple sclerosis. Arch Neurol 1999;56:1484–7.

65. Ramagopalan SV, DeLuca GC, Degenhardt A, et al. The genetics of clinical outcome in multiple sclerosis. J Neuroimmunol 2008;201(202):183–99.

66. The IFNB Multiple Sclerosis Study Group. Interferon beta-1b is effective in relapsing-remitting multiple sclerosis. I. Clinical results of a multicenter, randomized, double-blind, placebo-controlled trial. Neurology 1993;43:655–61.

67. Randomised double-blind placebo-controlled study of interferon β-1a in relapsing/remitting multiple sclerosis. PRISMS (Prevention of Relapses and Disability by Interferon β-1a Subcutaneously in Multiple Sclerosis) Study Group. Lancet 1998;352:1498–504.

68. Johnson KP, Brooks BR, Cohen JA, et al. Copolymer 1 reduces relapse rate and improves disability in relapsing-remitting multiple sclerosis: results of a phase III multicenter, double-blind, placebo-controlled trial. Neurology 1995;45: 1268–76.

69. Polman CH, O'Connor PW, Havrdova E, et al. A randomized, placebo-controlled trial of natalizumab for relapsing multiple sclerosis. N Engl J Med 2006;354: 899–910.

70. Rudick RA, Stuart WH, Calabresi PA, et al. Natalizumab plus interferon beta-1a for relapsing multiple sclerosis. N Engl J Med 2006;354:911–23.

71. Hartung HP, Gonsette R, Konig N, et al. Mitoxantrone in progressive multiple sclerosis: a placebo-controlled, double-blind, randomised, multicentre trial. Lancet 2002;360:2018–25.

72. Ramsaransing GS, DeKeyser J. Predictive value of clinical characteristics for "benign" multiple sclerosis. Eur J Neurol 2007;14:885–9.

73. Phadke JG. Clinical aspects of multiple sclerosis in north-east Scotland with particular reference to its course and prognosis. Brain 1990;113:1597–628.

74. Weinshenker BG, Bass B, Rice GP, et al. The natural history of multiple sclerosis: a geographically based study. 2. Predictive value of the early clinical course. Brain 1989;112:1419–28.

75. Confavreux C, Vukusic S, Adeleine P. Early clinical predictors and progression of irreversible disability in multiple sclerosis: an amnesic process. Brain 2003;126: 770–82.
76. Binquet C, Quantin C, Le Teuff G, et al. The prognostic value of initial relapses on the evolution of disability in patients with relapsing-remitting multiple sclerosis. Neuroepidemiology 2006;27:45–54.
77. Langer-Gould A, Popat RA, Huang SM, et al. Clinical and demographic predictors of long-term disability in patients with relapsing-remitting multiple sclerosis. Arch Neurol 2006;63:1686–91.
78. Koch M, Kingwell E, Rieckmann P, et al. The natural history of primary progressive multiple sclerosis. Neurology 2009;73:1996–2002.

Natural History of Multiple Sclerosis: Long-Term Prognostic Factors

Christel Renoux, MD, PhD

KEYWORDS

• Multiple sclerosis • Prognosis • Prognostic factors
• Disability • Epidemiology

Multiple sclerosis (MS) is a chronic neurologic disease with onset occurring predominantly in young adults. As such, the disease evolves throughout several decades and the affected individuals will be faced with the perspective of disability for a large part of their life. Such characteristics may explain why this disease has received so much attention and is among the most well described chronic diseases in terms of its natural history. The now well characterized natural history of MS has been complemented with numerous studies designed to delineate potential prognostic indicators of an unfavorable long-term prognosis. This aspect was already of importance years ago for counseling patients at a time when they had to make most of their personal and professional choices as young adults. It has become even more crucial nowadays when, with the so-called disease-modifying drugs now available, enlightened and weighted decisions regarding the initiation of treatment must be made.

Studying prognostic factors can achieve two goals: (1) helping to predict the long-term course and disability at the individual level, and (2) giving some insights about the pathogenesis of MS. The latter goal has definitely given more results, whereas the individualized prediction remains limited. The most scrutinized and earliest identified potential predictors are clinical characteristics at onset and during the early course of the disease, because they are easily obtained and more relevant if identified earliest in the course of the disease. Efforts are being made to supplement these indications with imaging data, as well as with biologic parameters and genetic or environmental factors. These additional factors will probably grow in importance as predictors as our knowledge of the pathogenesis of the disease increases. After a brief description

Disclosure: Dr Renoux is the recipient of a postdoctoral fellowship from the Multiple Sclerosis Society of Canada.
Center for Clinical Epidemiology, Jewish General Hospital, McGill University, 3755 Cote Ste-Catherine, H464, Montreal, QC H3T 1E2, Canada
E-mail address: christel.renoux@mail.mcgill.ca

Neurol Clin 29 (2011) 293–308
doi:10.1016/j.ncl.2011.01.006
0733-8619/11/$ – see front matter © 2011 Elsevier Inc. All rights reserved.

neurologic.theclinics.com

of the methodological concepts and material available for studying such factors, the authors first review the main demographic and clinical characteristics that influence the long-term course of MS, then describe the potential paraclinical information that may help predict the long-term evolution of MS.

THE PROGNOSIS OF MS
General Considerations: Definition of Prognosis

MS causes the accumulation of irreversible disability over time whereas survival is only slightly affected. Therefore, when concerned with prognosis, the interest is usually toward the potential for accrual of disability milestones. Disability can encompass various aspects as originally defined by the World Health Organization, and corresponds to limitation or inability in performing tasks. However, studies of MS prognosis have tended to focus mainly on physical disability and particularly on ambulation. This focus is not surprising, because difficulty with walking represents one of the first and most visible manifestations of the disease. Cognitive dysfunction has received comparatively less interest until recently.[1] Severe cognitive impairment and dementia are rare in MS.[2] Cognitive performances are rather affected by subtle changes but the prevalence of such alterations may be high, as figures most frequently reported vary between 40% and 60%.[1–4] Studies on the long-term evolution and prognosis of such cognitive changes are lacking, therefore this subject is not further reviewed here.

Several scales are available to measure disability in MS. The most widely used in prognostic studies as well as in clinical trials is the Disability Status Scale (DSS) or its extended version, the Expanded Disability Status Scale (EDSS), proposed by Kurtzke.[5,6] The EDSS is an ordinal scale based on the results of the neurologic examination and the patient's ability to walk. Scores range from zero (no neurologic abnormality) to 10 (death from MS), with increments of 0.5 points. Some drawbacks of the scale are that it actually combines impairment (in the lower scores) and disability (in the higher scores), and relies heavily on ambulation.[7] It is quite insensitive to cognitive and upper limb dysfunction. Despite these well-recognized limitations, no other scale has yet gained such acceptance, probably because of the lack of better psychometric properties and the difficulties in designing a scale that measures all aspects of the impact of MS.[8] Moreover, the requirements of a particular scale for the purpose of studying long-term outcomes may differ from the properties needed in short-term evaluation such as in clinical trials. Also, some outcomes relevant in the short term may be less relevant in the long term. Consequently, natural history studies, including those mentioned here, use the DSS or EDSS as a clinical outcome, focusing on disability scores both clinically relevant and readily identified, even in retrospect.

Natural History Cohorts

Numerous cohort studies have described the natural course of MS, including the accrual of irreversible disability over time. A complete description of the characteristics of these studies has been made elsewhere.[9] Major cohorts have been characterized by a well-defined and representative population, and essentially prospective, standardized and long-term follow-up. Of note, the majority of patients in these cohorts were untreated, or treated with drugs with no proven benefit and for a short time as compared with the duration of the disease, which gives little doubt about the absence of impact on the course of the disease. Such cohorts have allowed the estimation of the time from MS onset to the assignment of clinically relevant disability landmarks using survival analysis. From the London, Ontario, Canada cohort, median time from onset of MS to the assignment of a DSS score of 3 (defined as moderate disability) has been estimated to be 7.7 years, and time to DSS 6 (defined by the investigators as ambulatory but requiring walking aids) and DSS 8 (restricted to bed but with effective use of arms) to be 15.0 and 46.4 years.[10] From the Lyon, France cohort, estimated median times to reach irreversible DSS 4 (limited walking ability but ability to walk more than 500 m without aid or rest), 6 (ability to walk with unilateral support no more than 100 m without rest), and 7 (ability to walk no more than 10 m without rest while using a wall or furniture for support) were 8.4, 20.1, and 29.9 years, respectively.[11,12] From the Göteborg, Sweden cohort, median time to DSS 6 was 18 years.[13] Few recent studies found longer times to reach disability milestones[14,15] although others found estimates closer to those of earlier cohorts, notably for time to reach DSS 6.[16] The reasons for these discrepancies are not clear and may include methodological problems,[17] but also differences in the interpretation of the definition of the same DSS score, and possibly some inherent cohort factors influencing disease progression, such as race or vitamin D status.

These large cohorts of patients have constituted the basis for the study of prognostic factors associated with time to reach these clinically relevant disability milestones.

Methodological Insights

A detailed discussion of methods is beyond the scope of this article, but a few points deserve attention. One common consideration is that a study should be representative of the population of patients with MS. Some investigators describe their study population as population-based whereas others are clinic-based or hospital-based. Although in theory a hospital-based cohort would be more prone to selection toward more severe cases and therefore to the problem of selection bias, the reality is less straightforward. In practice, many patients with MS are likely to be seen at least once in a referral center for MS, and depending on the geographic location and relation with other neurology facilities, even a tertiary referral center may well capture virtually all MS patients of a particular region. Even if this is not the case, patients may still be referred in a manner that leads to an unbiased sample. Knowledge of the setting and organization of health care for a particular study helps to judge if the study population is reasonably well representative, or if the recruitment of patients with MS is complete or near complete. On the other hand, the population-based label is sometimes assigned based on loose criteria that do not protect with certainty against bias.

Potentially more problematic, although often neglected, are the quality and completeness of information available in databases. The increasing implementation of computerized files and access to technology allows rapid and easier collection of data. However, a database dedicated to research purposes is more than accumulation of computerized data. Without a coherent, standardized, and systematic collection of information from all patients by each participating physician, as well as recording of data by qualified personnel and regular maintenance and checking of quality and completeness, results obtained may be surprisingly divergent between studies. The constantly increasing number of observational studies performed using computerized databases not only in MS but in virtually every field of medicine must raise the awareness of the potential flaws attached to data quality. In this respect, major natural history studies that have established the description of the long-term course and prognosis of MS have gathered clinical information during regular and frequent follow-up in a standardized way. The long-term purpose of these studies is to build a complete description of the natural course of the disease, and as such, particular attention has been paid to the avoidance of potential bias related to assembly and follow-up of the cohort. Patients with MS are often seen some time after the first symptoms, and the retrospective assessment of the patient's history before the first visit is unavoidable and even crucial to ensure accurate description of the course of the disease. Solutions that consist of selecting only patients seen from onset, or taking into account only data collected prospectively after the first visit because the efforts to collect the history have not been made must be avoided, and results drawn from such methods regarded with circumspection. Similarly, avoiding the retrospective assignment of some disability scores and considering only scores assigned when a patient is seen at the clinic may be a source of bias. Indeed, when substantial gaps occur between visits, which is not so infrequent in practice, a subsequent disability score may have been reached during this time period. In this case, assigning the date of the visit for the date of assignment of disability will systematically overestimate the time to reach disability milestones. This factor is particularly problematic in databases only containing clinical information collected at the time of the visit with no information on clinical history between visits, because this problem cannot be fixed. Follow-up can be a major challenge for a disease that evolves over decades, and loss to follow-up is probably one of the major threats to validity if it is related to the outcome of interest, namely disability. This can be true even if the percentage lost to follow-up is low, although this information is often less well identified in natural history studies for two main reasons: first, because it may prove difficult to define at which point a particular patient is considered lost to follow-up, and the definition is somewhat arbitrary; second, it is not easy to determine whether the reason is related to the outcome of interest.

In the particular context of the study of prognostic factors in MS, it must be acknowledged that many of the characteristics studied are not independent but rather highly associated, particularly regarding clinical variables. Consequently, depending on which variables are studied and included in multivariate analysis, different and sometimes divergent findings may result, an important fact to keep in mind when interpreting results of different studies. Also, the interpretation of the respective importance of different potential prognostic factors may be difficult, and is best achieved when supported by extensive knowledge of the pathogenesis of the disease and clinical experience in order to avoid misinterpretation of the results. Simply stated, association is not causation, and the fact that a clinical characteristic is associated with prognosis does not mean that modifying this characteristic will necessarily change the long-term prognosis. Finally, the quality of measurement of the variables of interest is a prerequisite, as already mentioned, because no statistical techniques can correct for questionable data.

LONG-TERM PROGNOSTIC FACTORS OF IRREVERSIBLE DISABILITY
Demographic and Clinical

The following description of the potential prognostic factors mirrors the process in place in clinical practice where the prognosis is reevaluated regularly, taking into account all information available at a point in time, beginning with the most accessible information, which is demographic and clinical (**Fig. 1**). Preference is given to results from studies having achieved a substantial cohort follow-up, that is, around a decade or more, and using survival analysis when dealing with time-to-event data.

At onset of MS
While it is well established that the risk of developing MS varies with race and ethnic background, being highest for Caucasian individuals, possible variation in the severity of the disease course is also suspected. Several studies suggest that African Americans with MS have a more aggressive course than Caucasian Americans with MS.[18–21] In a recent retrospective cohort study, patients with MS of African American

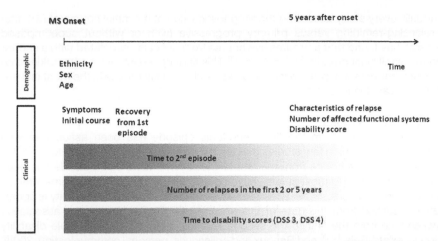

Fig. 1. Demographic and clinical characteristics associated with time to assignment of long-term irreversible disability in patients with MS along the course of the disease.

origin had a higher risk of ambulatory disability even after adjustment for other clinical variables such as age at onset.[18] It was also suggested that they may be at greater risk of disability in other domains such as hand and visual function.[20] Similarly, a retrospective cohort study conducted in France showed that patients of North African origin with MS had shorter time to irreversible disability (DSS 4 and 6) compared with patients from Europe.[22] In these studies ethnicity was self-defined and may be related to variable genetic ancestry.

The influence of sex on the long-term prognosis of MS has been assessed in numerous studies. Many have found that male sex is associated with a less favorable outcome than female sex in terms of time to major disability landmarks.[12,13,23,24] However, some have found no effect.[25–27] More importantly, overall it was found that sex did not have a strong influence on the long-term prognosis of MS when taking other factors into account, that is, in multivariable analysis.

How the age at onset of MS is placed in the list of relevant prognostic factors is quite different. Age at onset of MS exerts a strong influence on the long-term evolution of MS. A younger age at onset has been associated with a longer time to reach disability landmarks in most studies,[12,13,23,24,26,28] with some exceptions.[25,27] Moreover, the younger the age at onset, the more pronounced this phenomenon becomes.[28,29] However, the overall impact of age at onset can be seen from another perspective. Despite a longer time to reach disability landmarks, younger individuals at onset still reach these landmarks at a younger age than individuals with first symptoms at an older age.[15,29] Therefore, they reach the same level of disability earlier in life and are disabled for a longer part of their life, which leads to the conclusion that a younger age at onset cannot be considered a good prognosis.

The initial symptomatology in the form of motor, cerebellar, or sphincter dysfunction has been associated with a worse prognosis,[12,13,23–26] in contrast with an optic neuritis usually associated with longer time to disability.[12,13,24,26] However, the prognostic value was weak when taking other clinical information into account. A higher number of functional systems involved or, using another definition and terminology, a polyregional onset as opposed to symptoms from one region of the central nervous system, have also been mentioned as an indicator of worse prognosis by some investigators.[13,25]

Virtually every study assessing the prognostic value of the initial course of MS, that is, relapsing-remitting versus primary progressive (with or without superimposed relapses), has found that a progressive course from onset is associated with a shorter time to disability landmarks.[11–13,23–25,27,28] This finding persists even after taking into account other potential prognostic variables, and the initial course is the most influential clinical variable at onset.

During the course of MS

Incomplete recovery from the first neurologic episode has been associated with a worse prognosis in the few studies that have assessed this clinical variable.[12,13,25,26]

The influence of the time from the first to the second neurologic episode has been intensively studied, and most studies have concluded that the longer this time interval, the better the prognosis.[12,24,25,27,28,30] However, when the impact on disability is appropriately assessed from the date of this second neurologic episode, the association between time from the first to the second episode and time to irreversible disability no longer exists (Refs.[13,26] and Renoux and colleagues, personal communication, 2008).

Similarly, several studies have assessed the impact of relapses during the early course of the disease on long-term disability. A higher number of relapses during the first 2 or 5 years of the disease is associated with a higher risk of disability,[12,23,24,28,30] with few exceptions.[25] When appropriately (and logically) taking the end of the fifth year after onset of MS as a starting point in the survival analysis to evaluate prognosis value of relapses in the first 5 years of the disease, it was shown that relapses had either no long-term impact or only influenced prognosis for a relatively high number of relapses (5 relapses or more in the last 5 years).[13,26] A similar conclusion was reached when studying the impact of relapses after a certain threshold of irreversible disability had been reached, in which case early relapses had no influence on subsequent accrual of irreversible disability.[12] From another perspective, studying the impact of all relapses and not only of early relapses, and using a time-dependent analysis, there was a minimal impact of relapses on long-term disability.[31]

Clinical characteristics and accrual of disability in the early course may also provide information on the long-term prognosis. A higher DSS score in the first 2 and 5 years of the disease and a shorter time from MS onset to the assignment of DSS 3 or DSS 4 have been associated with a faster rate to subsequent disability scores.[12,24,30] Studying only patients with a relapsing-remitting onset, a high number of affected neurologic systems, a poor recovery from the last relapse, and a higher disability score, all characteristics evaluated at 5 years from onset, also best predicted an unfavorable long-term prognosis.[13,26] By contrast, some of the significant prognostic factors measured at onset such as sex, age, and symptoms were no longer associated with a worse long-term prognosis.[13,26] When assessed at the time when a certain detectable threshold of irreversible disability had been reached (DSS 4 in their study), Confavreux and colleagues[11,12] also showed that those demographic and clinical characteristics measured at onset no longer predicted time to subsequent disability milestones, and suggested that the disease then enters a final common pathway where accrual of irreversible disability is a self-perpetuating process, amnesic of the earlier clinical history.

Finally, time interval from MS onset to secondary progression was found to predict the time to DSS 7 but, secondary progression being a remote event in the course of the disease, it is a less useful predictor in practice.[26]

As expected, prognostic factors of time from onset to secondary progression in the subgroup of patients with relapsing-remitting onset are virtually one and the same as those described for the whole population, age at onset playing the major role in most studies.[13,16,25,26,28,32–35] In patients with a primary progressive onset, very few and sometimes contradictory prognostic factors associated with a worse outcome have been found, including the involvement of 3 or more functional systems at onset and a shorter time to reach DSS 3,[36] or the presence of motor, sensory, or brainstem symptoms at onset.[34] In a recent study, however, sensory symptoms at onset were associated with a longer time (and therefore an older age) to DSS 6 compared with the absence of such symptoms; younger age at onset was also associated with a longer time to disability.[37] For others, the number of functional systems involved 3, 4, and 5 years after disease onset, and bowel and bladder involvement 4 and 5 years after the onset of the first symptom rather than characteristics at onset, were correlated with progression to EDSS scores of 6.0 and 6.5.[38]

To conclude, it must be realized that the aforementioned demographic and clinical characteristics have been determined at the population level, contrasting with a great interindividual variability in the course of the disease. It is acknowledged that most of these characteristics are of limited value in clinical practice when making a reliable prognosis for a particular patient. To date, a few studies have attempted to validate models for the purpose of prognosis, but they have dealt mainly with short-term prognosis or have included too few patients to be reliable.[39–41] On the other hand, as described below, important concepts in the understanding of MS have been brought forth by prognostic studies.

Lessons drawn from epidemiology: implications for pathogenesis
Aside from the importance of identifying prognostic factors for the purpose of counseling patients and guiding the choice of treatment, natural history studies have proved useful for giving some clues about the pathogenesis of MS. In this respect, understanding the role of relapses in the accrual of irreversible disability is of utmost importance, because the impact of currently approved disease-modifying therapies relies mainly on the reduction of relapses rate with the underlying assumption that the demonstrated short-term effect on relapses will delay or deflate the accrual of long-term disability. The same reasoning has prevailed when testing the effect of disease-modifying therapies on delaying the time from the first to the second demyelinating neurologic episode and hence, conversion to clinically definite MS. Although the effect of currently approved treatments on relapses is not disputed, with a possible influence on short-term disability, uncertainty remains regarding their potential long-term effect on the course of the disease.[42] Indeed, disability worsening as assessed in the short-term clinical trials is not similar to truly irreversible disability as assessed in long-term natural history cohorts over many years.

The progression and accumulation of irreversible disability is believed to reflect the diffuse cumulative axonal loss. Therefore, questioning the relationship between relapses and accumulation of irreversible disability comes down to examination of the relation between acute focal inflammation and chronic axonal loss. Increasing evidence supports the view of a limited effect of relapses on long-term irreversible disability and therefore of acute focal inflammation on neurodegeneration.[9,43]

For instance, the rate of progression of disability from MS onset has been shown to be similar in progressive forms from onset with or without superimposed relapses.[38,44,45] Confavreux and colleagues[11,12] also showed that once a clinically detectable threshold of irreversible disability has been reached, namely DSS 4, the subsequent accrual of irreversible disability is not influenced by relapses irrespective of when they occur, before or during the progressive phase of MS. Taking a different approach, other investigators showed that time from onset of the progressive phase (when identified at DSS 2 or less for the purpose of the study) to long-term disability was similar whether numerous relapses, an isolated relapse, or no relapses preceded the onset of progression.[46]

From a different perspective, looking at age of assignment of disability instead of time to disability milestones, the initial course of MS, whether relapsing-remitting or progressive, had minor influence on the age at assignment of irreversible disability.[29] Similarly, age at onset of the progressive phase was found to be similar in primary and secondary progressive MS, that is, whether the progressive phase was preceded by relapses or not.[44,46] Aside from giving further credit to the limited influence of relapses on long-term disability and the dissociation between relapses and progression, these latter observations suggest that the progressive phase and the accrual of irreversible disability are rather, at least partly, under the influence of current age, along with age at onset as previously described. These factors may interact with each other to influence the rate of disability accrual.[47]

Complementary information on the relationship between focal inflammation and progression has been provided by neuropathology. Some investigators found that the progressive phase of MS, whether progressive from onset or secondary progressive, was characterized by diffuse white matter injury consisting in diffuse axonal injury on a background of a global inflammatory response compartmentalized behind the blood-brain barrier.[48,49] These characteristics were present in patients with relapsing-remitting MS, but to a lesser extent. No significant correlation was found between axonal damage in the normal-appearing white matter and the focal lesions load,[49] suggesting an independent development of diffuse white matter injury from focal demyelinated plaques. The timing of progression of this diffuse injury in the early phase of the disease remains to be fully determined, and the exact relation between focal inflammation, global inflammation, and neurodegeneration at the very onset of the disease is opened to speculation.

Paraclinical Prognostic Factors

The contribution of paraclinical data to the evaluation of the risk of long-term disability is currently limited, but this situation is likely to change owing to the growing interest in supplementing the information provided by clinical data, in parallel with the improvements in genetic, imaging, and biological techniques.

To date, there is no evidence to support the use of genetic information to predict the long-term course of MS. For instance, although the susceptibility to MS conferred by the human leukocyte antigen (HLA) class II is not disputed, its influence on the severity of the disease has been examined in several large studies, with conflicting results. As such, no convincing association between HLA DR15, or any other HLA allele, and long-term disability has been shown to date.[50–53] The role of the apolipoprotein E gene, in particular the ε4 allele, has also been studied in relation to the severity of MS; whereas some earlier studies suggested an association of the ε4 allele with a more severe disease evolution,[54–59] or a protective effect of ε2 allele,[59–61] some recent large studies and a meta-analysis did not confirm these results.[62–66] Various other genetic traits have been proposed as disease-modifying genes, but these studies await replication.[67] The difficulty in revealing consistent effects across studies may lie in part in the search for a small effect size of candidate genes on the long-term disease severity.

The utility of magnetic resonance imaging (MRI) in predicting the occurrence of a second neurologic episode and, therefore, conversion to clinically definite MS in patients with a first demyelinating event, is well established. The place and contribution of imaging in evaluating the long-term prognosis is less obvious, as illustrated in a prospective cohort study of 140 patients with a first neurologic episode suggestive of MS.[68,69] Among the 107 mostly untreated patients reevaluated after a mean follow-up of 20 years, brain T2 lesion volume at all time points, namely, baseline and 5, 10, 14, and 20 years, correlated moderately with EDSS at the end of follow-up.[69] Similar conclusions were reached when analysis was restricted to the subgroup of patients with clinically definite MS. The change in T2 lesion volume on brain MRI over the first 5 years of the disease also correlated with concurrent change in EDSS and weakened thereafter. While patients with a higher number of T2 lesions at baseline on brain imaging were more likely to be disabled 20 years later, about one-third of patients with more than 10 T2 lesions at baseline had minimal disability at the end of follow-up, and the investigators acknowledged that lesion counts provided limited prediction for long-term disability.[69] It is unclear whether the T2 lesion on cord imaging would correlate more strongly with the long-term disability.

Other paraclinical investigations performed at onset, such as the search for oligo-clonal immunoglobulin G bands (OCB) in the cerebrospinal fluid, have led to contradic-tory results regarding prognosis value. Whereas some investigators found that the presence of OCB carried no prognostic significance,[70,71] others found that patients with OCB had a higher risk of long-term disability than patients without OCB[25,72–74] and an earlier age at assignment of DSS 6.[75] The small number of patients without OCB combined with methodological disparities, including different control groups or various adjustments for other prognostic factors, may explain these findings. More-over, the frequent lack of information on characteristics such as type of clinical course or duration of follow-up hampers comparison between some studies. In any case, the small percentage of patients without OCB in MS raises questions about the usefulness of this biological parameter for prognostic purposes in practice. By contrast, further investigations of differences between patients with and without OCB may shed new light on some aspects of the pathogenesis of the disease. Recently, in a small group of 29 patients with MS with mean disease duration of 11 years, those with IgM oligo-clonal bands (n = 11) had a shorter time to secondary progression and DSS 6 than the 18 patients without IgM (17 patients with IgG OCB and 1 patient without OCB).[76] The investigators further showed that IgM directed against myelin lipids were more specif-ically associated with a worse prognosis.[77] Other markers, such as glial or axonal biomarkers, which may be relevant with respect to long-term prognosis and may improve the prediction based solely on previously described demographic and clinical characteristics, have yet to be found.

Pregnancy

The impact of pregnancy on the course of MS has been the subject of several studies. The absence of influence of pregnancy on the short-term course of the disease has been well characterized.[78] There is some question as to whether pregnancy has no effect,[79–83] or even a favorable effect in a few studies on the long-term course,[84–86] and thus should not be discouraged. The difficulty in interpreting these results comes from the fact that women with less severe disease are more likely to decide to get pregnant than women with a more active disease. Despite efforts to adjust for differ-ences in terms of demographic or clinical factors, residual confounding cannot be excluded and may, at least in part, explain these findings.

Environmental Factors

The influence of external factors on the course of MS, not to mention the long-term prognosis, is not well documented. Smoking is one exception, with an increasing amount of evidence indicating an adverse effect of smoking on the course of MS and, consequently, on the prognosis. Despite the debatable methodology of the available studies, which includes the source population not being the most appropriate for studying a clinical outcome,[87] and the imprecision in measurement or the modeling of smoking exposure, virtually all studies found that smoking increased the rate of conversion to secondary progression in patients with relapsing-remitting MS,[87–89] with one exception.[90] In cross-sectional analysis, smokers were also more likely to have primary progressive MS and to have more severe disease overall than nonsmokers.[88,89] However, an association with disability after a few years of follow-up has not been consistently found, and one study showed the difficulty of disentangling the effects of smoking from other factors that influence the course of the disease such as gender, age, and duration of the disease. All of these factors are often associated with smoking duration or intensity, and may confound the association.[89] No dose effect has been found that can be related to methodological problems cited earlier. In summary, smoking likely influences the course of the disease but the potential impact, if any, on the long-term disability is difficult to quantify. Evidence regarding other extraneous factors is either weak or anecdotal.

CHILDHOOD-ONSET MS

The subpopulation of patients with MS onset in childhood has received great attention recently, and an increasing number of studies are devoted to the delineation of the characteristics of the disease in this group. As an illustration of the influence of age at onset, it has been shown that patients with childhood-onset MS take longer to reach disability landmarks than patients with adult-onset MS. In the KIDMUS study, characteristics of a cohort of 394 patients who had MS with an onset at 16 years of age or younger and a group of 1775 patients who had MS with an onset after 16 years were compared.[91] For patients with childhood-onset MS, the estimated median time from onset to DSS scores of 4, 6, and 7 were 20.0, 28.9, and 37.0 years, respectively, and the corresponding median ages were 34.6, 42.2, and 50.5 years for later onset. In comparison with patients with adult-onset disease, those with childhood onset took approximately 10 years longer to irreversible disability. However, they reached these landmarks at an age approximately 10 years younger. Using the same cohort, potential prognostic factors of assignment to the same disability scores were assessed from 3 different time points during the early course of the disease: at MS onset, at the time of the second neurologic episode, and finally 2 years after onset of MS. At MS onset, a progressive onset was associated with shorter times to reach irreversible disability (DSS 4, 6, and 7) compared with a relapsing-remitting onset. At the time of the second neurologic episode, the time interval from onset of the disease to reach this second neurologic episode did not influence the time to reach irreversible disability. Two years after MS onset, a progressive course at onset remained the main prognostic factor associated with the highest increased risk of disability. The other significant prognostic factor was the number of relapses during the first 2 years of the disease. Each additional relapse increased the rate of disability, although to a lesser extent than the initial course. Sex, age at onset, and initial symptoms were not associated with times to disability scores in any analysis. Age at assignment of irreversible disability (DSS 4, 6, and 7) was only influenced by the initial course of the disease: a progressive initial course was associated with a younger age at development of disability. Others assessed the predictors of the assignment of an EDSS score of 4 in a cohort of 83 patients, all with a relapsing-remitting onset of MS and onset before the age of 16 (median disease duration 14.1 years).[92] In multivariate analysis, only sphincter symptoms at onset of the disease and a secondary progressive evolution were associated with a higher risk of EDSS 4. Age at onset and time between first and second neurologic episode were not prognostic factors.

In conclusion, useful clinical predictors of long-term disability are lacking in childhood-onset MS because the most influential predictor, a primary progressive presentation, is rare in children. For the majority of patients, individualized prognostic is currently limited.

SUMMARY

Several prognostic factors of long-term irreversible disability have been described in MS, mostly of demographic and clinical types. At onset, these prognostic factors are ethnicity, sex, age, type of symptoms, and initial course. Later on, they include recovery from the initial symptoms, delay to the second neurologic episode, number of relapses in the first few years, and clinical characteristics in the early phase of the disease. This apparent profusion of predictors hides two essential facts: most predictors have a minor influence on the long-term prognosis, and its corollary, which is that they are of limited value when applied at the individual level, even in combination. Consequently, from a clinical perspective, efforts are currently shifting toward finding relevant paraclinical predictors and developing validated prognostic models to improve the accuracy of individual prognosis. By contrast, the study of prognostic factors has given some insights into the pathogenesis of MS with the emergence of the following concepts. Relapses that are the clinical manifestation of acute focal inflammation have a minor impact on the accrual of long-term irreversible disability, which reflects chronic axonal loss. Rather, neurodegeneration seems to be, at least partly, an age-dependent process. From a therapeutic perspective, elucidating the exact mechanisms underlying neurodegeneration will hopefully lead to the development of new therapeutic targets, aside from those currently directed toward the control of relapses and acute inflammation.

REFERENCES

1. Hoffmann S, Tittgemeyer M, von Cramon DY. Cognitive impairment in multiple sclerosis. Curr Opin Neurol 2007;20:275–80.
2. Chiaravalloti ND, DeLuca J. Cognitive impairment in multiple sclerosis. Lancet Neurol 2008;7:1139–51.
3. Peyser JM, Rao SM, LaRocca NG, et al. Guidelines for neuropsychological research in multiple sclerosis. Arch Neurol 1990;47:94–7.
4. Rao SM, Leo GJ, Bernardin L, et al. Cognitive dysfunction in multiple sclerosis. I. Frequency, patterns, and prediction. Neurology 1991;41:685–91.
5. Kurtzke JF. On the evaluation of disability in multiple sclerosis. Neurology 1961; 11:686–94.
6. Kurtzke JF. Rating neurologic impairment in multiple sclerosis: an expanded disability status scale (EDSS). Neurology 1983;33:1444–52.
7. Sharrack B, Hughes RA. Clinical scales for multiple sclerosis. J Neurol Sci 1996; 135:1–9.
8. Thompson AJ, Hobart JC. Multiple sclerosis: assessment of disability and disability scales. J Neurol 1998;245:189–96.
9. Confavreux C, Compston A. The natural history of multiple sclerosis. In: Compston A, editor. McAlpine's multiple slerosis. 4th edition. London: Churchill Livingstone Elsevier; 2006. p. 183–272.

10. Weinshenker BG, Bass B, Rice GP, et al. The natural history of multiple sclerosis: a geographically based study. I. Clinical course and disability. Brain 1989; 112(Pt 1):133–46.
11. Confavreux C, Vukusic S, Moreau T, et al. Relapses and progression of disability in multiple sclerosis. N Engl J Med 2000;343:1430–8.
12. Confavreux C, Vukusic S, Adeleine P. Early clinical predictors and progression of irreversible disability in multiple sclerosis: an amnesic process. Brain 2003;126: 770–82.
13. Runmarker B, Andersen O. Prognostic factors in a multiple sclerosis incidence cohort with twenty-five years of follow-up. Brain 1993;116(Pt 1):117–34.
14. Pittock SJ, Mayr WT, McClelland RL, et al. Disability profile of MS did not change over 10 years in a population-based prevalence cohort. Neurology 2004;62: 601–6.
15. Tremlett H, Paty D, Devonshire V. Disability progression in multiple sclerosis is slower than previously reported. Neurology 2006;66:172–7.
16. Debouverie M, Pittion-Vouyovitch S, Louis S, et al. Natural history of multiple sclerosis in a population-based cohort. Eur J Neurol 2008;15:916–21.
17. Confavreux C. Defining the natural history of MS: the need for complete data and rigorous definitions. Mult Scler 2008;14:289–91.
18. Cree BA, Khan O, Bourdette D, et al. Clinical characteristics of African Americans vs Caucasian Americans with multiple sclerosis. Neurology 2004; 63:2039–45.
19. Kaufman MD, Johnson SK, Moyer D, et al. Multiple sclerosis: severity and progression rate in African Americans compared with whites. Am J Phys Med Rehabil 2003;82:582–90.
20. Marrie RA, Cutter G, Tyry T, et al. Does multiple sclerosis-associated disability differ between races? Neurology 2006;66:1235–40.
21. Weinstock-Guttman B, Jacobs LD, Brownscheidle CM, et al. Multiple sclerosis characteristics in African American patients in the New York state multiple sclerosis consortium. Mult Scler 2003;9:293–8.
22. Debouverie M, Lebrun C, Jeannin S, et al. More severe disability of North Africans vs Europeans with multiple sclerosis in France. Neurology 2007;68:29–32.
23. Kantarci O, Siva A, Eraksoy M, et al. Survival and predictors of disability in Turkish MS patients. Turkish Multiple Sclerosis Study Group (TUMSSG). Neurology 1998; 51:765–72.
24. Weinshenker BG, Rice GP, Noseworthy JH, et al. The natural history of multiple sclerosis: a geographically based study. 3. Multivariate analysis of predictive factors and models of outcome. Brain 1991;114(Pt 2):1045–56.
25. Amato MP, Ponziani G. A prospective study on the prognosis of multiple sclerosis. Neurol Sci 2000;21:S831–8.
26. Eriksson M, Andersen O, Runmarker B. Long-term follow up of patients with clinically isolated syndromes, relapsing-remitting and secondary progressive multiple sclerosis. Mult Scler 2003;9:260–74.
27. Myhr KM, Riise T, Vedeler C, et al. Disability and prognosis in multiple sclerosis: demographic and clinical variables important for the ability to walk and awarding of disability pension. Mult Scler 2001;7:59–65.
28. Confavreux C, Aimard G, Devic M. Course and prognosis of multiple sclerosis assessed by the computerized data processing of 349 patients. Brain 1980;103: 281–300.
29. Confavreux C, Vukusic S. Age at disability milestones in multiple sclerosis. Brain 2006;129:595–605.

30. Weinshenker BG, Bass B, Rice GP, et al. The natural history of multiple sclerosis: a geographically based study. 2. Predictive value of the early clinical course. Brain 1989;112(Pt 6):1419–28.
31. Tremlett H, Yousefi M, Devonshire V, et al. Impact of multiple sclerosis relapses on progression diminishes with time. Neurology 2009;73:1616–23.
32. Bergamaschi R, Berzuini C, Romani A, et al. Predicting secondary progression in relapsing-remitting multiple sclerosis: a Bayesian analysis. J Neurol Sci 2001;189:13–21.
33. Tremlett H, Yinshan Z, Devonshire V. Natural history of secondary-progressive multiple sclerosis. Mult Scler 2008;14:314–24.
34. Trojano M, Avolio C, Manzari C, et al. Multivariate analysis of predictive factors of multiple sclerosis course with a validated method to assess clinical events. J Neurol Neurosurg Psychiatry 1995;58:300–6.
35. Vukusic S, Confavreux C. Prognostic factors for progression of disability in the secondary progressive phase of multiple sclerosis. J Neurol Sci 2003;206:135–7.
36. Cottrell DA, Kremenchutzky M, Rice GP, et al. The natural history of multiple sclerosis: a geographically based study. 5. The clinical features and natural history of primary progressive multiple sclerosis. Brain 1999;122(Pt 4):625–39.
37. Koch M, Kingwell E, Rieckmann P, et al. The natural history of primary progressive multiple sclerosis. Neurology 2009;73:1996–2002.
38. Andersson PB, Waubant E, Gee L, et al. Multiple sclerosis that is progressive from the time of onset: clinical characteristics and progression of disability. Arch Neurol 1999;56:1138–42.
39. Bergamaschi R, Quaglini S, Trojano M, et al. Early prediction of the long term evolution of multiple sclerosis: the Bayesian Risk Estimate for Multiple Sclerosis (BREMS) score. J Neurol Neurosurg Psychiatry 2007;78:757–9.
40. de Groot V, Beckerman H, Uitdehaag BM, et al. Physical and cognitive functioning after 3 years can be predicted using information from the diagnostic process in recently diagnosed multiple sclerosis. Arch Phys Med Rehabil 2009;90:1478–88.
41. Mandrioli J, Sola P, Bedin R, et al. A multifactorial prognostic index in multiple sclerosis. Cerebrospinal fluid IgM oligoclonal bands and clinical features to predict the evolution of the disease. J Neurol 2008;255:1023–31.
42. Compston A, Coles A. Multiple sclerosis. Lancet 2008;372:1502–17.
43. Vukusic S, Confavreux C. Natural history of multiple sclerosis: risk factors and prognostic indicators. Curr Opin Neurol 2007;20:269–74.
44. Confavreux C, Vukusic S. Natural history of multiple sclerosis: a unifying concept. Brain 2006;129:606–16.
45. Kremenchutzky M, Cottrell D, Rice G, et al. The natural history of multiple sclerosis: a geographically based study. 7. Progressive-relapsing and relapsing-progressive multiple sclerosis: a re-evaluation. Brain 1999;122(Pt 10):1941–50.
46. Kremenchutzky M, Rice GP, Baskerville J, et al. The natural history of multiple sclerosis: a geographically based study 9: observations on the progressive phase of the disease. Brain 2006;129:584–94.
47. Trojano M, Liguori M, Bosco ZG, et al. Age-related disability in multiple sclerosis. Ann Neurol 2002;51:475–80.
48. Frischer JM, Bramow S, Dal-Bianco A, et al. The relation between inflammation and neurodegeneration in multiple sclerosis brains. Brain 2009;132:1175–89.
49. Kutzelnigg A, Lucchinetti CF, Stadelmann C, et al. Cortical demyelination and diffuse white matter injury in multiple sclerosis. Brain 2005;128:2705–12.

50. Barcellos LF, Sawcer S, Ramsay PP, et al. Heterogeneity at the HLA-DRB1 locus and risk for multiple sclerosis. Hum Mol Genet 2006;15:2813–24.
51. Hensiek AE, Sawcer SJ, Feakes R, et al. HLA-DR 15 is associated with female sex and younger age at diagnosis in multiple sclerosis. J Neurol Neurosurg Psychiatry 2002;72:184–7.
52. Masterman T, Ligers A, Olsson T, et al. HLA-DR15 is associated with lower age at onset in multiple sclerosis. Ann Neurol 2000;48:211–9.
53. Smestad C, Brynedal B, Jonasdottir G, et al. The impact of HLA-A and -DRB1 on age at onset, disease course and severity in Scandinavian multiple sclerosis patients. Eur J Neurol 2007;14:835–40.
54. Chapman J, Vinokurov S, Achiron A, et al. APOE genotype is a major predictor of long-term progression of disability in MS. Neurology 2001;56:312–6.
55. Evangelou N, Jackson M, Beeson D, et al. Association of the APOE epsilon4 allele with disease activity in multiple sclerosis. J Neurol Neurosurg Psychiatry 1999;67:203–5.
56. Fazekas F, Strasser-Fuchs S, Kollegger H, et al. Apolipoprotein E epsilon 4 is associated with rapid progression of multiple sclerosis. Neurology 2001;57:853–7.
57. Hogh P, Oturai A, Schreiber K, et al. Apolipoprotein E and multiple sclerosis: impact of the epsilon-4 allele on susceptibility, clinical type and progression rate. Mult Scler 2000;6:226–30.
58. Pinholt M, Frederiksen JL, Andersen PS, et al. Apo E in multiple sclerosis and optic neuritis: the apo E-epsilon4 allele is associated with progression of multiple sclerosis. Mult Scler 2005;11:511–5.
59. Schmidt S, Barcellos LF, DeSombre K, et al. Association of polymorphisms in the apolipoprotein E region with susceptibility to and progression of multiple sclerosis. Am J Hum Genet 2002;70:708–17.
60. Kantarci OH, Hebrink DD, Achenbach SJ, et al. Association of APOE polymorphisms with disease severity in MS is limited to women. Neurology 2004;62:811–4.
61. Savettieri G, Andreoli V, Bonavita S, et al. Apolipoprotein E genotype does not influence the progression of multiple sclerosis. J Neurol 2003;250:1094–8.
62. Burwick RM, Ramsay PP, Haines JL, et al. APOE epsilon variation in multiple sclerosis susceptibility and disease severity: some answers. Neurology 2006;66:1373–83.
63. Masterman T, Zhang Z, Hellgren D, et al. APOE genotypes and disease severity in multiple sclerosis. Mult Scler 2002;8:98–103.
64. Santos M, do Carmo CM, Edite RM, et al. Genotypes at the APOE and SCA2 loci do not predict the course of multiple sclerosis in patients of Portuguese origin. Mult Scler 2004;10:153–7.
65. Van der Walt A, Stankovich J, Bahlo M, et al. Apolipoprotein genotype does not influence MS severity, cognition, or brain atrophy. Neurology 2009;73:1018–25.
66. Weatherby SJ, Mann CL, Davies MB, et al. Polymorphisms of apolipoprotein E; outcome and susceptibility in multiple sclerosis. Mult Scler 2000;6:32–6.
67. Kantarci OH, de AM, Weinshenker BG. Identifying disease modifying genes in multiple sclerosis. J Neuroimmunol 2002;123:144–59.
68. Brex PA, Ciccarelli O, O'Riordan JI, et al. A longitudinal study of abnormalities on MRI and disability from multiple sclerosis. N Engl J Med 2002;346:158–64.

69. Fisniku LK, Brex PA, Altmann DR, et al. Disability and T2 MRI lesions: a 20-year follow-up of patients with relapse onset of multiple sclerosis. Brain 2008;131: 808–17.
70. Imrell K, Landtblom AM, Hillert J, et al. Multiple sclerosis with and without CSF bands: clinically indistinguishable but immunogenetically distinct. Neurology 2006;67:1062–4.
71. Siritho S, Freedman MS. The prognostic significance of cerebrospinal fluid in multiple sclerosis. J Neurol Sci 2009;279:21–5.
72. Joseph FG, Hirst CL, Pickersgill TP, et al. CSF oligoclonal band status informs prognosis in multiple sclerosis: a case control study of 100 patients. J Neurol Neurosurg Psychiatry 2009;80:292–6.
73. Stendahl-Brodin L, Link H. Relation between benign course of multiple sclerosis and low-grade humoral immune response in cerebrospinal fluid. J Neurol Neurosurg Psychiatry 1980;43:102–5.
74. Zeman AZ, Kidd D, McLean BN, et al. A study of oligoclonal band negative multiple sclerosis. J Neurol Neurosurg Psychiatry 1996;60:27–30.
75. Imrell K, Greiner E, Hillert J, et al. HLA-DRB115 and cerebrospinal-fluid-specific oligoclonal immunoglobulin G bands lower age at attainment of important disease milestones in multiple sclerosis. J Neuroimmunol 2009;210:128–30.
76. Villar LM, Masjuan J, Gonzalez-Porque P, et al. Intrathecal IgM synthesis is a prognostic factor in multiple sclerosis. Ann Neurol 2003;53:222–6.
77. Villar LM, Sadaba MC, Roldan E, et al. Intrathecal synthesis of oligoclonal IgM against myelin lipids predicts an aggressive disease course in MS. J Clin Invest 2005;115:187–94.
78. Confavreux C, Hutchinson M, Hours MM, et al. Rate of pregnancy-related relapse in multiple sclerosis. Pregnancy in Multiple Sclerosis Group. N Engl J Med 1998; 339:285–91.
79. Ghezzi A, Caputo D. Pregnancy: a factor influencing the course of multiple sclerosis? Eur Neurol 1981;20:115–7.
80. Poser S, Poser W. Multiple sclerosis and gestation. Neurology 1983;33:1422–7.
81. Roullet E, Verdier-Taillefer MH, Amarenco P, et al. Pregnancy and multiple sclerosis: a longitudinal study of 125 remittent patients. J Neurol Neurosurg Psychiatry 1993;56:1062–5.
82. Thompson DS, Nelson LM, Burns A, et al. The effects of pregnancy in multiple sclerosis: a retrospective study. Neurology 1986;36:1097–9.
83. Weinshenker BG, Hader W, Carriere W, et al. The influence of pregnancy on disability from multiple sclerosis: a population-based study in Middlesex County, Ontario. Neurology 1989;39:1438–40.
84. D'hooghe MB, Nagels G, Uitdehaag BM. Long-term effects of childbirth in MS. J Neurol Neurosurg Psychiatry 2010;81:38–41.
85. Runmarker B, Andersen O. Pregnancy is associated with a lower risk of onset and a better prognosis in multiple sclerosis. Brain 1995;118(Pt 1):253–61.
86. Verdru P, Theys P, D'hooghe MB, et al. Pregnancy and multiple sclerosis: the influence on long term disability. Clin Neurol Neurosurg 1994;96:38–41.
87. Hernan MA, Jick SS, Logroscino G, et al. Cigarette smoking and the progression of multiple sclerosis. Brain 2005;128:1461–5.
88. Healy BC, Ali EN, Guttmann CR, et al. Smoking and disease progression in multiple sclerosis. Arch Neurol 2009;66:858–64.
89. Pittas F, Ponsonby AL, van der Mei IA, et al. Smoking is associated with progressive disease course and increased progression in clinical disability in a prospective cohort of people with multiple sclerosis. J Neurol 2009;256:577–85.

308   Renoux

90. Koch M, van HA, Uyttenboogaart M, et al. Cigarette smoking and progression in multiple sclerosis. Neurology 2007;69:1515–20.
91. Renoux C, Vukusic S, Mikaeloff Y, et al. Natural history of multiple sclerosis with childhood onset. N Engl J Med 2007;356:2603–13.
92. Simone IL, Carrara D, Tortorella C, et al. Course and prognosis in early-onset MS: comparison with adult-onset forms. Neurology 2002;59:1922–8.

Natural History of Multiple Sclerosis: Have Available Therapies Impacted Long-Term Prognosis?

Maria Trojano, MD*, Damiano Paolicelli, MD, Carla Tortorella, MD,
Piero Iaffaldano, MD, Guglielmo Lucchese, MD, Vita Di Renzo, MD,
Mariangela D'Onghia, MD

KEYWORDS

- Multiple sclerosis • Long-term prognosis
- Disease-modifying drugs • Randomized trial
- Observational study • Propensity score

Multiple sclerosis (MS) is a lifelong, progressively disabling disease of the central nervous system, which mainly affects young adults. The clinical course of MS evolves over 30 years or more, and its prognosis is highly variable. The vast majority of patients experience an initial relapsing-remitting phase (RRMS). As the disease progresses, recovery tends to be incomplete, level of disability begins to increase steadily, even in the absence of relapses, and the disease transitions, with a median time of about 20 years, to the secondary progressive stage (SPMS). Natural history studies,[1,2] which typically followed cohorts of MS patients not treated with any disease-modifying drug (DMD), reported median times from onset to reach irreversible limitation in ambulation (Disability Status Scale [DSS] 4), requirement for unilateral aid for walking (DSS 6), and wheelchair-bound stage (DSS 7) of approximately 8, 20, and 30 years, respectively. Long-term disability progression represents the major issue with MS; thus, the most important goal of preventative therapy is to limit the development of this irreversible

Potential conflicts of interest: M.T. received consultancy or speaker honoraria from Biogen, Sanofi-Aventis, Merck Serono, and Bayer-Schering, and has received research grants from Merck Serono, Biogen, and Novartis. D.P. received speaker honoraria from Merck Serono; C.T. received speaker honoraria from Biogen and Sanofi-Aventis. The other authors declare that they have no conflicts of interest.
Department of Neurological and Psychiatric Sciences, University of Bari, Policlinico di Bari, Piazza Giulio Cesare 11, 70124 Bari, Italy
* Corresponding author.
E-mail address: mtrojano@neurol.uniba.it

Neurol Clin 29 (2011) 309–321
doi:10.1016/j.ncl.2010.12.008
0733-8619/11/$ – see front matter © 2011 Elsevier Inc. All rights reserved.

limitation. Before the early 1990s, management of MS patients was limited to acute and symptomatic treatment that had no impact on the disease course. Since the mid-1990s, several DMDs, such as β-interferons (IFNβ) and glatiramer acetate (GA), have become available to treat patients with RRMS. These therapies have known short- and medium-term (2–5 years) benefit in reducing relapses, disability progression, and accrual of new inflammatory lesions on magnetic resonance imaging (MRI).[3–13] However, the short duration of the randomized pivotal MS trials have provided little to no information about benefit from such treatment over periods of extended (>5 years) use. Whether DMDs may significantly alter the development of long-term disability remains uncertain, thus it remains challenging how to best approach the issue of long-term benefits from these treatments.

Only long-term randomized trials that remain blinded using an untreated control group might definitively answer this question. Such long-term placebo-controlled trials are impractical, expensive, and unethical.

In the last years, results from several open-label extensions of short-term random-ized controlled trials (RCTs)[14–22] and from postmarketing studies[23–29] have consis-tently suggested that DMDs affect long-term disability and prognosis in MS. In this article the authors review the results of these studies, and highlight study designs and/or statistical analyses to be considered for improving the validity of long-term observations of DMD effectiveness in MS populations.

IMPACT OF DMDs ON SHORT- AND MEDIUM-TERM DISABILITY COURSE

Several RCTs have shown that some DMDs can alter favorably the short- and medium-term course of RRMS[3–8] and clinically isolated syndrome (CIS).[9–13] Although these RCTs have typically evaluated relapse rate and MRI measures of disease activity, rather than disability outcome, a trend toward improvement or significant reductions of short-term disability progression have been reported in most of them (**Table 1**). The pivotal clinical trial of IFNβ-1b in RRMS[3] demonstrated a trend toward a risk reduc-tion, of about 29%, in the confirmed 1-point EDSS progression, after 3 years of treat-ment, in favor of the high dose treated group (8-MIU). After a median follow-up of 46 months,[4] this trend was confirmed because 56 out of 122 patients (46%) in the placebo arm progressed compared with 43 out of 122 (35%) in the 8-MIU group.

The pivotal phase 3 RCT of intramuscular (i.m.) IFNβ-1a[5] was the first to use delayed disability progression, as measured by time to progression of 1 point on the EDSS, sustained for 6 months, as the primary outcome measure. Although only 57% (n = 151/301) of patients completed the 2-year follow-up, a 37% reduction ($P = .02$) in disability progression was demonstrated in the IFNβ-1a group compared with the placebo group.

The placebo-controlled, double-blind Prevention of Relapses and Disability by Interferon β-1a Subcutaneously (s.c.) in MS (PRISMS) study[6] demonstrated that 2 years of treatment with both low (22 μg s.c. three times weekly [t.i.w.]) and high (44 μg s.c. t.i.w.) doses of IFNβ-1a produced a 30% reduction ($P = .01$) in the 1-point EDSS progression rate, confirmed at 3 months, compared with placebo. The initial PRISMS study was extended to 4 years, PRISMS-4, and patients initially receiving placebo were rerandomized to either low- or high-dose IFNβ-1a.[7] At the end of the 4 years, confirmed progression of disability was the lowest in patients who took a high dose for 4 years and the highest in those who received placebo for 2 years fol-lowed by low-dose IFNβ-1a for the next 2 years.

The original 2-year RCT of GA, 20 mg s.c. daily, showed a nonsignificant 12% reduction in the confirmed 1-point EDSS progression rate, and a significant 28%

Table 1
Randomized controlled trials and extension-phases of DMDs in RRMS

Therapy	RCT			Extension Phase		
	No. of Patients	Duration[Ref.]	Risk Reduction 1-Point EDSS Score Progression	No. of Patients (Retention Rate %)	Length of Follow-up[Ref.]	Disability Progression Outcome
IFNβ-1a intramuscularly, weekly	301	2 y[5]	37% (P = .02)	168 (56) 122 (40)	8 y[14] 15 y[15]	Risk reduction of progression to EDSS 6.0 30% 48% (30 μg vs placebo/30 μg)
IFNβ-1a subcutaneously, 3 times weekly	560	2–4 y[6,7]	30% (P = .01)	382 (68)	8 y[16]	Time to EDSS 6.0 3.5 y (44 μg) 2.0 y (22 μg) 1,7 y (placebo/44-22 μg)
IFNβ-1b subcutaneously, every other day	372	2–5 y[3,4]	29% (P not significant)	328 (88)	16 y[17,18]	Risk reduction of progression to EDSS 6.0 no difference (high vs low exposure)
Glatiramer acetate subcutaneously, daily	251	2 y[8]	12% (P not significant)	150 (60)	15 y[19]	Risk reduction of progression to EDSS 6.0 33% (ongoing vs withdrawn cohort)

reduction in the same unconfirmed outcome, in the GA recipients compared with placebo recipients.[8]

The BENEFIT study[11] conducted in patients with CIS was the first trial designed to capture the effect of early initiated IFNβ-1b therapy on later disability levels. CIS patients treated continuously over 3 years[12] with IFNβ-1b, 250 μg s.c. every other day, had a reduced risk (−40%; P = .022) of progression of 1 point on the EDSS score, confirmed at 6 months, compared with those treated with placebo for the first 1 or 2 years. The results from the 5-year analysis[13] of the BENEFIT study recently demonstrated a continued advantage for early compared with delayed treatment; however, the difference between the proportion of patients who experienced confirmed EDSS progression was no longer statistically significant between the early (25%) and delayed (29%) treatment groups.

IMPACT OF DMDs ON LONG-TERM DISABILITY

Several open-label extensions of short-term RCTs and postmarketing observational studies have been conducted to assess the efficacy of DMDs in delaying the appearance of permanent neurological disability.

Extensions of Short-Term RCTs of DMDs

In all the published extension studies of short-term RCTs the differences in clinical outcomes were compared in patients who received treatment from the study inception versus those who began the therapy approximately 2 to 3 years later (ie, patients originally randomized to placebo).

An open-label, 8-year follow-up evaluation[14] was obtained for about 56% of RRMS patients originally enrolled in the pivotal phase 3 trial of i.m. IFNβ-1a.[19] At the 8-year follow-up, 42.0% of the original placebo patients and 29.1% of the original IFNβ-1a patients reached an EDSS of 6.0, an observed treatment effect of approximately 30% that only trended toward significance (P = .09). Disability status was also ascertained after 15 years[15] in about 40% of the patients who were originally enrolled in phase 3. Patients who continued to use i.m. IFNβ-1a treatment (n = 56) had a lower mean EDSS score (4.4 vs 5.7; P = .011), a smaller mean increase from baseline EDSS scores (2.3 vs 3.3; P = .011), and less progression to EDSS 6.0 (32% vs 62%; P = .007) and 7.0 (9% vs 33%; P = .008) compared with patients who discontinued treatment (n = 66).

An unblinded retrospective long-term follow-up (LTFU) at 7 to 8 years was offered to all patients enrolled in PRISMS,[16] whether or not they had completed PRISMS-2[6] or PRISMS-4.[7] Sixty-eight percent (382/560) of patients returned for a single visit at the seventh or eighth anniversary of their enrollment into the trial. At that time, the overall progression to SPMS was 20%. Although comparisons must be interpreted cautiously, this conversion rate is notably lower than in the pre-DMD era natural history studies,[1] which would predict that approximately 40% of PRISMS patients would have progressed to SPMS after 6 to 10 years from disease onset. Patients receiving the higher dose showed a trend toward a greater effect in delaying disability progression. Increase of disability by 2 EDSS points was reached by 10% of patients in 2.3 years in the IFNβ-1a 44-μg group compared with 1 year in the combined late-treatment group. Progression to an EDSS score of 4.0 occurred in fewer patients in the 44-μg group than in the 22-μg or late-treatment (24%, 29%, and 28%, respectively) groups, and progression to an EDSS score of 6.0 was slower in the 44-μg group (3.5 years) than in the late-treatment group (1.7 years).

The IFNβ-1b 16-year LTFU study[17] was a multicenter, observational study aimed at evaluating the long-term safety and efficacy outcomes of IFNβ-1b treatment in RRMS patients using cross-sectional data collection from patients who had participated in the original pivotal trial. The results were analyzed by stratification according to the original assignment of the pivotal trial (placebo, 50 μg and IFNβ-1b, 250 μg) and according to the duration of treatment exposure during 16 years of follow-up (<20%; 20%–80%; >80% of exposure). About 88% (328/372) of patients in the original double-blind, placebo-controlled trial were recruited 16 years later for participation in this LTFU and 69.9% of them (260/372) had available case report forms. Patients remaining on long-term IFNβ-1b had a slower, even if not statistically significant, progression to EDSS 6.0 compared with those who received the treatment for a short period only. Of those patients who received IFNβ-1b for more than 80% of the 16-year interval, approximately 44% reached EDSS 6.0 and 29% reached EDSS 8.0. The median time to EDSS 6.0 in the same patients was approximately 13 years. For those patients on IFNβ-1b for a period between 10% to 80% of the 16-year interval, 46.9% of them reached EDSS 6.0 and 31% reached EDSS 8.0, respectively. Most importantly, the mortality rates among patients originally treated with IFNβ-1b were lower than in the original placebo group (18.3% for placebo, vs 8.3% for IFNβ-1b 50 μg and 5.4% for IFNβ-1b 250 μg).[18]

A prospective, open-label, extension study was conducted to evaluate the neurologic status and EDSS scores in patients from the original pivotal trial of GA[8] who had used GA, as a sole therapy, for up to 15 years. Clinical efficacy results were reported at 6,[19] 8,[20] 10,[21] and 15 years[22] after randomization to GA therapy. At the last observation, 232 patients received at least one GA dose (modified intention-to-treat [mITT] cohort; mean disease duration of 17 years and average of 8.6 years on GA treatment since study initiation), and 100 continued as of February 2008 (ongoing cohort; mean disease duration of 20 years and average of 13.6 years on GA treatment) while 132 left the study, 50 of whom were available for LTFU (withdrawn cohort; mean disease duration of 13 years and average of 4.8 years on GA treatment). The proportions of patients reaching EDSS milestones of 4.0, 6.0, and 8.0 were 38%, 18%, and 3% for ongoing and 40%, 27%, and 6% for withdrawn patients, respectively. LTFU visit of patients who had withdrawn from the pivotal trial showed that these patients had a trend for a greater disability than those who had continued on GA.

All the results from LTFU of short-term RCTs, on the whole, suggest that sustained early treatment might delay progression of disability, and support the concept that delaying early disability may have long-lasting effects. There are, however, some potential limitations of LTFU studies that deserve discussion. Despite efforts to retain study participants, the ascertainment was often incomplete due to accumulating dropouts. Patients' retention rate ranged between 88% and 40% in these studies (see **Table 1**). After completion of the respective RCTs, patients were managed in clinical practice by their physicians outside the context of a research protocol. For most of them data were collected retrospectively, after considerable intervals in which patients were not monitored and during which they may have discontinued for long periods, switched, or added other DMDs to the immunomodulatory therapy under study. Therefore, all these methodological restrictions limit the interpretation of the results from these studies.[30]

Postmarketing Studies of DMDs

Observational studies bear the benefit of relatively easy long-term monitoring and can supply data on the behavior of large cohorts of patients during extended treatment periods. These studies serve a wide range of purposes such as monitoring long-term effectiveness and safety, including the detection of rare side effects of drugs and drug-drug interactions, and also the collection of suitable information that may be predictive of treatment response.[31–34] A major issue is that observational studies are more exposed to biases in comparison with RCTs.[35–38] These biases can partly be addressed through rigorous study designs or statistical analyses. Several methodological improvements (matching, stratification, partitioning, adjustment, restriction and propensity score [PS]-adjusted analysis)[39–41] have been recently proposed and are available to enhance validity when randomization is absent.

Several postmarketing studies have been conducted in the last years to evaluate long-term effectiveness of DMDs in MS patients.

The risk of long-term disability progression according to the length of exposure to IFNβ was assessed in a large cohort of 2090 MS patients prospectively collected by the Italian MS Database Network.[23] A total of 44,140 patient visits were evaluated during a median follow-up period of 8.4 years, and a Cox proportional hazards regression adjusted for PS[40] was used for the analysis. The risk of 1-point EDSS score progression, confirmed at the end of treatment follow-up, was reduced by about 4 to 5 times (P<.001) in patients exposed to IFNβ for more than 4 years, compared with patients exposed for up to 2 years.

In a more recent study,[24] the long-term impact (for up to 7 years) of IFNβ treatment on times from first visit and from date of birth to reach an irreversible clinical disability, corresponding to EDSS scores 4.0 and 6.0, and to reach the SP phase, was prospectively evaluated in a large cohort of untreated (n = 401) and IFNβ-treated (n = 1103) RRMS patients, using an inverse weighting-PS-adjusted Cox proportional hazards regression.[42,43] The untreated control group, concurrent with the treated group, consisted of RRMS patients who voluntarily refused DMD treatment, who planned a pregnancy, who had concomitant diseases (ie, neoplasm, psychiatric diseases, or severe depression) that prevented them from receiving DMDs, who discontinued DMD treatment in the first 3 to 6 weeks because of clinical and hematological adverse events, or who had low disease activity at first presentation. The results of this observational study demonstrated that patients selected to receive IFNβ treatment have a better outcome than those who choose not to be treated or who are not selected for therapy. The IFNβ-treated group showed a substantial reduction in the incidence of conversion to SP, and reaching EDSS scores 4.0 and 6.0 (**Fig. 1**) when compared with untreated patients. SP and EDSS scores of 4.0 and 6.0 were reached with significant delays estimated by time from first visit (3.8, 1.7, and 2.2 years, respectively) and time from date of birth (8.7, 4.6, and 11.7 years, respectively) in favor of treated patients. The percentage of patients in the untreated group who converted to SP (20.2%) up to 7 years of follow-up (about 11 years from onset) was in line with the estimated mean rate of conversion to SP of 2% to 3% per year evaluated in previously published natural history studies,[44] whereas the proportion of treated patients who converted to SP was significantly lower (8%). A delay in age at SP and at EDSS 4.0 and 6.0 associated with IFNβ treatment was also demonstrated.

Similar conclusions were drawn from an observational, nonrandomized study,[25] using another interesting approach for analyzing DMD effectiveness on MS disability progression. A pre-post treatment analysis of change in EDSS was conducted in a cohort of 590 RRMS patients collected in a large database in Nova Scotia. Instead of an untreated control group, the investigators used DMD-treated patients as their own controls. DMD effectiveness was examined by comparing individuals' estimated annual changes on EDSS score during the treatment years with those in the years preceding and following the treatment. This study demonstrated an impact of DMDs on disability progression and, in particular, a more rapid EDSS increase in

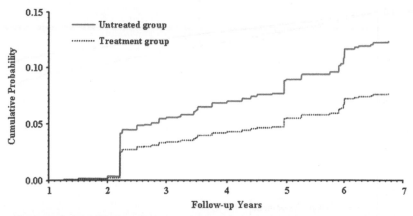

Fig. 1. Propensity score–adjusted survival curve for time from first visit to reach confirmed Expanded Disability Status Scale 6.0 score. Seven-year cumulative probability of reaching the end point in never-treated and interferon-β–treated MS patient groups. Red line indicates untreated group; blue line indicates treatment group. Cumulative probability represents the estimated proportion of patients reaching the end point. (*From* Trojano M, Pellegrini F, Fuiani A, et al. New natural history of interferon beta-treated relapsing multiple sclerosis. Ann Neurol 2007;61:304; with permission.)

the years following drug switches and treatment stops. So far, no clinical trial has been able to provide this last information.

The impact of early versus delayed IFNβ treatment on disability progression was evaluated in a large cohort of 2570 RRMS prospectively followed for up to 7 years in 15 Italian MS Centers.[26] The main objective of this study was to assess the optimal time to initiate IFNβ with regard to when the greatest benefit on clinical outcomes was observed. A Cox proportional hazards regression model adjusted for PS quintiles[45] was used to assess differences between groups of patients with early versus delayed IFNβ treatment on risk of reaching 1-point progression on EDSS score, and the EDSS 4.0 and 6.0 milestones. A set of PS-adjusted Cox hazards regression models was calculated according to different times of treatment initiation (within 1 year up to within 5 years from disease onset). The lowest hazard ratios for the 3 PS quintiles adjusted models were obtained by a cut-off of treatment initiation within 1 year from disease onset. Early treatment significantly reduced the risk of reaching the EDSS 4.0 milestone and 1-point progression in EDSS score (**Fig. 2**).

More interestingly, the results suggested that the greatest difference in treatment benefit was observed in RRMS patients who received DMDs within the first year from disease onset compared with those who received the treatment after this time. Moreover, the results of this observational study confirmed, in a population with definite RRMS and a longer period of follow-up (7 years), those shown in the extension phase of the original BENEFIT study in CIS patients (at 3 years).[12]

Several observational studies have assessed the efficacy of long-term GA therapy, suggesting a positive effect on disability progression. Three of them described experiences in France,[27] Argentina,[28] and the United States.[29] The data obtained in France[27] came from a compassionate use program. Two hundred and five RRMS patients were followed for 3.5 to 8 years on treatment. Mean EDSS scores remained stable over the course of the study, and only 5.7% of patients progressed by at least 1 point on the EDSS after 5 years. The data from Argentina[28] come from a large

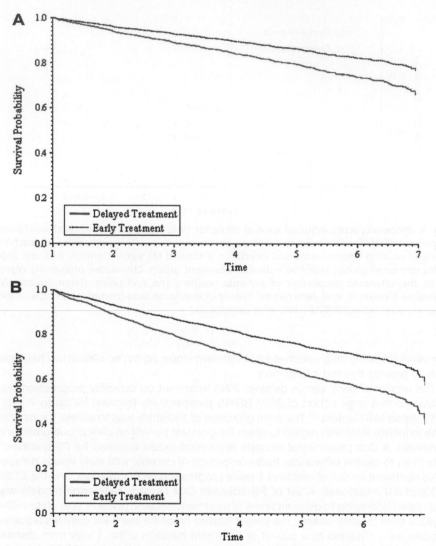

Fig. 2. Propensity score-adjusted survival curves for time from treatment initiation to reach confirmed EDSS 4.0 score (*A*), and 1-point progression on EDSS score (*B*). Seven year cumulative probability of reaching the end points in early treatment and delayed treatment MS patient groups. Survival probability represents the estimated proportion of patients who did not reach the end point. Red line indicates delayed treatment group; blue line indicates early treatment group. (*From* Trojano M, Pellegrini F, Paolicelli D, et al. Real-life impact of early interferon-β therapy in relapsing multiple sclerosis. Ann Neurol 2009;66:517; with permission.)

national registry collecting data on DMD-treated patients. The study evaluated 174 patients treated with GA, and the outcome was compared with a concurrent untreated cohort of 360 patients. All patients were evaluated prospectively every 6 months. During the entire follow-up period, about 22% of GA-treated patients improved by at least 1 point on the EDSS 6, 2.5% remained stable, and 15% worsened by at least

1 point. The median time from diagnosis to reach EDSS 6.0 was 15 years in GA-treated patients compared with 9 years in untreated patients. A very long-term (up to 22 years), open-label, compassionate-use study of GA was conducted in the United States[29] although on a small cohort of 46 RRMS patients. EDSS was measured every 6 months. Most of the patients (57%) displayed improved or unchanged EDSS scores. Only 10 of 28 (36%) patients with baseline EDSS les than 4.0 had a last observed value of 4 or greater, and 8 of 34 (24%) with entry EDSS less than 6.0 reached EDSS 6.0 or greater.

All the results from these observational studies seem to suggest a positive long-term impact of DMD on the natural course of MS when compared with nontreated patients over the same period, in a clinical practice setting, or when compared with historical cohorts. Until now, the only contrasting results derive from the recently published nonblinded, nonrandomized, 2-year interim analysis of the United Kingdom MS risk-sharing scheme.[46] In fact, these results do not provide reliable evidence on cost-effectiveness of DMD, showing that patients taking DMDs acquired, in the short-term, more disability than an untreated historical control group.[47] However a longer follow-up and analyses of additional data sets are awaited and are needed to confirm these preliminary findings.

Several limitations of observational studies merit discussion. Methodological issues may hinder the analysis of observational studies, including the lack of randomization, variation in duration of treatment, incomplete data collection, dropouts, unaccounted drug switches, and inherent difficulty with historical comparators. In particular, the internal validity of observational studies may be undermined by previously either known or unknown confounding factors, which may not be evenly distributed between intervention groups and may influence the measured association between the exposure of interest and outcome. However, the introduction of the recently proposed PS-adjusted analysis[48] and sensitivity analysis,[49] as already used in some postmarketing studies in MS populations,[23,24,26] has allowed, in the last years, a step forward in reducing the bias in treatment comparisons[50] in observational studies. In fact PS analysis,[48] taking into consideration parameters of interest that would likely affect the outcome, creates balanced groups that have a similar likelihood of receiving a therapy and resembles randomized cohorts of patients. In addition, sensitivity analysis allows determination of the magnitude of a potential unmeasured confounder that could erase the observed association or would need to be present to materially alter the conclusions of a study.[49]

SUMMARY

There is a need for a continued follow-up of MS patients who receive DMDs for several years, but the most reliable method to assess whether the treatment influences the long-term course is still under debate.

Despite the inherent limitations of follow-up studies, the results from long-term extensions of the RCTs and from observational studies, published in the last years, both support the evidence that currently available DMDs have, at least partially, impacted the long-term prognosis of RRMS patients, especially when they are administered at an early stage and for a prolonged period of time. Moreover, while the extensions of the RCTs[14–22] demonstrated these effects on restricted and highly selected subgroups of RRMS patients originally enrolled in pivotal trials, on the other hand and most importantly, observational studies[23–29] extended the findings from RCTs by reporting these effects in large MS cohorts exposed to DMDs. In other words, the results from RCTs and observational studies do complement each other, and both studies are necessary to provide a comprehensive picture of drug benefits.

However, each approach has strengths and weaknesses that can threaten external (whether or not the study results are generalizable to other populations) or internal (how the data are gathered and assigned) validity.[50]

Future methodological improvements to enhance the quality of both extensions of RCTs and observational studies are mandatory. Moreover, because RCTs of adequate size and with a very long period of follow-up remain the best approach to prove long-term benefits from treatments, greater efforts need to be made for minimizing obstacles (ethical, economic, regulatory, or political) that inappropriately may prevent their implementation.

Recommendations for the planning of future LTFU studies have recently been provided[51] that include, above all, the plan of adequate study designs that take into account the need for long-term data at the time of the original study, the selection of sites with capacity to maintain long-term contact and follow-up, and a continued care to original trial participants to maximize retention.

Phase 4 and observational studies should be designed to foresee careful enrollment criteria and a longitudinal, rigorously prospective, collection of data. Proper statistical analyses aimed at reducing bias in treatment comparisons should be used.[52] There are several methods to overcome the potential biases introduced by the lack of randomization. PS-adjusted analyses, which can create groups of patients who have similar likelihood of receiving a therapy, and sensitivity analyses[48,49] are the most common methods currently used for this purpose. However, PS methodology has led to many findings that would otherwise not be available, although it is not a replacement for RCTs. Therefore the conclusions from an observational study may not be considered as strong as those from RCTs. Failure in recognizing the limitations of extensions of RCTs and observational studies in the assessment of treatment effects may have serious consequences, including both the use of ineffective or dangerous treatments and the inappropriate withdrawal from effective treatments.[34,53]

REFERENCES

1. Weinshenker BG, Bass B, Rice GP, et al. The natural history of multiple sclerosis: a geographically based study. I. Clinical course and disability. Brain 1989; 112(Pt 1):133–46.
2. Confavreux C, Vukusic S, Moreau T, et al. Relapses and progression of disability in multiple sclerosis. N Engl J Med 2000;343(20):1430–8.
3. The IFNB Multiple Sclerosis Study Group. Interferon beta-1b is effective in relapsing-remitting multiple sclerosis. I. Clinical results of a multicenter, randomized, double-blind, placebo controlled trial. Neurology 1993;43:655–61.
4. The IFNb Multiple Sclerosis Study Group and The University of British Columbia MS/MRI Analysis Group. Interferon beta-1b in the treatment of multiple sclerosis: final outcome of the randomized controlled trial. Neurology 1995;45:1277–85.
5. Jacobs LD, Cookfair DL, Rudick RA, et al. Intramuscular interferon beta-1a for disease progression in relapsing multiple sclerosis. Ann Neurol 1996;39:285–94.
6. PRISMS (Prevention of Relapses and Disability by Interferon b-1a Subcutaneously in Multiple Sclerosis) Study Group. Randomised double-blind placebo-controlled study of interferonb-1a in relapsing/remitting multiple sclerosis. Lancet 1998;352:1498–504.
7. PRISMS Study Group and the University of British Columbia MS/MRI Analysis Group. PRISMS-4: long-term efficacy of interferon-beta-1a in relapsing MS. Neurology 2001;56:1628–36.

8. Johnson KP, Brooks BR, Cohen JA, et al. Copolymer 1 reduces relapse rate and improves disability in relapsing remitting multiple sclerosis: results of a phase III multicenter, double-blind placebo-controlled trial. The Copolymer 1 Multiple Sclerosis Study Group. Neurology 1995;45:1268–76.

9. Jacobs LD, Beck RW, Simon JH, et al. Intramuscular interferon beta-1a therapy initiated during a first demyelinating event in multiple sclerosis. CHAMPS Study Group. N Engl J Med 2000;343:898–904.

10. Comi G, Filippi M, Barkhof F, et al. Effect of early interferon treatment on conversion to definite multiple sclerosis: a randomized study. Lancet 2001;357:1576–82.

11. Kappos L, Polman CH, Freedman MS, et al. Treatment with interferon beta-1b delays conversion to clinically definite and McDonald MS in patients with clinically isolated syndrome. Neurology 2006;67:1242–9.

12. Kappos L, Freedman MS, Polman CH, et al. Effect of early versus delayed interferon beta-1b treatment on disability after a first clinical event suggestive of multiple sclerosis: a 3-year follow-up analysis of the BENEFIT study. Lancet 2007;370:389–97.

13. Kappos L, Freedman MS, Polman CH, et al. Long-term effect of early treatment with interferon beta-1b after a first clinical event suggestive of multiple sclerosis: 5-year active treatment extension of the phase 3 BENEFIT trial. Lancet Neurol 2009;8:987–97.

14. Rudick RA, Cutter GR, Baier M, et al. Estimating long term effects of disease-modifying drug therapy in multiple sclerosis patients. Mult Scler 2005;11:626–34.

15. Bermel RA, Weinstock-Guttman B, Bourdette D, et al. Intramuscular interferon beta-1a therapy in patients with relapsing-remitting multiple sclerosis: a 15-year follow-up study. Mult Scler 2010;16(5):588–96.

16. Kappos L, Traboulsee A, Constantinescu C, et al. Long-term subcutaneous interferon beta-1a therapy in patients with relapsing-remitting MS. Neurology 2006;67:944–53.

17. Ebers GC, Rice G, Konieczny A, et al. The interferon beta-1b 16-year long-term follow-up study: the final results. Neurology 2006;66(Suppl 2):A32.

18. Ebers GC, Traboulsee A, Li D, et al. Analysis of clinical outcomes according to original treatment groups 16 years after the pivotal IFNB-1b trial. J Neurol Neurosurg Psychiatry 2010;81(8):907–12.

19. Johnson KP, Brooks BR, Ford CC, et al. Glatiramer acetate (Copaxone): comparison of continuous versus delayed therapy in a six-year organized multiple sclerosis trial. Mult Scler 2003;9:585–91.

20. Johnson KP, Ford CC, Lisak RP, et al. Neurologic consequence of delaying glatiramer acetate therapy for multiple sclerosis: 8-year data. Acta Neurol Scand 2005;111:42–7.

21. Ford CC, Johnson KP, Lisak RP, et al. A prospective open-label study of glatiramer acetate: over a decade of continuous use in multiple sclerosis patients. Mult Scler 2006;12(3):309–20.

22. Ford C, Goodman AD, Johnson K, et al. Continuous long-term immunomodulatory therapy in relapsing multiple sclerosis: results from the 15-year analysis of the US prospective open-label study of glatiramer acetate. Mult Scler 2010;16(3):342–50.

23. Trojano M, Russo P, Fuiani A, et al. The Italian Multiple Sclerosis Database Network (MSDN): the risk of worsening according to IFNb exposure in multiple sclerosis. Mult Scler 2006;12:1–8.

24. Trojano M, Pellegrini F, Fuiani A, et al. New natural history of interferon beta-treated relapsing multiple sclerosis. Ann Neurol 2007;61:300–6.

25. Brown MG, Kirby S, Skedgel C, et al. How effective are disease modifying drugs in delaying progression in relapsing-onset MS? Neurology 2007;69:1498–507.
26. Trojano M, Pellegrini F, Paolicelli D, et al. Real-life impact of early interferonβ-therapy in relapsing multiple sclerosis. Ann Neurol 2009;66:513–20.
27. Debouverie M, Moreau T, Lebrun C, et al. A longitudinal observational study of a cohort of patients with relapsing remitting multiple sclerosis treated with glatiramer acetate. Eur J Neurol 2007;14:1266–74.
28. Carra A, Onaha P, Halfon J, et al. The impact of glatiramer acetate on progression of disability over a decade of continuous therapy. Mult Scler 2007;13(Suppl 2):S68.
29. Miller A, Spada V, Beerkircher D, et al. Long-term (up to 22 years), open-label, compassionate-use study of glatiramer acetate in relapsing remitting multiple sclerosis. Mult Scler 2008;14:494–9.
30. Noseworthy JH. How much can we learn from long-term extension trials in multiple sclerosis? Neurology 2006;67:930–1.
31. McKee M, Britton A, Black N, et al. Methods in health services research. Interpreting the evidence: choosing between randomised and nonrandomised studies. BMJ 1999;319:312–5.
32. Dobre D, van Veldhuisen DJ, DeJongste MJL, et al. The contribution of observational studies to the knowledge of drug effectiveness in heart failure. Br J Clin Pharmacol 2007;64:406–14.
33. Black N. Why we need observational studies to evaluate the effectiveness of health care. BMJ 1996;312:1215–8.
34. MacMahon S, Collins R. Reliable assessment of the effects of treatment on mortality and major morbidity, II: observational studies. Lancet 2001;357:455–62.
35. Feinstein AR. Clinical biostatistics. London: Mosby; 1977. p.16–20.
36. Matthews DE, Farewell VT. Using and understanding medical statistics. revised 2nd edition. Basel (Switzerland): Karger; 1988.
37. Rochon PA, Gurwitz JH, Sykora K, et al. Reader's guide to critical appraisal of cohort studies:1. Role and design. BMJ 2005;330:895–7.
38. Wolfe RA. Observational studies are just as effective as randomized clinical trials. Blood Purif 2000;18:323–6.
39. Normand SLT, Sykora K, Li P, et al. Readers guide to critical appraisal of cohort studies: 3. Analytical strategies to reduce confounding. BMJ 2005;330:1021–3.
40. Rosenbaum PR, Rubin DB. The central role of the propensity score in observational studies for causal effects. Biometrika 1983;70:41–55.
41. Rosenbaum PR, Rubin DB. Reducing bias in observational studies using subclassification on the propensity score. J Am Stat Assoc 1984;79:516–24.
42. Hirano K, Imbens GW. Estimation of causal effects using propensity score weighting: an application to data on right heart catheterization. Health Serv Outcomes Res Methodol 2001;2:259–78.
43. Lunceford JK, Davidian M. Stratification and weighting via the propensity score in estimation of causal treatment effects: a comparative study. Stat Med 2004;23:2937–60.
44. Vukusic S, Confavreux C. Prognostic factors for progression of disability in the secondary progressive phase of multiple sclerosis. J Neurol Sci 2003;206:135–7.
45. D'Agostino RB Jr. Propensity score methods for bias reduction in the comparison of a treatment to a non-randomized control group. Stat Med 1998;17:2265–81.
46. Boggild M, Palace J, Barton P, et al. Multiple sclerosis risk sharing scheme: two year results of clinical cohort study with historical comparator. BMJ 2009;339:b4677.

47. Ebers G. Natural history of multiple sclerosis. In: Compston A, Ebers G, Lassmann H, et al, editors. McAlpine's multiple sclerosis. 3rd edition. London: Churchill Livingstone; 1998. p. 191–221.
48. D'Agostino RB Jr, D' Agostino RB Sr. Estimating treatment effects using observational data. JAMA 2007;297(3):314–6.
49. Lin DY, Psaty BM, Krommal RA. Assessing the sensitivity of regression results to unmeasured confounders in observational studies. Biometrics 1998;54:948–63.
50. Rubin DB. The design versus the analysis of observational studies for causal effects: parallels with the design of randomized studies. Stat Med 2007;26:20–36.
51. Ebers GC, Reder AT, Traboulsee A, et al. Long-term follow-up of the original interferon-β1b trial in multiple sclerosis: design and lessons from a 16-year observational study. Clin Ther 2009;31:1724–36.
52. Trojano M, Pellegrini F, Paolicelli D, et al. Observational studies: propensity score analysis of non-randomized data. Int MS J 2009;16(3):90–7.
53. Hennekens CH, Buring JE, Manson JE, et al. Lack of effect of longterm supplementation with beta carotene on the incidence of malignant neoplasms and cardiovascular disease. N Engl J Med 1996;334:1145–9.

Demographic, Genetic, and Environmental Factors That Modify Disease Course

Ruth Ann Marrie, MD, PhD

KEYWORDS
- Multiple sclerosis • Prognosis • Race • Comorbidity
- Socioeconomic status • Genetics • Smoking

Multiple sclerosis (MS) is considered to be a complex disease; that is, one in which one or multiple environmental factors act on a genetically susceptible individual to cause disease. Similarly, multiple factors may also contribute to the well-recognized, yet poorly understood heterogeneity in disease outcomes observed in MS, although most studies have evaluated the impact of only a single factor or set of closely related factors.

As discussed by Mowry and colleagues, elsewhere in this issue, numerous cross-sectional and longitudinal studies have described the natural history and prognostic factors for MS.[1–6] Attempts to predict long-term outcomes generally focused on disease-related factors, such as age at onset, onset symptoms, early relapse rate, interval between first and second relapses, and other clinical characteristics related exclusively to MS.[3,4,7–10] Findings conflicted regarding the influence of sex, relapse rate, and age at onset.[4,6,8,11]

The ability to prognosticate early in the disease course remains poor, although prognostication improves when information regarding the first 5 years of the clinical course is available.[7,12] Using clinical characteristics in the first 2 years after onset, Weinshenker and colleagues[7] predicted the median time to a Disability Status Scale (DSS) score of 6 (needing an assistive device for walking). Their model correctly predicted the median time within 6 years for 55% of patients, but the median time to DSS 6 for the entire population was only 15 years. Adding the DSS score at 5 years to the model allowed correct prediction of the median time within 6 years for 65% of patients; still less than desired.

Funding: Supported in part by a Rudy Falk Clinician Scientist Award (University of Manitoba).
University of Manitoba, Health Sciences Center, GF-533, 820 Sherbrook Street, Winnipeg, Manitoba, R3A 1R9, Canada
E-mail address: rmarrie@hsc.mb.ca

Neurol Clin 29 (2011) 323–341
doi:10.1016/j.ncl.2010.12.004
0733-8619/11/$ – see front matter © 2011 Elsevier Inc. All rights reserved.

neurologic.theclinics.com

Instead of focusing on characteristics of the initial disease presentation, more recent studies considered the influence of a broader range of modifiable and nonmodifiable patient characteristics on disease outcome,[13–16] including genetic factors, race, ethnicity, socioeconomic status, comorbid diseases, and health behaviors.

GENETIC FACTORS

Although persons with sporadic and familial forms of MS do not differ with respect to age of symptom onset, clinical course, or severity of disability,[17] some studies suggest a higher degree of concordance than expected with respect to disease characteristics among persons with familial MS. Oturai and colleagues,[18] and Hensiek and colleagues[19] reported concordance for age of symptom onset and disease course among sibling pairs. Other investigators reported concordance for disease severity but not for age of symptom onset.[20] Inconsistent results may reflect small sample sizes or ascertainment methods,[21,22] but these findings suggest a genetic influence on disease course.

A growing literature describes the association between genetic factors and the age of MS symptom onset, clinical course, and disability progression. Initial studies focused on HLA-associated alleles, reflecting the recognized association between those alleles and susceptibility to MS; however, a broader range of factors have been examined in more recent studies including apolipoprotein E, tumor necrosis factor (TNF)-alpha, CCL5, CCR5, CTLA-4, CD28, MC1R, TYR, VDR, osteopontin, GSTM1, GSTM2, GSTT1, and GSTP1.[23–50] Many of these factors were examined previously as potential susceptibility factors for MS.

Several studies suggest that the presence of one or more HLA-DRB1 alleles is associated with an earlier age of onset. Weatherby and colleagues[29] evaluated 375 patients with clinically definite MS from Northwestern England and found that women with HLA-DRB1*15 had an average age of MS onset of 30 years, whereas women who were negative for HLA-DRB1*15 had an average age of MS onset of 33.2, a difference of 3 years ($P = .007$). Other studies reported a similar difference in the average age of onset, but in men and women.[32,48] Unfortunately, this finding has not been consistent across studies.[23,24,29,30,43,51,52]

Of particular interest has been the association of genetic factors with clinical course and disability, but the reported findings are inconsistent for HLA, apolipoprotein E (reviewed in Guerrero and colleagues[50]) and other factors studied. **Table 1** summarizes the results of some of these studies, selected to illustrate the range of genetic factors considered, populations studied, and their disparate results. Initial studies focused on disability progression, largely as measured by ambulatory disability, but more recent studies have examined cognitive disability, and neuroimaging abnormalities. For example, Sombekke and colleagues[46] found that 80 patients carrying HLA-DRB1*1501 had a median of 4 spinal cord lesions, whereas 70 patients who did not carry HLA-DRB1*1501 had a median of 2 lesions ($P<.001$). Zivadinov and colleagues[44] reported that HLA-DRB1 and HLA-DQB1 alleles were associated with T1 and T2 lesion volumes as well as brain atrophy. Van Veen and colleagues,[53] however, reported that there was no association between CTLA-4 or CD28 and brain atrophy or lesion volume in 96 patients with MS from the Netherlands.

Overall, the findings regarding genetic factors that may modify clinical course and disability progression are inconsistent, likely reflecting several factors. First, sample sizes in some studies have been small, reducing the power to detect an association. Second, characterization of genotype-phenotype associations requires very careful determination of phenotype, with consideration paid to the point in the disease course when this is being evaluated. Discussion continues regarding the best way to measure disability and disability progression in MS; existing measures have strengths and weaknesses. Studies focusing exclusively on ambulatory disability, for example, may fail to identify a relevant association between genotype and cognitive or other forms of disability. This is particularly important given the known dissociation of physical and cognitive disability in some patients, and the increasing recognition that some patients who are classified as having a benign course based on their level of physical disability suffer from significant cognitive disability.

Third, it is likely that gene-gene interactions or epistasis play a role in determining disease outcome. DeLuca and colleagues[54] examined 163 patients with sporadic MS and their nuclear family members (n = 625) reported that HLA-DRB1*01 and HLA-DRB1*15 alleles interact to influence MS clinical phenotypes, producing a milder disease course. Variation from one population to another in the frequency of the presence of interacting genetic factors other than the factor under study can lead to heterogeneous results. Fourth, environmental factors may also interact with genetic factors to influence phenotype. Ramagopalan and colleagues[55] recently reported that vitamin D may regulate the behavior of HLA-DRB1*15, and thus susceptibility to MS; these types of relationships may also modify disease course.

RACE AND ETHNICITY

The risk of MS varies across race and geographic region.[56] The disease occurs less often among non-whites than whites.[57] Using administrative health claims data from Alberta, Canada, the prevalence of MS in 2002 among First Nations people was 99.9 per 100,000 population, whereas it was 335.0 per 100,000 persons in the general population.[58]

Several studies suggest that race is also associated with clinical phenotype and severity of demyelinating disease.[13,59,60] Neuromyelitis optica (NMO) is a monophasic or relapsing-remitting inflammatory demyelinating disorder characterized by temporally linked optic neuritis and transverse myelitis.[61] NMO has a different underlying pathology from that of classical MS, and is associated with IgG antibodies to aquaporin-4.[62] It appears to overlap with the entity of opticospinal MS described in Asia, which is also characterized by predominant involvement of the optic nerves and spinal cord.[62,63] A relative excess of non-whites has been consistently recognized among patients with NMO relative to MS. In a study of 802 patients with demyelinating disease, NMO was more common among African American patients (16.8%) than among whites (7.9%, P<.001).[13] Mirsattari and colleagues[60] identified 7 Aboriginals from the Canadian province of Manitoba with demyelinating disease, of whom 5 had aggressive disease with predominant involvement of the optic nerves and spinal cord, consistent with NMO.

In both the adult and pediatric MS populations, race is associated with other clinical differences, although findings are not entirely consistent. Naismith and colleagues[64] suggested that African Americans are more likely to have primary progressive MS (PPMS) than whites. Although some studies report no significant difference in the age of symptom onset between African Americans and whites,[15] others suggest that African Americans have a later age of symptom onset,[13,65] and another suggests that African American males have an earlier age of symptom onset than white males.[66] These discrepancies may reflect the use of non–population-based samples or the difficulties inherent in using race to classify populations into subgroups with different underlying biologies.

Table 1
Selected examples of studies examining the associations between genetic factors and clinical characteristics of multiple sclerosis

Author (Year)	Study Population	Genetic Factor	Findings
Weatherby et al[29] 2001	375 persons with clinically definite MS from Northwestern England	HLA-DRB1	HLA-DRB1*15 associated with earlier age of onset in women HLA-DRB1*04 associated with PPMS No association with severity of disability
Hensiek et al[30] 2002	729 persons with MS from the United Kingdom	HLA-DR15	Earlier age of diagnosis No association with severity of disability
Masterman et al[27] 2000	815 persons with definite MS	HLA-DR15	Earlier age of onset in men and women
Villoslada et al[32] 2002	194 familial cases and 202 consecutive cases with clinically definite MS starting interferon-beta from Spain	HLA-DRB1, HLA-DQB1	Earlier age of onset (not significant) No association with disability
DeLuca et al[54] 2007	163 MS patients with "benign" or "malignant" MS	HLA-DRB1	HLA-DRB1*01 and HLA-DRB1*15 alleles interact to produce milder disease course Replicated findings in a Sardinian cohort and affected sibling pairs
Weinshenker et al[120] 1997	78 patients with MS from United States (Rochester County)	TNF-alpha	No association with clinical course or disability
Weinshenker et al[121] 1998	119 patients with MS from United States (Rochester County)	HLA-DR, HLA-DQ	No association with disability Suggestion that DR4-DQ8 and DR1-DQ5 associated with PPMS, and DR1-DQ5 associated with RRMS
McDonnell et al[24] 1999	102 patients with PPMS and 2002 with RRMS or SPMS from Northern Ireland	HLA-DR2	No association with clinical course or disability
Runmarker et al[23] 1994	308 MS patients from Sweden	HLA-DR, HLA-DQ	No association with clinical course DR17,DQ2 was significantly overrepresented in the quartile with the most malignant course
Cournu-Rebeix et al[45] 2008	651 MS patients from France	HLA-DRB1	No association with disease severity after stratification by clinical course Increased risk of SPMS (HLA-DR15)
Guerrero et al[50] 2008	82 MS patients from Spain	APOE	No association with disease severity

Study	Gene	Population	Findings
Okuda et al[48] 2009	HLA-DRB*1501	505 MS patients from the United States	Earlier age of onset, lower NAA concentrations in normal-appearing white matter, greater brain atrophy, and worse cognitive performance (PASAT)
Cree et al[49] 2009	HLA-DRB1	673 African Americans and 717 Caucasian Americans	HLA-DRB1*15 associated with earlier age of onset, "typical" MS rather than neuromyelitis optica; African American ancestry at HLA associated with increased disability
Zivadinov et al[44] 2007	HLA-DRB1, HLA-DQB1	41 Italian MS patients	HLA-DRB1*1501 associated with more brain atrophy and higher T1 lesion volumes; DQB1*0301 associated with higher T2 lesion volumes; DQB1*0302 associated with more gray matter atrophy and higher T1 and T2 lesion volumes; DQB1*0602 associated with more gray matter and brain atrophy; DQB1*0603 associated with higher T1 lesion volumes and more disability
Silva et al[51] 2007	HLA-DRB1	248 Portuguese patients	HLA-DRB1*15 negative patients had more rapid progression of disability
Van Veen et al[122] 2007	CCL5, CCR5	637 Dutch MS patients	CCR5 + 303*A associated with earlier age of onset; CCL5-403*A associated with more disability as measured by MSSS; CCR5 + 303*G was associated with reduced T2 hyperintense and T1 hypointense lesion volumes on MRI; CCR5Δ32 associated with reduced T2 lesion volume
Van Veen et al[53] 2003	CTLA-4, CD28	514 Dutch MS patients; 96–99 with imaging data	No association with lesion volume, brain atrophy
Partridge et al[40] 2004	MC1R, TYR, VDR	419 MS patients from Europe	Presence of ≥1 MC1R glu-encoding allele associated with greater disability

(continued on next page)

Table 1
(continued)

Author (Year)	Study Population	Genetic Factor	Findings
Kantor et al[37] 2003	256 MS patients from Israel	CCR5	The Δ32CCR5 mutation associated with slower progression of disability
Schreiber et al[34] 2002	70 Danish MS patients	HLA-DRB1*1501, Δ32CCR5, APOE	DRB1*1501 and APOE-e4 not associated with disability CCR5Δ32 associated with trend toward smaller lesion burden
Kantarci et al[39] 2004	221 persons with MS from the United States	APOE	Carriers of E4*e2 had a longer time to EDSS 6 (in 1 of 2 cohorts)
Smestad et al[43] 2007	1457 MS patients from Scandinavia	HLA-DR15, HLA-A	HLA-DR15 associated with earlier age of onset No association with disease course or disability
Hensiek et al[35] 2000	1056 persons with definite MS	Osteopontin gene (7 SNPs)	No association with disability
Caillier et al[36] 2003	821 patients with clinically definite MS from United States	Osteopontin (4 SNPs)	Presence of ≥1 wild-type osteopontin SNP 1284A allele less likely to have mild course, more likely SPMS [a]trend
Mann et al[26] 2000	400 persons with clinically definite MS	GSTM1, GSTM3, GSTT1, GSTP1	GSTM3 African American genotype associated with severe disability in patients with disease duration ≥10 years Homozygosity for both GSTM1*0 and GSTP1*Ile105 containing allele associated with severe disability in patients with disease duration ≥10 years
Sombekke et al[46] 2009	150 persons with MS from the Netherlands	HLA-DR	Increased number of spinal cord lesions
Vasconcelos et al[52] 2009	33 persons with PPMS from Brazil	DRB1*1501	More rapid disability progression

Abbreviations: MS, multiple sclerosis; PPMS, primary progressive MS; RRMS, relapsing/remitting MS; SNP, single-nucleotide polymorphism; SPMS, secondary progressive MS; TNF, tumor necrosis factor.
[a] Only one study.

As compared with whites, African Americans with optic neuritis more frequently have severe visual loss at baseline visual acuity (VA ≤20/200) and have less recovery at 1-year follow-up.[67] Among 330 patients with a clinically isolated syndrome who were at risk for MS or with early relapsing remitting MS followed for a median period of 633 days, non-whites had an increased risk of an early second relapse (hazard ratio [HR] 2.06; 95% confidence interval [CI]: 1.34, 3.17) after accounting for age of symptom onset, treatment status, and the severity of the initial presentation.[68] Non-whites also had a nonsignificant increase in the risk of having a more severe initial relapse (odds ratio [OR] 1.59; 95% CI: 0.85, 2.99). The non-white population included a mixture of African Americans, Asians, Hispanics or Latinos, and 13 participants of unknown race/ethnicity making it uncertain how this finding applies to the non-white subgroups.

In the study of 802 patients with MS by Cree and colleagues,[13] African Americans had an elevated risk of needing a cane to walk (HR 1.67; 95% CI: 1.29–2.15) after accounting for treatment status. Findings were similar in the New York State Multiple Sclerosis Consortium (NYSMSC) patient registry, which captures clinical data regarding patients from 18 MS centers.[66] African Americans constituted approximately 6% of the patients registered, but they had more severe gait and cognitive disability than non-African American registrants. However, disability progression was also reported to be similar among whites and African Americans once care was established at an MS center,[69] raising the question of whether some of the observed differences reflect differences in access to care or treatment. Wallin and colleagues[70] examined survival among 2500 veterans with service-connected MS from the time of MS onset. Median survival times from onset did not differ by race, being 43 years for white women, 30 years for black men, and 34 years for white men. A retrospective chart review of 46 children with MS found that the annualized relapse rate was higher among African Americans (mean 1.80; SD 1.14) than whites (mean 1.13; SD 0.50; P<.001).[71] Although the African Americans and whites did not differ in their mean time to initiation of disease-modifying therapy or in the proportion treated, this study did not adjust for age of symptom onset, use of disease-modifying therapy, or duration of follow-up.

In addition to possible differences in readily observable clinical characteristics, some investigators reported differences in immunologic measures and treatment responses. Rinker and colleagues[72] compared measures of cerebrospinal fluid humoral immunity between 66 African Americans and 132 whites. The median IgG synthesis rate was higher in African Americans (13.6 mg/d) than in whites (8.2 mg/d, P = .01). In a post hoc analysis of the EVIDENCE trial, which compared 2 formulations of interferon-beta-1a,[65,73] Cree and colleagues[65] compared relapse and imaging outcomes between 36 African American and 616 white participants. African Americans were less likely to be relapse free than whites at either 24 weeks (56% vs 70%) or at 48 weeks (47% vs 57%). Based on MRI, African Americans also had more new T2 lesions at 48 weeks. The investigators concluded that African Americans responded less to treatment, but such findings could also reflect similar response to treatment, but differential baseline disease severity. Further, the sample size was small.

The discrepancies in findings regarding the influence of race reflect differences in study design and ascertainment, the populations evaluated, and unmeasured confounders, but also highlight the limitations of using race to infer underlying biologic characteristics. Populations classified according to race remain heterogeneous. Historically, race has been defined as a group of persons who are relatively homogeneous with respect to biologic inheritance, a concept distinct from ethnicity, described as a "social group characterized by a distinctive social and cultural tradition, maintained within the group from generation to generation, a common history and origin, and a sense of identification with the group."[74] Genetic and environmental factors may vary with race,[75] and race is often used as a proxy for ancestry, which defines genetic relationships between individuals and populations. Use of race as a proxy for ancestry, and failure to consider ethnic and socioeconomic factors that co-vary with race may limit the ability to understand and identify biologic reasons for variation in MS outcomes.[75]

SOCIOECONOMIC STATUS

Numerous social determinants of health exist, including socioeconomic status (SES), culture, and social networks.[76] Socioeconomic status describes a person's position in society,[74,77] and usually is characterized by some combination of income and education, although these variables do not completely represent the construct.[78] Also essential to the construct are occupation, employment status, and wealth. Socioeconomic status is a fundamental determinant of health, and is associated with leading causes of death, reasons for hospital care, use of health care services, functional status, and health behaviors.[78–81]

Patients of lower SES are at higher risk of comorbidity, may undergo fewer investigations for MS-related symptoms, and receive fewer symptomatic therapies;[82–85] all factors that have the potential to influence long-term outcomes. In a study of the North American Research Committee on MS (NARCOMS; a large US-based self-report registry for persons with MS) population, differences in the severity of disability between African Americans and whites with MS were overestimated by up to 25% when SES was not considered.[15] Despite its potential importance, the impact of social factors on MS outcomes has received relatively little attention.

PREGNANCY

Several studies have examined the impact of pregnancy on MS, and consistently suggest an increased risk of relapse postpartum.[86,87] Most studies suggest that pregnancy does not adversely affect subsequent disability progression,[87–91] possibly because of a reported dissociation between relapses and disability progression.[92] Poser and Poser[88] suggested that pregnancy occurring after MS onset appeared to be associated with a better long-term prognosis until the younger age at onset of women who became pregnant after MS as compared with those who were pregnant before MS onset was considered. Runmarker and Andersen[90] and D'Hooghe and colleagues[93] suggested that pregnancy was associated with a better prognosis for disability progression. However, it is difficult to exclude the possibility that women with more active disease choose not to have children given the lower frequency of pregnancy among women with MS.[90] Further, these studies typically did not account for miscarriages and abortions. No long-term impact of breastfeeding on disability progression has been reported.[87]

COMORBIDITY

Comorbidity is usually defined as the total burden of illness other than the specific disease of interest,[94] and is distinct from disease-related complications. In other chronic diseases, comorbidity is recognized to adversely influence numerous health outcomes including disability, mortality, and health care use.[95–98] Increasingly, investigators are examining the influence of comorbidity on disability and disability progression in MS.

A study of 64 patients with definite or probable MS reported no association between comorbid autoimmune disease or isolated autoantibodies and age of MS onset, initial clinical presentation, or type of clinical course.[99] In this study, several different autoimmune diseases were grouped together in the analysis because of small sample size. In 2006, a study of participants in the NARCOMS Registry examined the association between comorbidity and disability at diagnosis of MS.[16] Disability was measured using Patient-Determined Disease Steps, patient-reported measures that assesses ambulatory disability and correlate highly with a physician-scored Expanded Disability Status Scale.[100] At diagnosis, the most common comorbidities reported were mental (such as depression, anxiety), vascular (such as hypertension, hyperlipidemia), and autoimmune disorders. More than 50% of participants were overweight or obese. The presence of vascular, musculoskeletal, or mental comorbidities or obesity at diagnosis was associated with greater disability at diagnosis. For example, participants with vascular comorbidity had 1.5-fold increased odds of moderate as compared with mild disability at diagnosis (OR 1.51; 95% CI: 1.12–2.05). Participants with obesity also had increased odds of moderate as compared with mild disability at diagnosis (OR 1.38; 95% CI: 1.02–1.87). Musculoskeletal (OR 1.81; 95% CI: 1.25–2.63) and mental (OR 1.62; 95% CI: 1.23–2.14) comorbidities were associated with increased odds of reporting severe as compared with mild disability at diagnosis. Autoimmune disease was not associated with the degree of disability at diagnosis.

Disability progression after diagnosis may also be influenced by comorbid disease. Kirby and colleagues[101] reviewed the medical records of 1730 patients followed at a population-based MS clinic and characterized the presence or absence of autoimmune diseases, asthma, and psychiatric syndromes. Autoimmune disease was not associated with disability progression, but asthma was associated with more rapid progression to an Expanded Disability Status Scale (EDSS) score of 3, equivalent to mild gait disability ($P = .028$). Finally, the presence of psychiatric syndromes was associated with more rapid progression of disability also, even after accounting for sex, clinical course, other comorbidities, age of MS onset, use of disease-modifying therapies, and initial clinical presentation.[102]

In a 3-year observational study of 146 patients with recently diagnosed MS, those with musculoskeletal comorbidities experienced a 5-point decline in the motor scale of the Functional Independence Measure, whereas those without such comorbidities experienced only a 2-point decline.[103] Marrie and colleagues[104] evaluated the association between vascular comorbidities, including hypertension, hyperlipidemia, heart disease, diabetes, and peripheral vascular disease, and disability progression among 8983 participants in the NARCOMS Registry. When compared with participants who did not report vascular comorbidities at diagnosis, those with vascular comorbidities had an increased risk of early gait disability (HR 1.70; 95% CI: 1.54–1.87), need for a unilateral assistive device to walk (HR 1.68; 95% CI: 1.51–1.87), and need for a bilateral assistive device to walk (HR 1.48; 95% CI: 1.26–1.74). Vascular comorbidities developing at any time during the disease course were also associated with an increased risk of early gait disability (HR 1.58; 95% CI: 1.48–1.68), unilateral assistance to walk (HR 1.54; 95% CI: 1.44–1.65), and bilateral assistance to walk (HR 1.38; 95% CI: 1.25–1.52).

Further work is needed to replicate and extend these findings regarding the impact of comorbidity on disease progression. As yet, the mechanisms for these findings are unknown, but could include influences at the pathophysiological level, or reflect the impact of multiple conditions simultaneously influencing a common outcome, such as mobility. No studies have examined the impact of more aggressive treatment of

Table 2
Studies examining the impact of smoking on disability progression and neuroimaging metrics

Author (Year)	Population	Smoking Definition	Outcome	Confounders Considered	Findings
Hernan et al[107] 2005	General Practice Research Database (UK)	Ever vs never smoker	Time to secondary progression	Age, sex, onset symptoms motor vs nonmotor	Ever smoking associated with higher risk of secondary progression HR 3.6 (95% CI 1.3–9.9)
D'Hooghe et al[110] 2005	160 MS patients	Ever, never, current smoking	MSSS	?none	Smoking status not associated with MSSS
Koch et al[109] 2007	364 MS patients from Netherlands	Smoker vs non-smoker	EDSS, MSSS	Age at onset, sex	Smoking status not associated
Di Pauli et al[114] 2008	129 patients with clinically isolated syndrome from Austria	Smoker vs non-smoker	Time to definite MS	Age at onset, sex, symptoms at onset	Smoking increased risk of progression to definite MS 2.0 (95% CI: 1.3–3.1)
Sundstrom and Nystrom[14] 2008	122 incident cases of MS from Sweden	Ever (early or later) smokers vs never smokers	Time to progressive MS, clinical course	Age at onset, sex	Onset smoking <15 years increased risk of PPMS; increased risk of progressive MS and disability, worse in smokers who started before age 15 years than after age 15 years
Pittas et al[108] 2009	203 patients with MS from Australia	Cumulative pack-years smoked	Disease progression	Time outside in previous 6 months, time in sun in previous 6 months, serum 25(OH)D, vigorous-moderate minimum exercise time per week, total exercise amount, marital status, socioeconomic occupational status at cohort entry, unemployed or not at study entry, total alcohol intake and total fish intake.	Smoking was associated with increased disability progression as measured by the MSSS

Healy et al[111] 2009	1465 patients from the United States	Current smoker vs ex-smoker vs never smoker	Clinical course, time to secondary progressive MS, T2 lesion volume, brain parenchymal fraction	Age, sex, disease duration, disease course	Current smokers more likely to have PPMS; smokers progressed from RRMS to SPMS faster than in never smokers (HR 2.50; 95% CI: 1.42–4.41) and had more rapid increases in T2-weighted lesion volume ($P = .02$), and brain parenchymal fraction decreased faster ($P = .02$)
Sena et al[113] 2009	205 women with MS from Portugal	Smoker vs nonsmoker		Age at onset	In women carrying the ApoE E4 isoform, smokers had a lower EDSS ($P = .033$) and MSS ($P = .023$) than nonsmokers.
Zivadinov et al[112] 2009	368 American patients with MS	Never smokers vs ever smokers	EDSS, brain atrophy, T2 lesion volume	Age, sex, disease, and treatment durations	Smoking associated with increased T1, T2, and contrast-enhancing lesions, decreased brain parenchymal fraction

Abbreviations: CI, confidence interval; EDSS, Expanded Disability Status Scale; HR, hazard ratio; MS, multiple sclerosis; MSSS, Multiple Sclerosis Severity Score; PPMS, primary progressive MS; RRMS, relapsing/remitting MS; SNP, single-nucleotide polymorphism; SPMS, secondary progressive MS.

comorbid disease as an avenue for improving outcome, nor considered the impact of therapies used for these conditions on disease course (such as antidepressants).

HEALTH BEHAVIORS

Health behaviors, such as tobacco use, alcohol consumption, and level of physical activity, substantially affect the risk and outcomes of chronic disease. Further, these behaviors account for some observed health disparities between ethnic groups.[105] Recognition is growing that these behaviors may influence health outcomes independent of comorbid diseases. For example, smokers with lung cancer have worse survival independent of smoking-associated comorbidities, cancer stage, and treatment.[106]

Of the health behaviors, smoking has been the subject of the greatest interest in MS. Several studies suggest that cigarette smoking is a risk factor for MS, whereas more recent studies suggest that it may also influence disease outcome (**Table 2**). In 2005, Hernan and colleagues[107] reported that smokers with relapsing remitting MS had a threefold increased risk of developing secondary progressive MS as compared with never smokers (HR 3.6; 95% CI 1.3–9.9). Only 20 patients had a secondary progressive course. Subsequent studies have had mixed results with 2 finding no association between smoking and disability progression, and 4 finding that smoking was associated with increased disability progression.[14,108–110] Two of these studies found that smokers had a greater T2-lesion burden and greater brain atrophy, as measured by brain parenchymal fraction, when compared with nonsmokers.[111,112] Neither study included a control group of smokers without MS. In contrast, Sena and colleagues[113] reported that smoking had a protective effect in women carrying the ApoE E4 isoform. Di Pauli and colleagues[114] followed 129 patients with a clinically isolated syndrome at high risk for developing MS based on the presence of multiple white matter lesions on MRI and positive oligoclonal bands. After 3 years, 75% of smokers developed MS, whereas only 51% of nonsmokers did so (HR 1.8; 95% CI: 1.2–2.8). Common to all but one of these studies was the failure to account for potential confounding effects owing to alcohol intake, obesity, or comorbid diseases associated with smoking.[108]

Overweight and obesity, alcohol intake, and physical activity are other health behaviors of potential interest but their influence on disability progression has not been studied. One study, however, suggested that patients who were obese when diagnosed with MS were more likely to have moderate rather than mild disability at diagnosis (OR 1.38; 95% CI: 1.02–1.87).[16] The influence of overweight and obesity on disease outcomes may become the subject of greater interest following a recent study of the Nurses Health Study cohorts, which suggested that adolescent obesity increases the risk of developing MS (in women); the relative risk of MS in a women who was obese at age 18 years was 2.25 (95% CI: 1.50–3.37) as compared with a woman of normal body weight.[115] Proposed mechanisms for the observed association were lower circulating levels of 25 hydroxy-vitamin D among those of higher body weight, and that adipose tissue secretes cytokines and adipokines, which may influence immune function; these may be relevant mechanisms to consider for disease progression as well. To date the influence of comorbid disease and health behaviors on responses to disease-modifying treatments has not been examined.

Sunlight exposure and vitamin D levels have gained significant attention for their potential etiologic role in MS.[116] These factors may also modulate the outcome of disease. In a population-based cohort of 142 patients with relapsing remitting MS, erythemal ultraviolet radiation levels were inversely associated with monthly relapse rates 1.5 months later (r = −0.32, P = .046), and 25-hydroxy vitamin D levels also inversely associated with monthly relapse rates (r = −0.31, P = .057).[117] However, relapse rates were also associated with upper respiratory tract infections, which are more common when vitamin D levels are low. Among 23 patients with MS from Finland, the serum levels of 25-hydroxy vitamin D and intact parathyroid hormone (iPTH) levels were lower during relapses than during periods of remission.[118] Although this suggests that lower vitamin D levels may influence the risk of relapses, the study design does not exclude the possibility that relapses reduce vitamin D levels. A more recent study of 110 children with a clinically isolated syndrome or relapsing remitting MS suggested that a 10 ng/mL increase in 25-hydroxy vitamin D level at baseline was associated with a 34% decrease in the number of subsequent relapses (incidence rate ratio 0.66; 95% CI: 0.46–0.95).[119] This study assumed that baseline vitamin D level was consistent throughout the duration of follow-up. Less is known about the influence of vitamin D on long-term disease progression.

REFERENCES

1. Patzold U, Pocklington PR. Course of multiple sclerosis. First results of a prospective study carried out of 102 MS patients from 1976–1980. Acta Neurol Scand 1982;65:248–66.
2. Poser S, Bauer HJ, Poser W. Prognosis of multiple sclerosis. Results from an epidemiological area in Germany. Acta Neurol Scand 1982;65:347–54.
3. Visscher BR, Liu K-S, Clark VA, et al. Onset symptoms as predictors of mortality and disability in multiple sclerosis. Acta Neurol Scand 1984;70:321–8.
4. Weinshenker BG, Bass B, Rice GP, et al. The natural history of multiple sclerosis: a geographically based study. 2. Predictive value of the early clinical course. Brain 1989;112:1419–28.
5. Trojano M, Avolio C, Manzari C, et al. Multivariate analysis of predictive factors of multiple sclerosis course with a validated method to assess clinical events. J Neurol Neurosurg Psychiatry 1995;58:300–6.
6. Confavreux C, Vukusic S, Moreau T, et al. Relapses and progression of disability in multiple sclerosis. N Engl J Med 2000;343:1430–8.
7. Weinshenker BG, Rice GP, Noseworthy JH, et al. The natural history of multiple sclerosis: a geographically based study. 3. Multivariate analysis of predictive factors and models of outcome. Brain 1991;114:1045–56.
8. Runmarker B, Andersen O. Prognostic factors in a multiple sclerosis incidence cohort with twenty-five years of follow-up. Brain 1993;116:117–34.
9. Miller DH, Hornabrook RW, Purdie G. The natural history of multiple sclerosis: a regional study with some longitudinal data. J Neurol Neurosurg Psychiatry 1992;55:341–6.
10. Hammond SR, McLeod JG, Macaskill P, et al. Multiple sclerosis in Australia: prognostic factors. J Clin Neurosci 2000;7:16–9.
11. Tremlett H, Paty D, Devonshire V. Male gender and an older age at onset do not indicate a worse outcome in multiple sclerosis: findings from the natural history of MS in British Columbia, Canada. Mult Scler 2005;11(Suppl 1):S106.
12. Eriksson M, Andersen O, Runmarker B. Long-term follow-up of patients with clinically isolated syndromes, relapsing-remitting and secondary progressive multiple sclerosis. Mult Scler 2003;9:260–74.
13. Cree BA, Khan O, Bourdette D, et al. Clinical characteristics of African Americans vs Caucasian Americans with multiple sclerosis. Neurology 2004;63:2039–45.

14. Sundstrom P, Nystrom L. Smoking worsens the prognosis in multiple sclerosis. Mult Scler 2008;14(8):1031–5.
15. Marrie RA, Cutter G, Tyry T, et al. Does multiple sclerosis-associated disability differ between races? Neurology 2006;66(8):1235–40.
16. Marrie RA, Horwitz RI, Cutter G, et al. Comorbidity delays diagnosis and increases disability at diagnosis in MS. Neurology 2009;72(2):117–24.
17. Ebers G, Koopman WJ, Hader W, et al. The natural history of multiple sclerosis: a geographically based study. 8. Familial multiple sclerosis. Brain 2000;123: 641–9.
18. Oturai AB, Ryder LP, Fredrikson S, et al. Concordance for disease course and age of onset in Scandinavian multiple sclerosis coaffected sib pairs. Mult Scler 2004;10:5–8.
19. Hensiek AE, Seaman SR, Barcellos LF, et al. Familial effects on the clinical course of multiple sclerosis. Neurology 2007;68(5):376–83.
20. Chataway J, Mander A, Robertson N, et al. Multiple sclerosis in sibling pairs: an analysis of 250 families. J Neurol Neurosurg Psychiatry 2001;71(6):757–61.
21. Weinshenker BG, Bulman D, Carriere W, et al. A comparison of sporadic and familial multiple sclerosis. Neurology 1990;40:1354–8.
22. Robertson NP, Clayton D, Fraser M, et al. Clinical concordance in sibling pairs with multiple sclerosis. Neurology 1996;47:347–52.
23. Runmarker B, Martinsson T, Wahlström J, et al. HLA and prognosis in multiple sclerosis. J Neurol 1994;241(6):385–90.
24. McDonnell GV, Mawhinney H, Graham CA, et al. A study of the HLA-DR region in clinical subgroups of multiple sclerosis and its influence on prognosis. J Neurol Sci 1999;165(1):77–83.
25. Celius EG, Harbo HF, Egeland T, et al. Sex and age at diagnosis are correlated with the HLA-DR2, DQ6 haplotype in multiple sclerosis. J Neurol Sci 2000; 178(2):132–5.
26. Mann CL, Davies MB, Boggild MD, et al. Glutathione S-transferase polymorphisms in MS: their relationship to disability. Neurology 2000;54:552–7.
27. Masterman T, Ligers A, Olsson T, et al. HLA-DR15 is associated with lower age at onset in multiple sclerosis. Ann Neurol 2000;48:211–9.
28. Fazekas F, Strasser-Fuchs S, Kollegger H, et al. Apolipoprotein E epsilon 4 is associated with rapid progression of multiple sclerosis. Neurology 2001;57: 853–7.
29. Weatherby SJ, Thomson W, Pepper L, et al. HLA-DRB1 and disease outcome in multiple sclerosis. J Neurol 2001;248(4):304–10.
30. Hensiek AE, Sawcer SJ, Feakes R, et al. HLA-DR 15 is associated with female sex and younger age at diagnosis in multiple sclerosis. J Neurol Neurosurg Psychiatry 2002;72(2):184–7.
31. Masterman T, Zhang Z, Hellgren D, et al. APOE genotypes and disease severity in multiple sclerosis. Mult Scler 2002;8:98–103.
32. Villoslada P, Barcellos LF, Rio J, et al. The HLA locus and multiple sclerosis in Spain. Role in disease susceptibility, clinical course and response to interferon-[beta]. J Neuroimmunol 2002;130(1/2):194–201.
33. Barcellos LF, Oksenberg JR, Begovich AB, et al. HLA-DR2 dose effect on susceptibility to multiple sclerosis and influence on disease course. Am J Hum Genet 2003;72(3):710–6.
34. Schreiber K, Otura AB, Ryder LP, et al. Disease severity in Danish multiple sclerosis patients evaluated by MRI and three genetic markers (HLA-DRB1*1501, CCR5 deletion mutation, apolipoprotein E). Mult Scler 2002;8:295–8.

35. Hensiek AE, Roxburgh R, Meranian M, et al. Osteopontin gene and clinical severity of multiple sclerosis. J Neurol 2003;250(8):943–7.
36. Caillier S, Barcellos LF, Baranzini SE, et al. Osteopontin polymorphisms and disease course in multiple sclerosis. Genes Immun 2003;4(4):312–5.
37. Kantor R, Bakhanashvili M, Achiron A. A mutated CCR5 gene may have favorable prognostic implications in MS. Neurology 2003;61(2):238–40.
38. Gade-Andavolu R, Comings D, MacMurray J, et al. Association of CCR5 [delta] 32 deletion with early death in multiple sclerosis. Genet Med 2004;6(3):126–31.
39. Kantarci OH, Hebrink DD, Achenbach SJ, et al. Association of APOE polymorphisms with disease severity in MS is limited to women. Neurology 2004; 62(5):811–4.
40. Partridge JM, Weatherby SJ, Woolmore JA, et al. Susceptibility and outcome in MS: associations with polymorphisms in pigmentation-related genes. Neurology 2004;62(12):2323–5.
41. Cocco E, Sotgiu A, Costa G, et al. HLA-DR, DQ and APOE genotypes and gender influence in Sardinian primary progressive MS. Neurology 2005;64(3):564–6.
42. Burwick RM, Ramsay PP, Haines JL, et al. APOE epsilon variation in multiple sclerosis susceptibility and disease severity. Some answers. Neurology 2006; 66:1373–83.
43. Smestad C, Brynedal B, Jonasdottir G, et al. The impact of HLA-A and -DRB1 on age at onset, disease course and severity in Scandinavian multiple sclerosis patients. Eur J Neurol 2007;14(8):835–40.
44. Zivadinov R, Uxa L, Bratina A, et al. HLA-DRB1*1501, -DQB1*0301, -DQB1*0302, -DQB1*0602, and -DQB1*0603 alleles are associated with more severe disease outcome on MRI in patients with multiple sclerosis International Review of Neurobiology. In: Minagar A, editor, The neurobiology of multiple sclerosis, Volume 79. Academic Press; 2007. p. 521–35.
45. Cournu-Rebeix I, Genin E, Leray E, et al. HLA-DRB1*15 allele influences the later course of relapsing remitting multiple sclerosis. Genes Immun 2008;9(6): 570–4.
46. Sombekke MH, Lukas C, Crusius JBA, et al. HLA-DRB1*1501 and spinal cord magnetic resonance imaging lesions in multiple sclerosis. Arch Neurol 2009; 66(12):1531–6.
47. Stankovich J, Butzkueven H, Marriott M, et al. HLA-DRB1 associations with disease susceptibility and clinical course in Australians with multiple sclerosis. Tissue Antigens 2009;74(1):17–21.
48. Okuda DT, Srinivasan R, Oksenberg JR, et al. Genotype-phenotype correlations in multiple sclerosis: HLA genes influence disease severity inferred by 1HMR spectroscopy and MRI measures. Brain 2009;132(1):250–9.
49. Cree BAC, Reich DE, Khan O, et al. Modification of multiple sclerosis phenotypes by African ancestry at HLA. Arch Neurol 2009;66(2):226–33.
50. Guerrero AL, Laherrán E, Gutiérrez F, et al. Apolipoprotein E genotype does not associate with disease severity measured by Multiple Sclerosis Severity Score. Acta Neurol Scand 2008;117(1):21–5.
51. Silva AM, Pereira C, Bettencourt A, et al. The role of HLA-DRB1 alleles on susceptibility and outcome of a Portuguese Multiple Sclerosis population. J Neurol Sci 2007;258(1/2):69–74.
52. Vasconcelos CCF, Fernández O, Leyva L, et al. Does the DRB1*1501 allele confer more severe and faster progression in primary progressive multiple sclerosis patients? HLA in primary progressive multiple sclerosis. J Neuroimmunol 2009;214(1/2):101–3.

53. van Veen T, Crusius JB, van Winsen L, et al. CTLA-4 and CD28 gene polymorphisms in susceptibility, clinical course and progression of multiple sclerosis. J Neuroimmunol 2003;140(1/2):188–93.
54. DeLuca GC, Ramagopalan SV, Herrera BM, et al. An extremes of outcome strategy provides evidence that multiple sclerosis severity is determined by alleles at the HLA-DRB1 locus. Proc Natl Acad Sci U S A 2007;104(52): 20896–901.
55. Ramagopalan SV, Maugeri NJ, Handunnetthi L, et al. Expression of the multiple sclerosis-associated MHC class II Allele HLA-DRB1*1501 is regulated by vitamin D. PLoS Genet 2009;5(2):e1000369.
56. Pugliatti M, Sotgiu S, Rosati G. The worldwide prevalence of multiple sclerosis. Clin Neurol Neurosurg 2002;104:182–91.
57. Noonan CW, Williamson DM, Henry JP, et al. The prevalence of multiple sclerosis in 3 US communities. Prev Chronic Dis 2010;7(1):A12.
58. Svenson LW, Warren S, Warren KG, et al. Prevalence of multiple sclerosis in First Nations people of Alberta. Can J Neurol Sci 2007;34:175–80.
59. Modi G, Mochan A, Modi M, et al. Demyelinating disorder of the central nervous system occurring in black South Africans. J Neurol Neurosurg Psychiatry 2001; 70:500–5.
60. Mirsattari SM, Johnston JB, McKenna R, et al. Aboriginals with multiple sclerosis: HLA types and predominance of neuromyelitis optica. Neurology 2001; 56:317–23.
61. Wingerchuk DM, Lennon VA, Pittock SJ, et al. Revised diagnostic criteria for neuromyelitis optica. Neurology 2006;66:1485–9.
62. Lennon VA, Wingerchuk DM, Kryzer TJ, et al. A serum autoantibody marker of neuromyelitis optica: distinction from multiple sclerosis. Lancet 2004;364: 2106–12.
63. Kira J. Neuromyelitis optica and Asian phenotype of multiple sclerosis. Ann N Y Acad Sci 2008;1142:58–71 The Year in Neurology 2008.
64. Naismith RT, Trinkaus K, Cross AH. Phenotype and prognosis in African-Americans with multiple sclerosis: a retrospective chart review. Mult Scler 2006;12(6):775–81.
65. Cree BA, Al-Sabbagh A, Bennett R, et al. Response to interferon beta-1a treatment in African American multiple sclerosis patients. Arch Neurol 2005;62: 1681–3.
66. Weinstock-Guttman B, Jacobs LD, Brownscheidle CM, et al. Multiple sclerosis characteristics in African American patients in the New York State Multiple Sclerosis Consortium. Mult Scler 2003;9:293–8.
67. Phillips PH, Newman NJ, Lynn MJ. Optic neuritis in African Americans. Arch Neurol 1998;55:186–92.
68. Mowry EM, Pesic M, Grimes B, et al. Clinical predictors of early second event in patients with clinically isolated syndrome. J Neurol 2009;256(7):1061–6.
69. Kaufman MD, Johnson SK, Moyer D, et al. Multiple sclerosis: severity and progression rate in African Americans compared with whites. Am J Phys Med Rehabil 2003;82:582–90.
70. Wallin MT, Page WF, Kurtzke JF. Epidemiology of multiple sclerosis in US veterans. VIII. Long-term survival after onset of multiple sclerosis. Brain 2000; 123:1677–87.
71. Boster AL, Endress CF, Hreha SA, et al. Pediatric-onset multiple sclerosis in African-American Black and European-Origin white patients. Pediatr Neurol 2009;40(1):31–3.

72. Rinker JR II, Trinkaus K, Naismith RT, et al. Higher IgG index found in African Americans versus Caucasians with multiple sclerosis. Neurology 2007;69(1):68–72.
73. Schwid SR, Thorpe J, Sharief M, et al. Enhanced benefit of increasing interferon beta-1a dose and frequency in relapsing multiple sclerosis: the EVIDENCE study. Arch Neurol 2005;62(5):785–92.
74. Last JM, editor. A dictionary of epidemiology. 2nd edition. New York: Oxford University Press; 1988. p. 44.
75. Bamshad M. Genetic influences on health: does race matter? JAMA 2005; 294(8):937–46.
76. Last JM. Social and behavioral determinants of health. In: Last JM, editor. Public health and human ecology. East Norwalk (CT): Appleton & Lange; 1987. p. 211–42.
77. Braveman PA, Cubbin C, Egerter S, et al. Socioeconomic status in health research: one size does not fit all. JAMA 2005;294:2879–88.
78. Kaplan GA, Keil JE. Socioeconomic factors and cardiovascular disease: a review of the literature. Circulation 1993;88:1973–98.
79. Steenland K, Hu S, Walker J. All-cause and cause-specific mortality by socio-economic status among employed persons in 27 US states, 1984–1997. Am J Public Health 2004;94:1037–42.
80. Stephansson O, Dickman PW, Johansson ALV, et al. The influence of socioeconomic status on stillbirth risk in Sweden. Int J Epidemiol 2001;30:1296–301.
81. Minkler M, Fuller-Thomson E, Guralnik JM. Gradient of disability across the socioeconomic spectrum in the United States. N Engl J Med 2006;355:695–703.
82. Marrie RA, Horwitz R, Cutter G, et al. Comorbidity, socioeconomic status, and multiple sclerosis. Mult Scler 2008;14(8):1091–8.
83. Shabas D, Hoffner M. Multiple sclerosis management for low-income minorities. Mult Scler 2005;11:635–40.
84. Minden SL, Hoaglin DC, Hadden L, et al. Access to and utilization of neurologists by people with multiple sclerosis. Neurology 2008;70(13_Part_2):1141–9.
85. Beatty PW, Hagglund KJ, Neri MT, et al. Access to health care services among people with chronic or disabling conditions: patterns and predictors. Arch Phys Med Rehabil 2003;84:1417–25.
86. Hellwig K, Brune N, Haghikia A, et al. Reproductive counselling, treatment and course of pregnancy in 73 German MS patients. Acta Neurol Scand 2008; 118(1):24–8.
87. Confavreux C, Hutchinson M, Hours MM, et al. Pregnancy in Multiple Sclerosis Group. Rate of pregnancy-related relapse in multiple sclerosis. N Engl J Med 1998;339:285–91.
88. Poser S, Poser W. Multiple sclerosis and gestation. Neurology 1983;33(11): 1422–7.
89. Weinshenker BG, Hader W, Carriere W, et al. The influence of pregnancy on disability from multiple sclerosis: a population-based study in Middlesex County, Ontario. Neurology 1989;39(11):1438–40.
90. Runmarker B, Andersen O. Pregnancy is associated with a lower risk of onset and a better prognosis in multiple sclerosis. Brain 1995;118(1):253–61.
91. Thompson DS, Nelson LM, Burns A, et al. The effects of pregnancy in multiple sclerosis: a retrospective study. Neurology 1986;36(8):1097–9.
92. Tremlett H, Yousefi M, Devonshire V, et al. Impact of multiple sclerosis relapses on progression diminishes with time. Neurology 2009;73(20):1616–23.
93. D'Hooghe MB, Nagels G, Uitdehaag BMJ. Long-term effects of childbirth in MS. J Neurol Neurosurg Psychiatry 2010;81(1):38–41.

94. Gijsen R, Hoeymans N, Schellevis FG, et al. Causes and consequences of comorbidity: a review. J Clin Epidemiol 2001;54:661–74.
95. Sprangers MAG, de Regt EB, Andries F, et al. Which chronic conditions are associated with better or poorer quality of life? J Clin Epidemiol 2000;53: 895–907.
96. Battafarano RJ, Piccirillo JF, Meyers BF, et al. Impact of comorbidity on survival after surgical resection in patients with stage I non-small cell lung cancer. J Thorac Cardiovasc Surg 2006;123:280–7.
97. Braunstein JB, Anderson GF, Gerstenblith G, et al. Noncardiac comorbidity increases preventable hospitalizations and mortality among Medicare beneficiaries with chronic heart failure. J Am Coll Cardiol 2003;42:1226–33.
98. Greenfield S, Apolone G, McNeil BJ, et al. The importance of co-existent disease in the occurrence of postoperative complications and one-year recovery in patients undergoing total hip replacement. Comorbidity and outcomes after hip replacement. Med Care 1993;31:141–54.
99. Tourbah A, Clapin A, Gout O, et al. Systemic autoimmune features and multiple sclerosis: a 5-year follow-up study. Arch Neurol 1998;55:517–21.
100. Hohol MJ, Orav EJ, Weiner HL. Disease Steps in multiple sclerosis: a simple approach to evaluate disease progression. Neurology 1995;45:251–5.
101. Kirby S, Brown MG, Murray TJ, et al. Progression of multiple sclerosis in patients with other autoimmune diseases. Mult Scler 2005;11(Suppl 1):S28–9.
102. Kirby S, Fisk JD, Brown MG, et al. Progression of multiple sclerosis in patients with psychiatric syndromes. Mult Scler 2005;11(Suppl 1):S28–9.
103. Dallmeijer AJ, Beckerman H, Groot VD, et al. Long-term effect of comorbidity on the course of physical functioning in patients after stroke and with multiple sclerosis. J Rehabil Med 2009;41(5):322–6.
104. Marrie RA, Rudick R, Horwitz R, et al. Vascular comorbidity is associated with more rapid disability progression in multiple sclerosis. Neurology 2010;74: 1041–7.
105. National Center for Health Statistics. Health, United States, 2005. With chartbook on trends in the health of Americans. Hyattsville (MD): U.S. Department of Health and Human Services; 2005.
106. Tammemagi CM, Neslund-Dudas C, Simoff M, et al. Smoking and lung cancer survival. The role of comorbidity and treatment. Chest 2004;125:27–37.
107. Hernan MA, Jick SS, Logroscino G, et al. Cigarette smoking and the progression of multiple sclerosis. Brain 2005;128(Pt 6):1461–5.
108. Pittas F, Ponsonby AL, van der Mei IA, et al. Smoking is associated with progressive disease course and increased progression in clinical disability in a prospective cohort of people with multiple sclerosis. J Neurol 2009;256(4):577–85.
109. Koch M, van Harten A, Uyttenboogaart M, et al. Cigarette smoking and progression in multiple sclerosis. Neurology 2007;69(15):1515–20.
110. D'Hooghe MB, Nagels G. Smoking behavior and multiple sclerosis severity. Mult Scler 2005;11(Suppl 1):S27.
111. Healy BC, Ali EN, Guttmann CRG, et al. Smoking and disease progression in multiple sclerosis. Arch Neurol 2009;66(7):858–64.
112. Zivadinov R, Weinstock-Guttman B, Hashmi K, et al. Smoking is associated with increased lesion volumes and brain atrophy in multiple sclerosis. Neurology 2009;73(7):504–10.
113. Sena A, Couderc R, Ferret-Sena V, et al. Apolipoprotein E polymorphism interacts with cigarette smoking in progression of multiple sclerosis. Eur J Neurol 2009;16(7):832–7.

114. Di Pauli F, Reindl M, Ehling R, et al. Smoking is a risk factor for early conversion to clinically definite multiple sclerosis. Mult Scler 2008;14(8):1026–30.
115. Munger KL, Chitnis T, Ascherio A. Body size and risk of MS in two cohorts of US women. Neurology 2009;73(19):1543–50.
116. Cantorna MT. Vitamin D and multiple sclerosis: an update. Nutr Rev 2008; 66(s2):S135–8.
117. Tremlett H, van der Mei IA, Pittas F, et al. Monthly ambient sunlight, infections and relapse rates in multiple sclerosis. Neuroepidemiology 2008;31(4):271–9.
118. Soilu-Hanninen M, Laaksonen M, Laitinen I, et al. A longitudinal study of serum 25-hydroxyvitamin D and intact PTH levels indicate the importance of vitamin D and calcium homeostasis regulation in multiple sclerosis. J Neurol Neurosurg Psychiatry 2008;79:152–7.
119. Mowry EM, Krupp LB, Milazzo M, et al. Vitamin D status is associated with relapse rate in pediatric-onset multiple sclerosis. Ann Neurol 2010;67(5):618–24.
120. Weinshenker BG, Wingerchuk DM, Liu Q, et al. Genetic variation in the tumor necrosis factor alpha gene and the outcome of multiple sclerosis. Neurology 1997;49(2):378–85.
121. Weinshenker BG, Santrach P, Bissonet AS, et al. Major histocompatibility complex class II alleles and the course and outcome of MS: a population-based study. Neurology 1998;51(3):742–7.
122. van Veen T, Nielsen J, Berkhof J, et al. CCL5 and CCR5 genotypes modify clinical, radiological and pathological features of multiple sclerosis. J Neuroimmunol 2007; 190(1/2):157–64.

Magnetic Resonance Imaging in Multiple Sclerosis: The Role of Conventional Imaging

Nancy L. Sicotte, MD

KEYWORDS

• Multiple sclerosis • Magnetic resonance imaging
• White matter lesions • Diagnosis

Magnetic resonance imaging (MRI) uses strong magnetic fields and radiofrequency energy to produce images of the central nervous system with exquisite anatomic detail. The ability to noninvasively assess the brain and spinal cord has transformed the approach to the diagnosis and treatment of multiple sclerosis (MS). The evolution of the diagnostic criteria for MS reflects the increasing importance of MRI findings in establishing the likelihood of the diagnosis, from examination-based to the currently used McDonald criteria in which MRI findings can be used to establish dissemination in both time and space.[1-3] The presence of typical MS lesions at the time of a clinically isolated event can allow the clinician to stratify individuals into low or high risk for conversion to MS.[4,5] All of the currently disease-modifying therapies (DMTs) approved by the Food and Drug Administration have demonstrated an ability to decrease the number and volume of inflammatory white matter lesions as detected on conventional MRI scans,[6-11] and clinicians routinely obtain clinical MRI scans in the course of managing patients with MS to aid in decision making regarding treatment efficacy and disease progression. In this article the clinical applications of MRI in MS are reviewed.

STANDARD "CLINICAL" MRI

Routine MR imaging of the brain and spinal cord includes sequences that produce a variety of tissue contrasts reflecting the varying responses of protons in different

This work was supported by Grants from the National Multiple Sclerosis Society RG3914, RG4716.
Multiple Sclerosis Program, Cedars-Sinai Medical Center, David Geffen School of Medicine at UCLA, 8730 Alden Drive, Thalians E216, Los Angeles, CA 90048, USA
E-mail address: Nancy.Sicotte@cshs.org

Neurol Clin 29 (2011) 343–356
doi:10.1016/j.ncl.2011.01.005
0733-8619/11/$ – see front matter © 2011 Elsevier Inc. All rights reserved.

tissue types. In almost every instance, an MS MRI protocol will include T1-weighted, T2-weighted, and postcontrast scans. T1-weighted scans (spin-lattice) produce images in which fat is bright and water is dark, providing good contrast between white and gray matter. In scans that are T2-weighted (spin-spin), fat is dark and water is bright, thus pathologic processes associated with edema will appear bright on T2-weighted scans. FLAIR (fluid-attenuated inversion recovery) is a T2-weighted scan with an added inversion pulse that nulls the water signal from cerebrospinal fluid (CSF)-filled spaces such as the ventricles, thus accentuating periventricular lesions and juxtacortical lesions typical of MS. The added conspicuity that FLAIR scans offer also facilitates the quantification of lesion numbers and volumes and in clinical trials of therapeutic agents.[12] A T2-weighted or FLAIR scan obtained in the sagittal plane is especially useful in demonstrating involvement of the corpus callosum and the presence of "Dawson's fingers" lesions that parallel the penetrating venous system.[13] Both of these findings are typical of demyelinating lesions and therefore are helpful in establishing the diagnosis of suspected MS.[14]

Also helpful in establishing a diagnosis of MS and for monitoring the effect of DMTs is the collection of a scan after the administration of intravenous contrast. Gadolinium-based contrast agents (GBCA) cause T1 shortening, and therefore appear bright on postcontrast T1-weighted scans. In cases where active inflammation is associated with an opening of the blood-brain barrier (BBB), Gd+ contrast will be detectable within the brain parenchyma as an area of abnormal enhancement. The presence of Gd+ lesions is helpful in establishing a likely diagnosis of MS[3] and in predicting short-term clinical activity[15] (see later discussion). In addition, unlike T2-weighted abnormalities, the presence of Gd+ lesions is a sign of recent activity, as these lesions show enhancement for a limited period of time, typically 6 to 8 weeks (**Fig. 1**).[16]

Although the types of clinical scans tend to be similar, the sequences can vary significantly across centers, reflecting local preferences and requirements for speed and image resolution as well as the limitations of the particular make and model of the scanner used. In most clinical settings, time is the most important factor in determining the specifics of the standard protocols that are implemented, and time can be saved by collecting fewer slices at a lower resolution. A standard protocol designed to determine whether an obvious abnormality such as a tumor or an MS plaque is present might be 5 mm thick and include gaps of up to 2.5 mm to survey the entire brain in the shortest period of time. This approach works for large-mass lesions, but can be counterproductive in establishing a diagnosis of MS in which the number and evolution of lesions detected on T2-weighted scans has become an important metric. To address this issue, the Consortium of MS Centers has developed a standardized MR protocol for use in assessing suspected MS at the time of diagnosis as well as for disease monitoring. The key issues identified are the use of an appropriate field strength (1.5 T or higher) and the use of thinner slices (3 mm) obtained at a standard angle without gaps.[13] These relatively simple suggestions, if routinely implemented, would enhance the clinical utility of routinely collected MR scans. Of importance, the adoption of these guidelines requires the cooperation of clinical radiologists who typically have the final say over the details of the imaging protocols that are adapted at a particular center. Neurologists can play an important role in educating their local neuroradiologists on the evolution of diagnostic approaches in MS and the need for consistent scan acquisition in the serial evaluation of patients with MS.

At the same time, advances in both the hardware and software of imaging technology have led to the adoption of innovative imaging approaches in clinical practice.

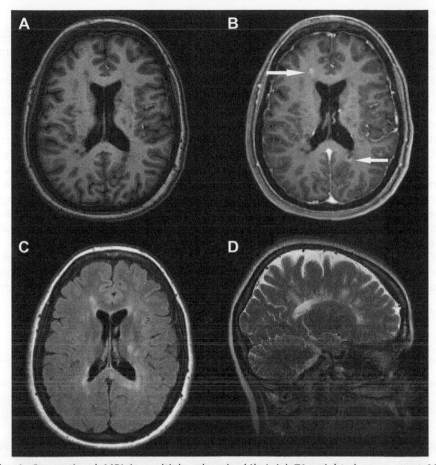

Fig. 1. Conventional MRI in multiple sclerosis. (*A*) Axial T1-weighted noncontrast MRI demonstrating presence of multiple hypointensities or "T1 black holes." Note also the ventricular enlargement and sulcal widening. (*B*) Axial T1-weighted MRI after the administration of gadolinium-based contrast agent. Contrast can be detected in white matter regions undergoing active inflammation leading to blood-brain barrier breakdown. Two areas of contrast enhancement are indicated by arrows. Note that both of these lesions appear hypointense on the precontrast scan. (*C*) Axial FLAIR scan demonstrating typical periventricular white matter lesions. (*D*) Axial T2-weighted MRI shows pattern of linear regions of high signal corresponding to perivenous demyelination, known as "Dawson's fingers."

An example of this is the rapid adoption of diffusion-weighted imaging (DWI), which is exquisitely sensitive to ischemic changes.[17] Multiple images can be collected rapidly with the use of echo-planar imaging (EPI), and this combination of sensitivity and rapid image acquisition has resulted in the inclusion of DWI into many imaging protocols, including routine MS scans. Higher field strength magnets (3.0 T) are now found in most centers, and provide improved signal to noise ratios, which in turn improves image quality while decreasing scan times but also makes it feasible to collect previously "nonconventional" sequences such as spectroscopy in clinically appropriate time periods. As imaging technology improves, these advanced techniques may find their way into clinical practice.

FINDINGS IN MS

Clinical MRI scans can be assessed for several features that are relevant to MS diagnosis or disease activity. White matter lesions are the most readily observable and most frequently described abnormality seen in MS. Best seen on T2-weighted scans, especially FLAIR, typically MS lesions have an ovoid shape, which are perpendicular to the long axis of the ventricles in the axial plane, or appear as longitudinal columns in the sagittal plane. Demyelinating lesions are larger (>3 mm) than the usually punctate nonspecific white matter lesions associated with ischemic risk factors and migraine. Over time they tend to become confluent, especially around the posterior aspects of the lateral ventricles. In addition to the periventricular locations, lesions associated with MS are found in juxtacortical and infratentorial locations.[14] Studies have established that these characteristics have good sensitivity and specificity for MS-related changes and have been incorporated into the most recent, widely accepted MS diagnostic criteria.[3] Subsequent modifications to the initial McDonald criteria emphasized the important role that spinal cord lesions play in establishing the diagnosis of MS (**Fig. 2**).[18]

Postcontrast T1-weighted images are used to detect the presence of BBB breakdown at the location of a T2 lesion, thus indicating active inflammation. The T1 precontrast scan provides useful information as well, and should be examined for the

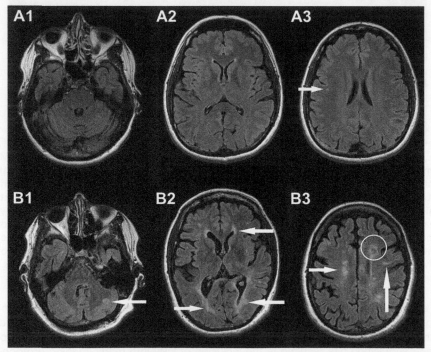

Fig. 2. White matter lesions on FLAIR MRI. (*A*) Axial FLAIR MRI images from a healthy control. Note the single punctuate white matter hyperintensity in image *A3* indicated by the area representing a nonspecific finding. (*B*) Axial FLAIR MRI images from an individual with MS, demonstrating features of the Barkhof criteria including infratentorial (*B1*), periventricular (*B2* and *B3*), and juxtacortical (*B3; perpendicular arrow*). Note area of low signal within a large confluent periventricular plaque, consistent with a severe black hole (*B3; circle*).

presence of T1 "black holes."[19] Black holes are areas of low signal within the white matter that represent of subset of T2 lesions that have more severe tissue destruction and axonal loss.[20] The number and volume of T1 black holes shows a better correlation with measures of disability than T2 lesion volumes, and has been proposed as a potential biomarker of neurodegeneration.[21] It is important to recognize that all acutely or recently enhancing lesions will appear as hypointense on the precontrast T1 scan, due to the effects of edema. Only a small percentage of these lesions will evolve into "chronic black holes" (CBHs) while the rest will resolve.[22] In addition, CBHs represent a spectrum of neuropathological change, in much the same way that T2 lesions are relatively nonspecific.[23] That said, some people with MS seem to have a propensity to form CBHs, which may reflect limited repair abilities and could be helpful in identifying those at greater risk for more severe disability progression.[24] A useful metric to capture this aspect is the T1/T2 ratio. Bakshi and colleagues[25] have found that individuals with high ratios are at higher risk for future neurologic worsening.

Spinal cord lesions in MS are most frequently detected in the cervical cord, but can also be found in the thoracic and conus regions.[26] Improvements in imaging technology have led to better detection of spinal cord lesions, but they remain difficult to detect especially in the axial plane. It is still useful to obtain spinal cord imaging, especially in cases where the diagnosis is in question, and to evaluate for MS variants.[27] In the case of primary progressive MS in which the course is usually characterized by a progressive myelopathy in the absence of relapse events, it is critical to obtain spinal cord imaging to eliminate the possibility of other structural disease and to rule out other MS mimics.[28]

Characteristic findings on cord imaging can also be seen in neuromyelitis optica (NMO), known also by the eponym Devic disease. Key features that distinguish NMO include large spinal cord lesions spanning several vertebral levels with the presence of severe edema and associated contrast enhancement, along with severe bouts of optic neuritis frequently affecting both eyes in turn.[29] Individuals with suspected NMO should be tested for the presence of the NMO antibody, detectable in serum and CSF.[30,31] Treatment options for NMO are different from typical relapsing forms of MS, as standard DMTs have been shown to be ineffective; therefore it is important to establish the diagnosis early in the course of suspected NMO. With the availability of the NMO antibody test as a biomarker, the spectrum of imaging findings in NMO is now recognized to frequently include lesions in the fourth ventricle and hypothalamic regions, areas rich in aquaporin-4, the target antigen of the NMO antibody (Fig. 3).[29,32,33]

Non–White Matter Abnormalities

Although the hallmark of MRI findings in MS is inflammatory lesions in the white matter, there are several other changes that can be detected on conventional MRI scans in passing. Note that these may not be reported by the reviewing neuroradiologist, and therefore will not be appreciated unless the scans are reviewed personally by the referring neurologist, thus providing another reason why it is always worthwhile to view patients' scan data to glean as much information as possible from these studies.

Atrophy

Most easily noted is the presence of diffuse global atrophy as reflected by enlargement of the ventricular system and sulcal widening, seen best on the noncontrast T1-weighted scan. An early and robust finding is enlargement of the third ventricle[34] that has been correlated with thalamic atrophy and associated with cognitive

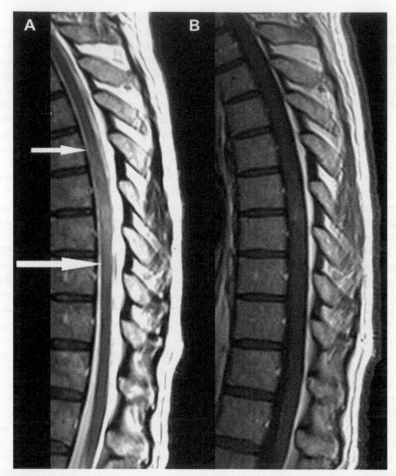

Fig. 3. Spinal cord imaging in neuromyelitis optica. (*A*) Sagittal T2-weighted MRI of the thoracic spine demonstrating a region of hyperintensity and cord swelling extending over multiple vertebral levels (*horizontal arrows*). (*B*) Sagittal postcontrast T1-weighted image reveals area of gadolinium enhancement consistent with active inflammation. On further testing, this individual was found to have abnormal visual evoked potentials bilaterally and a positive NMO antibody titer.

impairment.[35] In a similar way the temporal horns, which abut mesial temporal lobe structures including the hippocampus, may be enlarged early in the course of MS. There is evidence that hippocampal atrophy is detectable in early MS and is associated with verbal memory impairment.[36] Serial imaging often reveals the rapid pace of brain atrophy that occurs in MS, calculated to occur at an average rate of 0.8% per year, albeit with considerable variance,[37–39] but that can frequently be appreciated by visual inspection alone (**Fig. 4**).

Gray Matter Involvement

As previously described, the use of FLAIR scanning, especially at high field strength, has revealed the presence of high signal within cortical and juxtacortical regions that correspond to demyelinating lesions of varying types.[40] Cortical plaques appear to be more frequent in progressive MS, although they are detectable in early

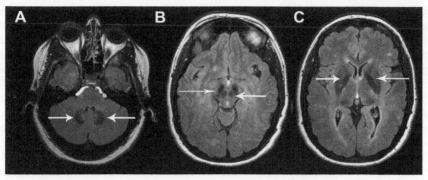

Fig. 4. Deep gray matter T2 hypointensity in MS. Axial FLAIR MRI scans show areas of low signal in deep gray matter structures in an individual with MS, including the dentate nucleus (*A*), red nucleus and substantia nigra (*B*), and basal ganglia (*C*) (*horizontal arrows*).

relapsing-remitting MS.[41,42] Their presence is associated with an increased risk of seizures and cognitive impairment,[43,44] but the specificity of these findings awaits better techniques to reliably detect the majority of cortical lesions.[45] The effectiveness of standard DMTs in reducing cortical plaques is also not certain at this time. In the clinical setting, the rapid accumulation of cortical plaques is a sign of continued disease progression in the same way that white matter lesion accumulation would be; however, significant cortical involvement is associated with a greater degree of disability, in particular cognitive impairment.[46]

In addition to areas of high signal on T2-weighted scans, MS patients frequently have regions of T2 signal hypointensity, especially in deep gray matter structures such as the putamen, globus pallidus, and thalamus.[47] Pathologically, these signal changes are associated with iron deposition, which has been posited as a marker of neurodegeneration.[48] Similar changes are also seen in other systemic disorders such as chronic liver disease,[49] and the clinical significance of these findings is still under investigation. Newer techniques such as susceptibility weighted imaging are currently under study for use as a quantitative measure of iron deposition,[50] and serial studies are under way to better understand the dynamics of this process in MS.[51] At a minimum, the presence of significant gray matter T2 hypointensity is consistent with a long-standing diagnosis of MS.

HOW TO USE CONVENTIONAL MRI IN MS
Diagnosis

The basis for a diagnosis of MS is involvement of the central nervous system occurring over time leading to neurologic dysfunction, either episodic (relapsing-remitting MS) or progressive (primary progressive MS). The hallmark is the occurrence of multiple areas of inflammation over multiple time points. In the past, clinical criteria were used to establish evidence of at least 2 separate events. A young woman presenting with an episode of optic neuritis was known to have a high risk of eventually developing MS, but if there was no evidence of other events, a diagnosis of MS could not be made with any certainty. In the days before any available DMT, there was little urgency to make a diagnosis. All this changed with the advent of the first generation of MS therapies, when the ability to accurately and more rapidly achieve diagnostic certainty gained importance. At the same time, findings from seminal longitudinal studies established that at the time of the first episode, or a clinically isolated syndrome (CIS), the presence of characteristic white matter lesions on MRI were associated with a high risk of eventually developing clinically definite MS.[52] Subsequent testing of the available DMTs in the setting of CIS with MRI lesions has shown a benefit in delaying the onset of a second clinical event as well as a reduction in the accumulation of white matter lesions.[53–55] However, a recent article with cohorts followed for 6 and 20 years suggests that up to 15% of CIS patients may have no further clinical events despite radiographic progression, and that radiographic features at baseline did not differ between those with and without subsequent clinical and/or radiographic progression.[56] These results suggest that further study of these cohorts is needed along with a search for possible genetic or other factors that may modify or mitigate the risk of MS disease progression.

Reflecting the increased role of MRI in the CIS setting, the McDonald criteria delineate the use of MRI findings to detect dissemination in both time and space, thus validating the use of serial MRI as a critical tool in establishing a diagnosis of MS.[3] This evaluation is most effective when applied using the scanning principles described previously, including the acquisition of 3.0-mm nongapped slices obtained at a consistent angle. As always, it is critical to assess for MS mimics, and the reader is referred to excellent reviews that are especially useful in cataloging "red flags" observed on MRI scans that should prompt consideration of other diagnoses and the pursuit of further testing as indicated.[57,58]

In these days of easy access to MR imaging, a common scenario arises in which a previously healthy individual undergoes a brain scan for a minor head injury or migraine headaches and is found to have white matter lesions that are consistent with demyelination and, in many cases, fulfill McDonald criteria for dissemination in space. The only missing variable is any episode or examination abnormality to validate a clinical event.[59] Recent studies have shed light on this situation, deemed the "radiologically isolated syndrome" (RIS).[60] Serial studies indicate that over a 2-year period, about one-third of these individuals will develop a CIS and two-thirds will demonstrate radiological progression.[59,60] The presence of gadolinium-enhancing lesions, spinal cord lesions, or typical CSF abnormalities is associated with a faster conversion from RIS to CIS or clinically definite MS,[61,62] but a substantial part of the cohort remains asymptomatic and/or clinically stable, prompting difficult questions regarding when and if to institute treatment.

Prognosis

MRI features at the time of MS diagnosis have not yielded especially useful markers that can reliably predict future disease progression; however, a more rapid accumulation of T2 lesion burden in the first 5 years after diagnosis has been associated with higher levels of disability at 20 years.[63] This finding fits nicely with the clinical observation that individuals with frequent relapses in the 5 years after diagnosis have a greater risk for future disability. It also seems that changes in white matter lesion burden become less important in the later stages of disease, whereas other measures such as cortical or gray matter atrophy become more important.[64–68]

Treatment Response

Although clearly useful in establishing a diagnosis of MS, the use of routine clinical MRI to monitor treatment response is less well defined. Clinical practice varies tremendously among neurologists who treat patients with MS, and there are relatively fewer data to help guide decision making, although there has been progress in this area. Most practitioners will obtain a new set of MRI scans at the time of diagnosis and before the initiation of a new treatment modality; when and whether to scan at other times is more controversial. Clinical activity reflects only a portion of ongoing disease activity, so periodic MRIs in clinically stable patients seems reasonable, but raises difficult questions. If subclinical activity is detected, should therapy be changed? Since none of the DMTs cures MS, how much new activity is "too much"? Should scans be obtained more frequently during the early years after diagnosis?

Defining "breakthrough disease"

Work has been done recently to establish some clinically relevant guidelines to aid in determining when to consider further evaluation and modification of treatment in the setting of continued disease activity, both clinically and radiologically defined.[69] MRI scanning, in particular the presence of Gd+ lesions indicating active inflammatory activity, plays an important role in this assessment.[70] Consideration should also be given to the routine acquisition of cervical MRI scans that frequently reveal clinically silent lesions.[71] Detailed algorithms combining clinical and radiological features suggesting breakthrough disease have been published.[72]

Serial Scanning

Findings from serial MRI scans should always be used in conjunction with clinical evaluation, following the adage "treat the patient, not the scan," given our limited understanding of how MR changes relate to individual disease progression. However, there are several markers of disease activity that can be assessed on a conventional MRI scan; these include the accumulation of white matter lesion volume as seen on T2-weighted/FLAIR scans, and the appearance of T1 black holes that indicate more severe tissue destruction. As a corollary, T1 holes that are particularly large and severe can be seen as areas of decreased signal on a FLAIR image, because the loss of tissue is complete, leaving only a fluid-filled space that mimics a mini "ventricle" with a nulling of the water signal occurring after the application of the inversion pulse as seen in Fig. 2. The volume of T1 holes shows a better correlation with disability measures than T2 volumes,[19] and the ratio of T1 hole volume to total T2 volume may be a useful measure of disease severity in MS as previously described.[25] Over time, areas of new T2 abnormality may be limited; however, some have suggested that progression is accompanied by increased tissue destruction within already established T2 lesion areas.[73]

Progressive gray matter changes can also be detected on serial T2-weighted images including the accumulation of cortical plaques and/or deep gray matter hypointensity.[51,74] Global and gray matter atrophy may be reflected by sulcal widening and enlarging ventricular spaces, including the third ventricle and the temporal horns. As previously mentioned, potential pitfalls in achieving relevant serial data include variations in the slice thickness, slice gaps, angle that scans were acquired, scanner hardware or software changes, or most commonly, no access to the prior scan to perform a useful comparison.

LIMITATIONS OF CLINICAL MRI SCANNING IN MS

There are several important shortcomings in the use of traditional MRI techniques to assess and monitor disease activity in MS. Most obvious is that abnormalities detected as areas of high signal on T2/FLAIR scans reflect increased water content and are as such histopathologically nonspecific, reflecting anything from edema to complete tissue loss. Including information on T1 holes helps to some degree, but T1 holes are themselves nonspecific and subject to evolution over time.[23,75]

More important, however, is the now well-documented realization that traditional MRI measures capture only a small fraction of MS disease-related changes that are detectable by other techniques and verified by pathology; these include subtle changes in the normal appearing white matter and normal appearing gray matter, and the presence of widespread cortical plaques.[76]

In addition, purely structural measures fail to account for adaptive functional changes in MS that limit the clinical expression of disease-related damage, at least initially, and therefore are likely important contributors to the radiological/clinical paradox in MS.[77]

SUMMARY

Despite limitations, conventional MR plays an important role in establishing the diagnosis of MS, as well as differentiating MS mimics and demyelinating disease subtypes. Clinical MR scans are effective in detecting the presence of white matter inflammatory lesions. Inflammatory lesions, in particular Gd+ lesions, are good predictors of clinical relapses in MS. These measures will continue to play an important role in clinical practice and in clinical trials, where they serve as useful biomarkers for short-term anti-inflammatory effects. Better markers for long-term outcomes in MS more closely linked to gray matter involvement, functional compensation, and diffuse white matter changes are still needed. Newer approaches that better capture these changes are described in detail in the following article of this issue by Fox and colleagues.

REFERENCES

1. Poser CM, Paty DW, Scheinberg L, et al. New diagnostic criteria for multiple sclerosis: guidelines for research protocols. Ann Neurol 1983;13(3):227–31.
2. Schumacher F, Beeve G, Kibler F, et al. Problems of experimental trials of therapy in multiple sclerosis. Ann N Y Acad Sci 1965;122:552–68.
3. McDonald WI, Compston A, Edan G, et al. Recommended diagnostic criteria for multiple sclerosis: guidelines from the International Panel on the diagnosis of multiple sclerosis. Ann Neurol 2001;50(1):121–7.
4. Optic Neuritis Study Group. Multiple sclerosis risk after optic neuritis: final optic neuritis treatment trial follow-up. Arch Neurol 2008;65(6):727–32.
5. Tintore M, Rovira A, Rio J, et al. Baseline MRI predicts future attacks and disability in clinically isolated syndromes. Neurology 2006;67(6):968–72.
6. Paty DW, Li DK. Interferon beta-1b is effective in relapsing-remitting multiple sclerosis. II. MRI analysis results of a multicenter, randomized, double-blind, placebo-controlled trial. UBC MS/MRI Study Group and the IFNB Multiple Sclerosis Study Group. Neurology 1993;43(4):662–7.
7. Simon JH, Jacobs LD, Campion M, et al. Magnetic resonance studies of intramuscular interferon beta-1a for relapsing multiple sclerosis. The Multiple Sclerosis Collaborative Research Group [see comments]. Ann Neurol 1998;43(1): 79–87.
8. Li DK, Paty DW. Magnetic resonance imaging results of the PRISMS trial: a randomized, double-blind, placebo-controlled study of interferon-beta1a in relapsing-remitting multiple sclerosis. Prevention of Relapses and Disability by Interferon-beta1a Subcutaneously in Multiple Sclerosis. Ann Neurol 1999;46(2): 197–206.
9. Ge Y, Grossman RI, Udupa JK, et al. Glatiramer acetate (Copaxone) treatment in relapsing-remitting MS: quantitative MR assessment. Neurology 2000;54(4): 813–7.
10. Miller DH, Khan OA, Sheremata WA, et al. A controlled trial of natalizumab for relapsing multiple sclerosis. N Engl J Med 2003;348(1):15–23.

11. Cohen JA, Barkhof F, Comi G, et al. Oral fingolimod or intramuscular interferon for relapsing multiple sclerosis. N Engl J Med 2010;362(5):402–15.
12. Filippi M, Yousry T, Baratti C, et al. Quantitative assessment of MRI lesion load in multiple sclerosis. A comparison of conventional spin-echo with fast fluid-attenuated inversion recovery. Brain 1996;119:1349–55.
13. Simon JH, Li D, Traboulsee A, et al. Standardized MR imaging protocol for multiple sclerosis: consortium of MS Centers consensus guidelines. AJNR Am J Neuroradiol 2006;27(2):455–61.
14. Barkhof F, Filippi M, Miller DH, et al. Comparison of MRI criteria at first presentation to predict conversion to clinically definite multiple sclerosis. Brain 1997; 120(Pt 11):2059–69.
15. Sormani MP, Bonzano L, Roccatagliata L, et al. Magnetic resonance imaging as a potential surrogate for relapses in multiple sclerosis: a meta-analytic approach. Ann Neurol 2009;65(3):268–75.
16. Miller DH, Rudge P, Johnson G, et al. Serial gadolinium enhanced magnetic resonance imaging in multiple sclerosis. Brain 1988;111(Pt 4):927–39.
17. Fisher M, Prichard JW, Warach S. New magnetic resonance techniques for acute ischemic stroke. JAMA 1995;274(11):908–11.
18. Polman CH, Reingold SC, Edan G, et al. Diagnostic criteria for multiple sclerosis: 2005 revisions to the "McDonald Criteria". Ann Neurol 2005;58(6):840–6.
19. Truyen L, van Waesberghe JH, van Walderveen MA, et al. Accumulation of hypo-intense lesions ("black holes") on T1 spin-echo MRI correlates with disease progression in multiple sclerosis. Neurology 1996;47(6):1469–76.
20. van Walderveen MA, Kamphorst W, Scheltens P, et al. Histopathologic correlate of hypointense lesions on T1-weighted spin-echo MRI in multiple sclerosis. Neurology 1998;50(5):1282–8.
21. Barkhof F, Calabresi PA, Miller DH, et al. Imaging outcomes for neuroprotection and repair in multiple sclerosis trials. Nat Rev Neurol 2009;5(5):256–66.
22. Cadavid D, Cheriyan J, Skurnick J, et al. New acute and chronic black holes in patients with multiple sclerosis randomised to interferon beta-1b or glatiramer acetate. J Neurol Neurosurg Psychiatry 2009;80(12):1337–43.
23. Li BS, Regal J, Soher BJ, et al. Brain metabolite profiles of t1-hypointense lesions in relapsing-remitting multiple sclerosis. AJNR Am J Neuroradiol 2003;24(1): 68–74.
24. Pozzilli C, Tomassini V, Marinelli F, et al. 'Gender gap' in multiple sclerosis: magnetic resonance imaging evidence. Eur J Neurol 2003;10(1):95–7.
25. Bakshi R, Neema M, Healy BC, et al. Predicting clinical progression in multiple sclerosis with the magnetic resonance disease severity scale. Arch Neurol 2008;65(11):1449–53.
26. Edwards LJ, Tench CR, Gilmore CP, et al. Multiple sclerosis findings in the spinal cord. Expert Rev Neurother 2007;7(9):1203–11.
27. Bot JC, Barkhof F, Polman CH, et al. Spinal cord abnormalities in recently diagnosed MS patients: added value of spinal MRI examination. Neurology 2004; 62(2):226–33.
28. Miller DH, Leary SM. Primary-progressive multiple sclerosis. Lancet Neurol 2007; 6(10):903–12.
29. Wingerchuk DM, Lennon VA, Lucchinetti CF, et al. The spectrum of neuromyelitis optica. Lancet Neurol 2007;6(9):805–15.
30. Lennon VA, Wingerchuk DM, Kryzer TJ, et al. A serum autoantibody marker of neuromyelitis optica: distinction from multiple sclerosis. Lancet 2004;364(9451): 2106–12.

31. Jarius S, Wildemann B. AQP4 antibodies in neuromyelitis optica: diagnostic and pathogenetic relevance. Nat Rev Neurol 2010;6(7):383–92.
32. Simon JH, Kleinschmidt-DeMasters BK. Variants of multiple sclerosis. Neuroimaging Clin N Am 2008;18(4):703–16, xi.
33. Li Y, Xie P, Lv F, et al. Brain magnetic resonance imaging abnormalities in neuromyelitis optica. Acta Neurol Scand 2008;118(4):218–25.
34. Benedict RH, Bruce JM, Dwyer MG, et al. Neocortical atrophy, third ventricular width, and cognitive dysfunction in multiple sclerosis. Arch Neurol 2006;63(9):1301–6.
35. Houtchens MK, Benedict RH, Killiany R, et al. Thalamic atrophy and cognition in multiple sclerosis. Neurology 2007;69(12):1213–23.
36. Sicotte NL, Kern KC, Giesser BS, et al. Regional hippocampal atrophy in multiple sclerosis. Brain 2008;131(Pt 4):1134–41.
37. Fisher E, Rudick RA, Simon JH, et al. Eight-year follow-up study of brain atrophy in patients with MS. Neurology 2002;59(9):1412–20.
38. Zivadinov R, Bakshi R. Central nervous system atrophy and clinical status in multiple sclerosis. J Neuroimaging 2004;14(Suppl 3):27S–35S.
39. De Stefano N, Giorgio A, Battaglini M, et al. Assessing brain atrophy rates in a large population of untreated multiple sclerosis subtypes. Neurology 2010; 74(23):1868–76.
40. Bakshi R, Ariyaratana S, Benedict RH, et al. Fluid-attenuated inversion recovery magnetic resonance imaging detects cortical and juxtacortical multiple sclerosis lesions. Arch Neurol 2001;58(5):742–8.
41. Calabrese M, Battaglini M, Giorgio A, et al. Imaging distribution and frequency of cortical lesions in patients with multiple sclerosis. Neurology 2010;75(14): 1234–40.
42. Mainero C, Benner T, Radding A, et al. In vivo imaging of cortical pathology in multiple sclerosis using ultra-high field MRI. Neurology 2009;73(12):941–8.
43. Kutzelnigg A, Lassmann H. Cortical demyelination in multiple sclerosis: a substrate for cognitive deficits? J Neurol Sci 2006;245(1–2):123–6.
44. Koch M, Uyttenboogaart M, Polman S, et al. Seizures in multiple sclerosis. Epilepsia 2008;49(6):948–53.
45. Geurts JJ, Bo L, Pouwels PJ, et al. Cortical lesions in multiple sclerosis: combined postmortem MR imaging and histopathology. AJNR Am J Neuroradiol 2005;26(3): 572–7.
46. Calabrese M, Agosta F, Rinaldi F, et al. Cortical lesions and atrophy associated with cognitive impairment in relapsing-remitting multiple sclerosis. Arch Neurol 2009;66(9):1144–50.
47. Bakshi R, Benedict RH, Bermel RA, et al. T2 hypointensity in the deep gray matter of patients with multiple sclerosis: a quantitative magnetic resonance imaging study. Arch Neurol 2002;59(1):62–8.
48. Brass SD, Chen NK, Mulkern RV, et al. Magnetic resonance imaging of iron deposition in neurological disorders. Top Magn Reson Imaging 2006;17(1):31–40.
49. Malecki EA, Devenyi AG, Barron TF, et al. Iron and manganese homeostasis in chronic liver disease: relationship to pallidal T1-weighted magnetic resonance signal hyperintensity. Neurotoxicology 1999;20(4):647–52.
50. Haacke EM, Makki M, Ge Y, et al. Characterizing iron deposition in multiple sclerosis lesions using susceptibility weighted imaging. J Magn Reson Imaging 2009; 29(3):537–44.
51. Neema M, Arora A, Healy BC, et al. Deep gray matter involvement on brain MRI scans is associated with clinical progression in multiple sclerosis. J Neuroimaging 2009;19(1):3–8.

52. O'Riordan JI, Thompson AJ, Kingsley DP, et al. The prognostic value of brain MRI in clinically isolated syndromes of the CNS. A 10-year follow-up. Brain 1998; 121(Pt 3):495–503.
53. Jacobs LD, Beck RW, Simon JH, et al. Intramuscular interferon beta-1a therapy initiated during a first demyelinating event in multiple sclerosis. CHAMPS Study Group. N Engl J Med 2000;343(13):898–904.
54. Comi G, Martinelli V, Rodegher M, et al. Effect of glatiramer acetate on conversion to clinically definite multiple\ sclerosis in patients with clinically isolated syndrome (PreCISe study): a\ randomised, double-blind, placebo-controlled trial. Lancet 2009;374(9700):1503–11.
55. Kappos L, Polman CH, Freedman MS, et al. Treatment with interferon beta-1b delays conversion to clinically definite and\ McDonald MS in patients with clinically isolated syndromes. Neurology 2006;67(7):1242–9.
56. Chard DT, Dalton CM, Swanton J, et al. MRI only conversion to multiple sclerosis following a clinically isolated syndrome. J Neurol Neurosurg Psychiatry 2011; 82(2):176–9.
57. Miller DH, Weinshenker BG, Filippi M, et al. Differential diagnosis of suspected multiple sclerosis: a consensus approach. Mult Scler 2008;14(9):1157–74.
58. Charil A, Yousry TA, Rovaris M, et al. MRI and the diagnosis of multiple sclerosis: expanding the concept of "no better explanation". Lancet Neurol 2006;5(10):841–52.
59. Lebrun C, Bensa C, Debouverie M, et al. Unexpected multiple sclerosis: follow-up of 30 patients with magnetic resonance imaging and clinical conversion profile. J Neurol Neurosurg Psychiatry 2008;79(2):195–8.
60. Okuda DT, Mowry EM, Beheshtian A, et al. Incidental MRI anomalies suggestive of multiple sclerosis. The radiologically isolated syndrome. Neurology 2009;72(9): 800–5.
61. Okuda DT, Crabtree F, Mowry EM, et al. Asymptomatic spinal cord lesions predict clinical progression in Radiologically Isolated Syndrome (RIS) subjects. Neurology 2010;74(Suppl 2):A119.
62. Lebrun C, Bensa C, Debouverie M, et al. Association between clinical conversion to multiple sclerosis in radiologically isolated syndrome and magnetic resonance imaging, cerebrospinal fluid, and visual evoked potential: follow-up of 70 patients. Arch Neurol 2009;66(7):841–6.
63. Fisniku LK, Brex PA, Altmann DR, et al. Disability and T2 MRI lesions: a 20-year follow-up of patients with relapse onset of multiple sclerosis. Brain 2008;131(Pt 3): 808–17.
64. Sormani MP, Rovaris M, Comi G, et al. A reassessment of the plateauing relationship between T2 lesion load and disability in MS. Neurology 2009;73(19): 1538–42.
65. Fisniku LK, Chard DT, Jackson JS, et al. Gray matter atrophy is related to long-term disability in multiple sclerosis. Ann Neurol 2008;64(3):247–54.
66. Fisher E, Lee JC, Nakamura K, et al. Gray matter atrophy in multiple sclerosis: a longitudinal study. Ann Neurol 2008;64(3):255–65.
67. Zhao Y, Petkau AJ, Traboulsee A, et al. Does MRI lesion activity regress in secondary progressive multiple sclerosis? Mult Scler 2010;16(4):434–42.
68. Li DK, Held U, Petkau J, et al. MRI T2 lesion burden in multiple sclerosis: a plateauing relationship with clinical disability. Neurology 2006;66(9):1384–9.
69. Rio J, Comabella M, Montalban X. Predicting responders to therapies for multiple sclerosis. Nat Rev Neurol 2009;5(10):553–60.
70. Rovaris M. The definition of non-responder to multiple sclerosis treatment: neuroimaging markers. Neurol Sci 2008;29(Suppl 2):S222–4.

71. O'Riordan JI, Losseff NA, Phatouros C, et al. Asymptomatic spinal cord lesions in clinically isolated optic nerve, brain stem, and spinal cord syndromes suggestive of demyelination. J Neurol Neurosurg Psychiatry 1998;64(3):353–7.

72. Freedman MS, Forrestal FG. Canadian treatment optimization recommendations (TOR) as a predictor of disease breakthrough in patients with multiple sclerosis treated with interferon beta-1a: analysis of the PRISMS study. Mult Scler 2008; 14(9):1234–41.

73. Sahraian MA, Radue EW, Haller S, et al. Black holes in multiple sclerosis: definition, evolution, and clinical correlations. Acta Neurol Scand 2010;122(1):1–8.

74. Calabrese M, Filippi M, Rovaris M, et al. Morphology and evolution of cortical lesions in multiple sclerosis. A longitudinal MRI study. Neuroimage 2008;42(4): 1324–8.

75. Bagnato F, Jeffries N, Richert ND, et al. Evolution of T1 black holes in patients with multiple sclerosis imaged monthly for 4 years. Brain 2003;126(Pt 8):1782–9.

76. Giacomini PS, Arnold DL. Non-conventional MRI techniques for measuring neuroprotection, repair and plasticity in multiple sclerosis. Curr Opin Neurol 2008; 21(3):272–7.

77. Filippi M, Agosta F. Magnetic resonance techniques to quantify tissue damage, tissue repair, and functional cortical reorganization in multiple sclerosis. Prog Brain Res 2009;175:465–82.

Advanced MRI in Multiple Sclerosis: Current Status and Future Challenges

Robert J. Fox, MD[a,b,]*, Erik Beall, PhD[c], Pallab Bhattacharyya, PhD[c],
Jacqueline T. Chen, PhD[d], Ken Sakaie, PhD[c]

KEYWORDS

- MRI • Imaging • Magnetization transfer imaging
- Spectroscopy • Functional MRI • Diffusion tensor imaging

MRI is a noninvasive imaging technique that provides excellent contrast between intact and demyelinated white matter (WM). MRI lesions typically persist for decades, providing a long-term record of multiple sclerosis (MS) injury within the brain and spinal cord. MRI was formally integrated into the MS diagnostic criteria in 2000 and can be used to demonstrate both of the classic demyelinating hallmarks of MS—dissemination in space and dissemination in time.[1] MRI also has been an important tool in the study of new MS agents, where reduction in new lesions is usually the primary outcome of phase II trials of anti-inflammatory therapies.

Conventional MRI modalities include T2-weighted (T2w), T1-weighted (T1w), and post-gadolinium (Gd) T1w images. Although useful in the diagnosis and management of MS, conventional imaging has several limitations. Lesions are nonspecific, indicating areas of inflammation, demyelination, ischemia, edema, cell loss, and gliosis. Conventional imaging is unable to differentiate between these different pathologies. Conventional imaging also poorly characterizes the degree of injury in demyelinated lesions. In addition, conventional imaging does not identify all of the pathology in MS: there are widespread abnormalities in the WM that appear normal on T2w and

This work was supported by RG 4091A3/1 (RJF), RG 3751B2 (EB), and RG 3753A1/2 (PB) from the National MS Society, and R21 EB005302-02 (PB).

[a] Mellen Center for Multiple Sclerosis, Neurological Institute, 9500 Euclid Avenue, U-10, Cleveland, OH 44195, USA
[b] Cleveland Clinic Lerner College of Medicine, Cleveland, OH, USA
[c] Mellen Imaging Center, Imaging Institute, Cleveland, OH, USA
[d] Department of Neurosciences, NC30, Lerner Research Institute, Cleveland Clinic, Cleveland, OH, USA
* Corresponding author. Mellen Center for Multiple Sclerosis, Neurological Institute, 9500 Euclid Avenue, U-10, Cleveland, OH 44195.
E-mail address: FOXR@ccf.org

Neurol Clin 29 (2011) 357–380
doi:10.1016/j.ncl.2010.12.011
0733-8619/11/$ – see front matter © 2011 Elsevier Inc. All rights reserved.

T1w images. Cortical demyelination is common in MS patients but is rarely seen on conventional imaging. Gradually progressive disability is common on the later stages of MS, even though conventional imaging usually shows no changes. To address these shortcomings, advanced imaging modalities have been developed and applied to MS. These advanced imaging methods provide a more sensitive and specific assessment of MS tissue injury. MRI is also useful in studying the pathophysiology of MS, with different imaging modalities providing pathologic insights into the MS injury and later recovery. This review describes some of the ways MRI is used to study MS.

BRAIN ATROPHY

Inflammatory injury in MS causes both demyelination and axonal loss.[2] The end result of this injury can be loss of tissue, and this loss of tissue can be measured by brain atrophy.[3] Brain atrophy begins early in the disease course and progresses throughout the different stages of MS. Although atrophy correlates only modestly with existing clinical disability, progression of atrophy more strongly predicts later disability progression.[4]

MS therapies might also have an impact on the progression of brain atrophy, although the relationship is not always straightforward.[5–7] The anti-inflammatory effect of MS therapies can reduce brain volume, called a pseudoatrophy effect.[8] Even patient hydration status can also affect atrophy measurements.[9] Brain atrophy is an attractive outcome metric for progressive MS trials using putative neuroprotective therapies, where conventional lesion measures do not characterize the underlying neurodegeneration.[10]

QUANTITATIVE ANALYSIS OF CONVENTIONAL IMAGING

Because new and enlarging lesions define active inflammation, sensitive and accurate quantitative measures of these lesions are a valuable research tool. Image analysis software has been helpful in measuring lesions accurately and reproducibly. Application of quantitative lesion measures to longitudinal studies can characterize changes in lesions over time, including new lesions and changes in overall lesion burden. Quantitative measures of conventional imaging are now standard outcome metrics in MS clinical trials. New Gd-enhancing or T2 lesions are typical primary outcome measures in phase II anti-inflammatory MS trials, whereas these lesion measures are relegated to secondary outcomes in phase III trials.

Although useful in many ways, quantitative measures have several limitations. The measures are relatively dependent on pulse sequence and other scanner settings. Changes in scanner settings, including scanner and pulse sequence upgrades, can have a significant impact on quantitative measures. Different software programs work differently, yielding different measures of lesion burden and atrophy.[11] Artifacts, such as patient motion, can also have an impact on quantitative measures. Because imaging abnormalities are not specific for MS, not all "lesions" seen on imaging represent actual MS lesions. Nonetheless, quantitative image analysis software provides powerful tools to assess the inflammatory components of MS injury.

MAGNETIZATION TRANSFER IMAGING

In vivo markers of myelin are essential for quantifying demyelination and remyelination in the brains of MS patients. Unfortunately, the protons associated with myelin have T2 relaxation times that are too short (<1 ms) to be directly detected by conventional brain MRI. Instead, the protons associated with myelin can be indirectly detected by harnessing a physical phenomenon called magnetization transfer (MT). MT ratio (MTR) imaging is one of the most promising MRI modalities with sensitivity and specificity to myelin and is widely available.

MT is a phenomenon in which protons of two or more environments (pools) with distinctly different magnetic resonance (MR) properties exchange magnetization. In a simple model of the brain, two pools of protons with distinctly different MR properties and biologic properties are liquid (or mobile) protons and macromolecular (or bound) protons. The protons associated with water (both intracellular and extracellular) contribute to the liquid pool of protons. The protons associated with myelin, cell membranes, and proteins contribute to the macromolecular pool of protons. To detect the macromolecular pool of protons, an off-resonance radiofrequency pulse (often referred to as the MT pulse) is used. This pulse preferentially excites the macromolecular pool of protons and is added immediately before a conventional (usually T1w or proton density–weighted [PDw]) MRI sequence. Adding this pulse induces the transfer of magnetization from the macromolecular protons to nearby liquid protons, yielding an MRI with intensities that have been modulated by the presence of myelin.

One type of MT imaging is quantitative MT (qMT) imaging. In a qMT imaging session, many different MRIs with different parameters (MRI modalities without the MT pulse, MRI with variable MT pulse duration or pulse offset frequency, and so forth) are acquired. After the acquisition, these MRIs are analyzed to completely characterize the two- (or more) pooled model of protons in the brain. One of the quantities that can be extracted from this analysis is a 3-D image of the fraction of macromolecular protons (f_B). The sensitivity and specificity of f_B to myelin density in lesional WM and normal-appearing WM (NAWM) has been demonstrated in a study that performed qMT imaging on unfixed brain slices, followed by histopathologic analyses.[12] Unfortunately, qMT imaging can only be performed at specialized centers and it typically yields low-resolution images if performed on the whole brain.[10,14]

Another type of MT imaging is MTR imaging (**Fig. 1**). To obtain an MTR image, two different MRIs are acquired in a single session: (1) an MT_{off} image, which is a conventional MRI (T1w or PDw), and (2) an MT_{on} image, which is the same conventional MRI acquired with the additional MT pulse. After acquisition, a 3-D MTR image is calculated by measuring the percentage difference in the MT_{on} image relative to the MT_{off} image ($MTR = 100 \times [MT_{off} - MT_{on}]/MT_{off}$). The sensitivity of MTR to myelin density has been demonstrated by postmortem imaging and histopathologic analyses in MS brains that revealed strong associations between myelin content and MTR in WM lesions and NAWM.[15,16] In addition, in vivo imaging and postmortem histopathology of MS brain are validated MTR metrics for remyelination and demyelination within an initially enhancing WM lesion.[17]

The relative specificity of MTR to myelin density in brain has been demonstrated by postmortem imaging and histopathologic analyses that revealed no significant associations with axonal count (after accounting for the correlation between myelin content and axonal count) or gliosis[16] and by in vivo imaging of acute MS lesions that revealed no significant effect of inflammation on the correlation of MTR with qMT-derived macromolecular content.[18] Although changes in brain MTR values underestimate demyelination in acute lesions due to edema,[18] several observations suggest that MTR imaging is a powerful tool for MS research: the strong correlation between MTR and qMT-derived macromolecular content over the 10-month evolution of acute lesions, the strong associations between MTR and histopathologically derived metrics of myelin density, and the clinical feasibility of performing whole-brain MTR imaging on most modern scanners at a clinically relevant resolution.

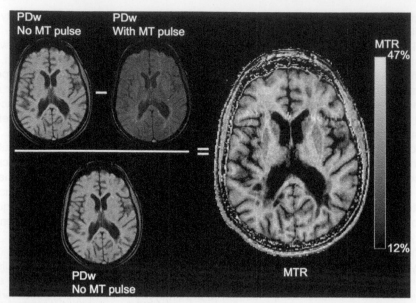

Fig. 1. MTR imaging in a secondary-progressive MS patient at 1.5 T: the 3-D MTR image is calculated by measuring the percentage difference in the MT_{on} image relative to the MT_{off} image. The MT pulse was applied to a 3-D fast low-angle shot PDw (repetition time = 30 ms, echo time = 11 ms, flip angle = 15°).

MTR in MS

MTR has provided many insights regarding the evolution of demyelination and remyelination in acute WM lesions. Decreased MTR before the appearance of a WM lesion on T2w MRI or Gd-enhanced T1w MRI suggests early myelin pathology not detectable by conventional MRI.[19–21] The evolution of MTR within new lesions varies from lesion to lesion: mean lesional MTR may recover over 1 to 5 months,[21–25] suggesting remyelination, or it may remain low[21,22,25] or decrease further,[22,25,26] suggesting ongoing demyelination. This variable MTR outcome for acute lesions is supported by postmortem observations of both remyelinated shadow plaques and demyelinated lesions in the same brain.[27] The evolution of MTR in individual lesion voxels (typically 1 to 3 mm^3) has also been shown to vary: within a given lesion there may be groups of voxels that remain stable with low MTR, suggesting static demyelination; increase significantly, suggesting remyelination; or decrease significantly, suggesting ongoing demyelination.[17,28] This variable MTR outcome for different regions of a lesion is supported by postmortem observations of inactive demyelinated WM lesions with variable peripheral remyelination[29] and in vivo MTR with postmortem histopathology validating that the spatial variability in MTR outcome was associated with demyelinated and remyelinated lesion regions.[17]

MTR of nonlesional brain tissue has also been found to be abnormally low in MS patients, in both NAWM[30] and normal-appearing gray-matter (NAGM).[30,31] MTR of nonlesional brain tissue has been shown to be associated with concurrent disability. Mean MTR of normal-appearing brain tissue was associated with existing cognitive impairment.[32] MTR in cortical regions was associated with the regionally relevant clinical disability scores.[33] Mean cortical MTR was significantly lower in cognitively impaired compared with cognitively preserved benign MS patients.[34]

MTR of nonlesional brain tissue predicts disability progression. Mean MTR in NAWM predicted disability progression over 5 years.[35] Peak height of the NAGM MTR histogram best predicted progression over 3 years.[36] Despite the clinical relevance of these MTR findings in brain regions without MRI-detectable WM lesions, studies of NAWM and NAGM using both MRI (including high-resolution MTR) and histopathology (including immunohistochemical analyses to determine myelin distribution and pathology and electron microscopy to investigate myelin and tissue ultrastructure) have not been performed to adequately understand the substrate for these MTR differences.

MTR of cervical spinal cord has also been found to be abnormally low in MS patients and associated with disability.[37] Performing MTR imaging in spinal cord is challenging, in part due to the motion of the cord during each scan and between the two scans. A new approach acquiring only the MT_{on} scan and normalizing the intensities using the cerebrospinal fluid (CSF) has demonstrated associations between column-specific CSF-normalized MT values and the relevant measures of sensorimotor impairment.[38]

Future Challenges to MTR Imaging

An important goal for MS therapies could be to enhance remyelination, yet there is no well-accepted MRI metric of remyelination. The sensitivity and specificity of MTR to myelin suggests that image processing of MTR may yield a metric of in vivo remyelination. As described previously, there is preliminary validation of MTR as useful metrics for remyelination and demyelination of acute WM lesions.[17] Another method of detecting significant changes in MTR within lesional and nonlesional brain voxels has also been proposed,[39] although further validation of all of these methods is still needed. An advantage with MTR is that most imaging systems have MTR easily available, making implementation in multicentered clinical trials more straightforward than other advanced imaging techniques. Additional advances in standardized image acquisition and analysis will help increase the application of MTR to assessing therapies that target remyelination. Several ongoing clinical trials are using MTR, and initial results seem promising.[40]

Cortical demyelination is commonly observed in MS brains through postmortem histopathology and the extent of demyelination can be great. Some cortical lesions can be observed by double inversion recovery (DIR),[41–43] fluid-attenuated inversion recovery and spoiled gradient-recalled echo,[44] DIR and phase-sensitive inversion recovery,[45] DIR and phase-sensitive inversion recovery and magnetization-prepared rapid acquisition with gradient echo (MPRAGE),[46] and MPRAGE and T2w imaging.[47] However, all of these methods identify only a small proportion of the overall cortical lesions seen on histopathology. The most common cortical lesions involve the layers nearest to the pial surface, and these are typically not visualized with current techniques, including MTR. Advanced image processing of MTR, however, may yield a metric of in vivo cortical demyelination that is not always visually apparent. As discussed previously, image processing of cortical MTR has detected abnormalities, but further MRI and histopathological studies are needed to determine the relationship between cortical lesions and abnormal cortical MTR.

DIFFUSION TENSOR IMAGING

Diffusion tensor imaging (DTI) is an advanced imaging method that describes the 3-D diffusion of water within tissue. In the 1960s Stejskal and Tanner found that a magnetic field gradient can be used to measure the ease by which molecules can diffuse.[48] Moseley and colleagues[49] recognized that adding diffusion weighting gradients

(DWGs), or a gradient in the magnetic field across the imaging plane, into an MRI acquisition could detect edema on acute ischemia, leading to the earliest clinical application of diffusion imaging.

DWG can be applied in only one direction per scan (or single-image acquisition), whereas DTI takes advantage of the fact that the direction of the DWG affects the signal contrast within tissues. When a DWG is parallel to the axons and myelin sheaths (the least restricted direction of diffusion), there is relatively more signal attenuation. When a DWG is perpendicular to myelin sheaths, the most restricted direction of diffusion, the signal is brighter (**Fig. 2**). By integrating the signal contrast when DWGs are applied in different directions over multiple scans, a 3-D characterization of water diffusion can be derived.

The diffusion ellipsoid provides an intuitive description of the diffusion tensor (**Fig. 3**). The shape of the ellipsoid corresponds with tissue microstructure, with the long (principal) axis parallel to fiber bundles. Although only 6 DWGs are needed to fully describe the ellipsoid, tensor estimates vary depending on the orientation of the ellipsoid with respect to the primary magnetic field if only 6 DWGs are used. Therefore, typically 30 or more noncollinear (ie, different directions) DWGs are used to reliably estimate the diffusion tensor.[50]

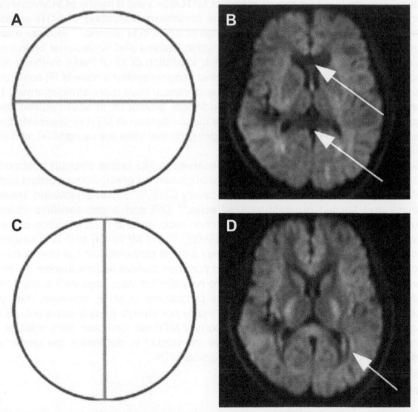

Fig. 2. An illustration of the contrast induced by DWGs. When the DWG is aligned left to right (*A*), signal attenuation is greatest in regions with highly organized bundles of myelin aligned left right (*B*) (*arrows*). When the DWG is aligned anterior to posterior (*C*), signal attenuation is greatest in regions with myelin sheaths aligned anterior posterior (*D*) (*arrow*).

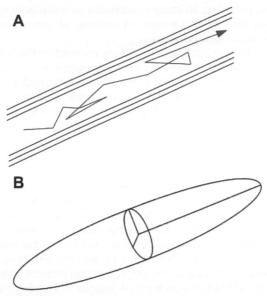

Fig. 3. (*A*) Cartoon of an axon with myelin sheaths (*blue lines*). A water molecule diffusing in this environment follows a path with movement preferentially aligned along the myelin sheath (*red arrow*). (*B*) Diffusion ellipsoid representation of diffusion tensor, with long axis aligned with preferred direction of water diffusion.

Several metrics can be derived from the tensor to correlate with degree and type of tissue injury. The two most commonly reported metrics are mean diffusivity, which reflects the overall amount of diffusion, and fractional anisotropy (FA), which represents the degree of elongation of diffusion. An increase of mean diffusivity can accompany loss of physiologic barriers to diffusion associated with cell loss or injury and is commonly observed in MS patients. FA is large in highly organized WM, because diffusion is relatively elongated; tissue injury (eg, demyelination) can, therefore, lead to a decrease in FA.

The individual components of the diffusion ellipsoid (called eigenvalues) can be evaluated separately, too. Longitudinal diffusivity (LD) is simply the largest of the 3 eigenvalues and is also known as axial diffusivity. Relative decreases in LD correlates with axonal injury at the acute stage of inflammatory injury,[51,52] and such abnormalities are found distal from site of injury.[53,54] This observation suggests a picture in which transection of axons reduces the ease by which water moves along axon bundles.[55,56] Transverse diffusivity (TD) is the mean of the smaller two eigenvalues and is also known as radial diffusivity. In highly organized fiber tracts, transverse diffusivity corresponds to diffusion across fibers. Relative increase of TD correlates with demyelination and suggests a picture in which fragmented or missing myelin leads to fewer barriers for water diffusion.[53,57]

DTI Tractography

Tractography is a diffusion analysis technique that aims to identify specific WM pathways and may enable association between WM injury and functional deficit. For example, measures of TD in the motor pathway have been found to correlate with arm function (the 9-hole peg test) in MS patients. Injury has been found in pathways distal to MS lesions, providing an imaging correlate to wallerian degeneration.[55,56,58] These changes may also explain advanced imaging abnormalities in WM regions that appear normal on conventional imaging.

The basic concept behind tractography entails connecting the orientation information at each voxel. In the most common implementation, the principal eigenvector, which is associated with the largest axis of the diffusion ellipsoid, is used. Streamlines are constructed by connecting principal eigenvectors in each voxel, thus creating whole-brain maps of fibers.[59,60] Unfortunately, such methods fail with small fibers, in regions of fiber crossings, and in the presence of tissue injury, such as MS lesions.[61] Several higher-order methods have been developed to model crossing fibers,[62–64] and more complex tractography methods have been introduced to capture more of the fascicle anatomy.[65,66]

Analysis of tractography results typically involves one of two approaches. One can measure tract-specific values, such as LD, TD, FA, and MD.[67] This approach has found correlation with clinical measures of disability in MS and with functional MRI (fMRI) measures of transcallosal inhibition. Another approach counts streamlines generated by the tractography algorithm. This counting approach and the related tract volume metric demonstrate relatively high variability and reduced sensitivity, however.[68]

Tract-based spatial statistics is an image processing method distinct from tractography that constructs a WM skeleton from FA images.[69] Imaging metrics associated with these skeletons can be compared between subjects, so tract-based spatial statistics shows promise for bridging the gap between imaging and clinical disability.[70,71]

DTI in MS

The sensitivity and physiologic interpretation of DTI suggest a range of applications relevant to MS. DTI is sensitive to abnormalities in NAWM, which appears normal on conventional imaging[72,73] and can differentiate different types of lesions.[74,75] DTI-related parameters have also been used to assess the impact of new drug therapies.[76,77] Correlation with several clinical, physiologic, and psychological scores suggest the potential of DTI for assessing and perhaps predicting patient-specific progression of disease and response to therapy.[67,78,79]

Future Challenges to DTI

Modeling water diffusion as a tensor is helpful in highly organized WM tracts, but the tensor models are a less accurate description of water diffusion in more complex tissues, including those with crossing fiber tracts, gray matter (GM), and tissue injury. Therefore, several methods have been proposed to model multicomponent diffusivity, which may provide additional information about tissue. Examples include diffusion spectrum imaging,[80] q-space imaging,[81] multiexponential modeling,[82] and diffusion kurtosis imaging.[83]

The wide dynamic range of measurement and the relative pathologic specificity of DTI to axonal and myelin integrity suggest that it may be useful in measuring the impact of MS therapies. As therapies emerge with potential remyelination and neuroprotection effects, DTI is an attractive metric to assess efficacy.[84] Methods to assure comparability of DTI measures across different magnet types and different centers are needed to effectively implement DTI in multicenter clinical trials.

SPECTROSCOPY

MR spectroscopy (MRS) is an imaging tool used to study the chemical characteristics of tissues. Where conventional MRI characterizes the physical characteristics of a region of tissue relative to surrounding regions, MRS characterizes the chemical properties of a region of tissue, most commonly focusing on cellular metabolites. The sensitivity of MRS measurements is proportional to $A\gamma^3$, where A is the natural abundance of the isotope of the MR active nucleus and γ is the gyromagnetic ratio, which is determined by the magnetic moment of the nucleus. The sensitivities of the isotopes commonly used in clinical MRS are listed in **Table 1**.

Of the 3 isotopes listed in **Table 1**, proton (^{1}H) spectroscopy is used most frequently in clinical practice. **Table 2** lists some of the major resonances appearing in in vivo MR spectra from cerebral imaging.[85,86] Imbalances in the relative amount of the metabolites measured in vivo indicate presence of diseases, so precise identification and accurate quantification of the peaks in MR spectra are sometimes necessary for diagnostic purposes.

MRS in MS

MRS has been used to study changes and imbalances in different cellular metabolites over the course of MS. MRS has also been explored as a diagnostic tool, although MRS is not considered a standard modality in the diagnosis of MS.[87]

N-Acetylaspartate
MS lesions usually have lower N-acetylaspartate (NAA), which is an indicator of axonal/neuronal loss or dysfunction. Significant reduction in NA (sum of NAA and NAA glutamate) was found in chronic WM lesions in relapsing-remitting (RR), secondary progressive (SP), and primary progressive (PP) MS patients, whereas no such reduction in NA was seen in benign MS patients.[88] The same study found a decrease in NA level in NAWM in PPMS, whereas no such effect was seen in benign MS. MRS has shown a decrease in NAA/Cr ratio in patients with moderate to severe chronic disease.[89] In a longitudinal study, transient changes of NAA level in acute plaques were observed, indicating that reduced NAA is not necessarily associated with axonal loss.[90] The average NAA level within the spectroscopic volume was found inversely correlated with the total lesion volume in the whole brain in the same study. Reduction in NAA level in cortical GM (CGM), NAWM, and lesion has been reported in mild RRMS, suggesting widespread neuronal loss or dysfunction early in the course of the disease.[91] Decrease in NA levels in CGM and NAWM has been reported in early RRMS.[92] Significant reduction in whole-brain NAA level has been reported in RRMS patients, where the observed decrease in NAA was higher in older than younger patients.[93]

Creatine
MRS has found mixed results for creatine (Cr) levels. Cr level was similar in NAWM and CGM between RRMS and healthy controls[94] and in NAWM between PPMS and controls.[95] In other studies, however, Cr level was modestly higher in MS NAWM than in controls,[96,97] although Cr concentration was similar within T1 isointense

Table 1
The abundance and sensitivity of isotopes commonly measured in clinical spectroscopy studies

Isotope	γ (MHz T^{-1})	Abundance (%)	%Sensitivity
^{1}H	42.58	99.98	1.00
^{31}P	17.25	100.0	6.65×10^{-2}
^{13}C	10.71	1.108	1.76×10^{-4}

Table 2	
Major resonance peaks in MR spectra	
Metabolite	Description
NAA	Predominantly present in cell bodies and acts as neuronal marker
Cr/PCr	PCr is converted to Cr during the conversion of ADP to the high-energy compound ATP
Cho-containing compounds	Usually grouped within the B-complex vitamins and are present in the synaptic ends of cholinergic neurons and cell membranes, and are part of lipid metabolism
Glu and Gln	Glu is the major excitatory neurotransmitter and Gln is a regulator of Glu metabolism
ml	Acts as glia cell markers in brain tissue
Lac and glucose	Lac is the final product of the anaerobic glycolysis cycle and is important in assessing ischemic tissue and tumors; glucose is important in energy metabolism of the brain
Ala	A glucogenic amino acid and is readily converted to pyruvate, which can enter the TCA cycle
GABA	A major inhibitory neurotransmitter
Macromolecules and lipids	Cellular components

Abbreviations: ADP, anenosine diphosphate; Ala, Alanine; Lac, Lactate; PCr, phosphocreatine; TCA, tricarboxylic acid cycle.

lesions and NAWM in RRMS. Cr levels in CGM correlated with clinical disability as measured by the MS functional composite (MSFC).[92]

Choline
No significant difference between choline (Cho) concentration in isointense lesions in T1w MRI and NAWM in RRMS was seen in MRS study, whereas NAWM Cho concentration was reported to be 14% higher in MS patients compared with controls.[96] The increase in Cho and Cr levels was interpreted as (1) attempted remyelination in isointense lesions and ongoing gliosis and (2) increased cellularity (gliosis, inflammation) along with membrane turnover. Significant increase in Cho level in MS plaques has been reported,[98] and a decrease in NAA/Cho ratio observed in the same study was speculated to be related either to axonal degeneration or gliosis. In a short-term serial study,[99] Cho levels in large demyelinating lesions was found to increase 3 days after the onset of symptoms, and at 8 months the level remained high at the center of the lesion. The Cho levels surrounding the lesion, however, normalized by 8 months. The abnormal Cho level was interpreted to indicate persistent demyelination. In a longer-term longitudinal study, Cho levels within NAWM that became a visible MS lesion 6 to 12 months later showed higher Cho compared with regions that did not become lesions.[100] Similarly, lesions that increased in size after 6 months had higher Cho/Cr ratio at baseline than lesions, which remained stable in size. Significant reduction in CGM Cho level was observed in RRMS.[92]

Glutamate and Glutamine
Elevated glutamate (Glu) has been reported in acute lesions and NAWM, whereas no significant elevation in Glu within chronic lesions was observed.[101] These observations suggest an alteration of Glu metabolism in MS. A significant reduction in Glx (combined Glu and glutamine [Gln]) levels has been observed in CGM, and a significant

correlation between CGM Glx level and disability (measured by MSFC) has also been reported in MS.[92] The correlation between clinical disability and CGM Cr and Glx levels but not between disability and NAWM NA is suggestive of close correlation between reduced NAA and neuronal metabolic dysfunction rather than neuronal loss in early RRMS.[92]

Myoinositol

MRS studies in MS patients have observed increased myoinositol (mI) levels in acute MS lesions and chronic T2 lesions.[91,102] mI levels are also elevated in NAWM, and these elevations are inversely correlated with disability as measured by MSFC.[92] This correlation is speculated to relate to glial proliferation and function in MS patients. mI levels are also elevated in NAWM and CGM of patients with either MS or clinically isolated syndromes suggestive of MS.[91,103]

Other metabolites

Elevated lactate levels have been reported in acute MS lesions.[102] Elevated levels of macromolecule have been observed in acute MS lesions compared with chronic lesions in MS patients and NAWM from healthy controls, indicating that macromolecule resonances may be a useful marker of acute MS lesions.[104] Lipid resonances were observed to be elevated in enhancing MS lesions, which probably represented lipid products of myelin breakdown. These lipid levels remained elevated for a mean of 5 months.[105] Elevated lipid peaks have also been observed in chronic T2 lesions, suggesting possible alternative pathophysiologic processes leading to demyelination.[90] Strong lipid resonances in GM and NAWM have been reported in PPMS even in the absence of lesions, which is suggestive of regionally altered myelin macromolecular structure.[106]

MRS to measure the impact of MS therapies

Because MRS is thought to provide a quantitative (relative and absolute) measure of many different metabolites, it is reasonable to hypothesize that MRS may measure the efficacy of MS therapies. To date, however, only a few studies have used MRS to evaluate the effect of MS therapies, with mixed results.[87]

Future Applications and Challenges of MRS

With the recent development of improved hardware (higher strength clinical scanners, multichannel phased array coils, and so forth) and software (improved pulse sequences for scans and data analysis software), MRS is becoming a more useful tool than ever in the understanding of MS. These developments should allow increased understanding of MS pathophysiology and its relationship with brain function.

Spinal cord MRS

Most MRS research in MS has focused on the brain. Although the spinal cord is known to be involved in the disability associated with MS,[107,108] few MRS studies have focused on this region. ^{1}H MRS could provide useful information on axonal damage in spinal cord. Spinal cord MRS, however, is technically challenging due to the small size of the cord, susceptibility artifacts at tissue-bone interfaces, artifacts from cardiac and respiratory motion, and cerebrospinal fluid pulsations; hence, only a few spinal cord MRS studies have been performed. Nonetheless, the feasibility of cervical cord MRS and metabolite quantification has recently been demonstrated using 3T magnets in healthy controls.[109] Significant differences in NA, Cr, Cho, and mI concentrations were observed between spinal cord and brainstem. A study in MS patients found reduced level of NAA in the cervical spinal cord in MS supporting the presence of axonal loss and damage in normal-appearing spinal cords of MS patients.[110] Significant correlations were also observed between Cr, Cho, and mI levels in the cervical cord and disability, as measured by Expanded Disability Status Scale and 9-hole peg test.[111]

Identifying cortical marker of MS

Damage to CGM in MS has long been acknowledged in pathologic studies.[112,113] MRS can be explored as a potential cortical marker of the disease. For this purpose, it would be most appropriate to study metabolites contained within neurons, which are present primarily in GM. γ-aminobutyric acid (GABA) is an inhibitory neurotransmitter, which is present in GM at a much higher level than in WM.[114,115] Although pathologic study has explored the role of GABA in MS,[116] MRS of cortical GABA in MS is largely not explored. In vivo cortical GABA measurement by MRS is technically challenging due to very low cerebral GABA level and presence of stronger overlapping resonances. Nonetheless, a recent preliminary study of MRS of GABA in MS is encouraging.[117]

Motion

A significant problem in MRS studies is subject motion. A single scanning session is 30 to 45 minutes or longer, and it is difficult for a subject to stay still throughout such a long session. Patient motion can result in scanning the wrong brain region and thus can lead to inaccurate results.[118] The advent of multicoil technology and parallel imaging has reduced the total scan time, but it remains important for subjects to remain still for each 5 to 10 minutes and this is often difficult for MS patients. Moreover, identification of motion from final spectrum is not always possible,[119] so it is important to have other mechanisms to identify motion during the scan. Although several studies have proposed methods of addressing the issue of subject motion,[119–122] the problem can persist with patient populations for longer scans.

FUNCTIONAL MRI

fMRI techniques take advantage of the relationship between brain activity and small changes in MRI signal. This effect, called the blood oxygen level–dependent (BOLD) effect, is the result of a cascade of physiologic events that link neural activity to MRI signal changes.[123,124] Upon initiating a task, the neurons in the brain regions involved in that task increase neuronal firing. This neural activity leads to increased metabolic demand, to which the brain responds. Through a combination of metabolic and synaptic signaling, cerebral blood flow (the hemodynamic response) is increased in the local blood capillaries within approximately 1 mm of the neural activity. This increased blood flow results in increased total blood oxygen content. In appropriately tuned MR acquisitions, the increased blood oxygen produces an increase in the MRI signal. The BOLD signal change is typically only a few percentage points of the baseline signal, which can make it difficult to differentiate from background variability or noise.

The BOLD effect has been used to identify and study brain activity in response to various tasks or stimuli by looking at the time evolution of changes in signal across the brain.[125,126] The typical MRI pulse sequence for fMRI is the echo planar imaging sequence. This pulse sequence allows fast (2–3 seconds per whole-brain sample) imaging of the BOLD effect across the entire brain with spatial resolution of 10–100 cubic millimeters. Neuroimaging fMRI studies typically involve the performance of some task during the scan session. The subject's response to the task in the scanner is compared with the MR signal to obtain various parameters relating to the neural activity, such as 3-D maps of BOLD activation. The task or stimuli can be designed to stimulate a particular domain, such as motor, sensory, emotional, or cognitive. The overall study design typically measures activation during a task and compares that between two groups of subjects. Comparison can be between MS patients and healthy controls or between different MS subgroups (**Fig. 4**). Functional connectivity MRI is a newer fMRI technique which measures low-frequency oscillations in BOLD signals across the entire brain.[127,128] The same type of data as acquired with fMRI is acquired in functional connectivity MRI studies, but the subject is usually resting in a scanner instead of performing a task. Functional connectivity analysis depicts the strength of networks between cortical regions.

fMRI in MS

fMRI of MS has produced a range of insights into the progression of the disease. Early studies of fMRI in MS began through evaluations of the visual and motor systems. The first use of fMRI in MS was a case report of a patient fully recovered from an acute episode of homonymous hemianopsia.[129] During the fMRI scan, hemifield visual stimulation was presented, and the resulting activation maps were compared with those of controls. They found that the recovered visual cortex behaved similarly to controls. Several years later, motor and visual tasks were used to evaluate changes in fMRI in MS patients.[130] This study found MS patients with motor weakness experienced larger motor activation than controls whereas patients with optic neuritis experienced smaller visual activation than controls. The reduced visual activation in optic neuritis was confirmed shortly after and shown to correlate with increased latency of visual evoked potentials recorded in the cortex of the affected eye.[131] Subsequent studies explored attention and arithmetic performance using the paced serial addition test (PASAT),[132,133] working memory (Sternberg task),[134] attention processes,[135,136] and verbal working memory,[137] among other tests.

Compensation and reorganization

The majority of the fMRI studies in MS have examined compensatory processes and reorganization of functional tissue. Observations of cortical reorganization support the hypothesis that compensatory processes in brain tissue limit the correspondence between pathology and apparent disability.[100,139] The most common finding is increased extent or strength of activation in MS patients compared with controls,

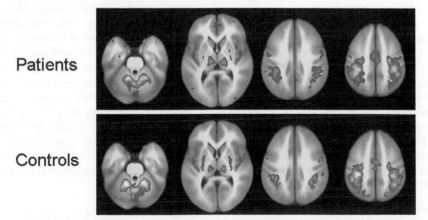

Patients

Controls

Fig. 4. Group-averaged BOLD activation to a complex finger-tapping task in MS patients and controls. MS patients showed 5% larger cortical volume of activation.

implying compensation or reorganization of neuronal activation.[140,141] Later studies investigated how the limits of the adaptive cortical changes may play a role in clinical progression.[136] The basis for these limits were seen in studies that showed regions recruited by MS patients during simple motor tasks are components recruited by healthy controls in more difficult tasks.[142] Reorganization of sensory circuits to sensorimotor integration circuits (eg, putamen) was seen in a passive motor movement fMRI study.[143] These studies of adaptive reorganization suggest that clinical disability is dependent on some combination of tissue damage, repair, and cortical reorganization.[144] Longitudinal fMRI studies are needed to further understand this complex relationship and provide clinical benefit to MS patients.[145]

Rehabilitation and longitudinal studies

Longitudinal studies have been used to evaluate how fMRI findings relate to disease evolution and clinical recovery. Initial longitudinal studies found reduced ipsilateral motor activation correlated with disease progression.[146] Later studies found adaptive plasticity in bilateral visual cortex and lateral geniculate nucleus after recovery from acute unilateral optic neuritis.[147] A change in cognitive activation in the lateral prefrontal cortices in MS patients correlated with change in PASAT scores over 1 year.[148] The use of serial administration of PASAT suffers from the potential confound of practice effects.[149] These training effects were explored by pre and post-training fMRI motor task sessions, with a reduced effect of training seen in MS patients, implying reduced capacity to adapt.[150] Administration of the cholinesterase inhibitor, rivastigmine, in MS patients causes a normalization of fMRI activation on an attention fMRI task (Stroop test).[135,151] Further studies are needed to clarify how fMRI may be helpful in guiding specific rehabilitation methods.[152]

Fatigue

Fatigue is a common but incompletely understood symptom in MS. fMRI studies have observed a relationship between cortical activation and fatigue severity.[153] Fatigue Severity Scale scores correlated inversely with right hand finger flexion-extension motor activation in several motor-associated regions: greater fatigue was associated with less relative activation in these regions. Subsequent studies indicate that nonmotor functions of the basal ganglia may be involved in fatigue processes, where greater activation over time in MS patients was observed over repeated sessions of a processing speed task.[154] Performance of a cognitively fatiguing mental task (PASAT) between motor fMRI scans led to an increase in activation to a paced finger task in primarily nonmotor areas of MS patients but a decrease in controls. This observation implies that the presence of fatigue may suggest an increased level of neuronal reorganization required to perform a particular task.[155] Furthermore, newly recruited tissue may not habituate or respond in the same way as older ingrained circuitry in the presence of fatigue. In a similar study, performance of a physically fatiguing motor task between motor fMRI scans showed little change in activation in MS patients in the second (postfatigue) scan but an increase in control subject activation.[156] A group comparison showed, however, that MS patients had significantly greater activation in the prefatigue scan, such that postfatigue level of activation was already at maximum for MS patients. These studies all point to fatigue in MS patients being associated with reaching the limit of neuronal compensation. Further exploration in the area of fatigue in MS is needed.

Connectivity

Imaging biomarkers of MS progression historically relied on T2 and contrast-enhanced lesions, with the assumption that structural connections between brain regions were reduced in MS. Studies correlating structural damage (T2 lesion load) and functional changes support this hypothesis.[157,158] Transcranial magnetic stimulation and motor fMRI showed that loss of transcallosal inhibitory motor fibers is correlated with increased ipsilateral motor activation.[159] MS patients with damage to the superior longitudinal fasciculus had bilateral activation to a serial addition task, which results in lateralized (language-dominant hemisphere) activation in controls and MS patients without superior longitudinal fasciculus damage (no difference in task performance).[160] A study of functional connectivity and DTI structural connectivity between motor cortices found a direct correlation between the two modes of connectivity in MS patients and controls.[161]

Future Directions

Several areas of research remain for fMRI studies. More longitudinal studies are needed to evaluate adaptive plasticity and rehabilitation.[145,162] Specifically, the current imaging biomarkers of disease progression have a poor prospective correlation with eventual outcomes.[163] Improved understanding of the reorganization process (including natural tissue repair, natural reorganization, rehabilitation-induced reorganization, and pharmacologic-induced reorganization) and the limits of cortical adaptability to various cognitive demands could improve the ability to predict outcomes in MS. A single fMRI scan, however, is typically specific to 1 or 2 pathways, but MS deficits may arise from injury or dysfunction to a number of different pathways. The pathway-specific nature of fMRI may limit its application in predicting general MS outcomes. Functional connectivity and structural connectivity, however, can be determined for many different pathways in a practical scan time, which may overcome that limitation. Longitudinal connectivity studies and other fMRI biomarker studies are needed to better understand the ability of fMRI to measure overall disease progression.

An often underappreciated issue in BOLD fMRI is bias and improper design. fMRI and connectivity techniques have been shown to be susceptible several potential confounds that could bias results, and many were not recognized in previous studies.[164] These include the effect of motion,[165] physiologic noise,[166,167] vasoreactivity, and blood flow,[164] among others. Sensitive behavioral measures of performance also need to be recognized. For example, bilateral fiber optic gloves to monitor hand movements are preferable over visual inspection, because visual inspection often misses subtle motor activation that may have an impact on fMRI results. MS patients differ from healthy subjects in several ways: increased motion, altered cerebral blood flow, and reduced ability to perform behavioral tasks. A failure to account for these differences in a population-based study may call into question whether or not the results are only nondisease-related artifacts of the patient population. Even within a single MS patient population, a change in these variables over time may mask an underlying change in fMRI or masquerade as altered activation. These shortcomings notwithstanding, fMRI has become a powerful tool in understanding cortical function and the connectivity between different brain regions. The data provided by fMRI complement those obtained by conventional imaging in understanding the impact of MS disease injury.

SUMMARY

MRI has rapidly become a leading research tool in the study of MS. Advances in imaging are providing a more accurate characterization of tissue injury, including demyelination, axonal injury, and its functional and metabolic consequences. Not only are these tools providing greater insight into MS pathophysiology but also several may be useful in measuring the potential benefit of remyelinating and neuroprotective therapies.

REFERENCES

1. McDonald WI, Compston A, Edan G, et al. Recommended diagnostic criteria for multiple sclerosis: guidelines from the international panel on the diagnosis of multiple sclerosis. Ann Neurol 2001;50:121.
2. Trapp BD, Peterson J, Ransohoff RM, et al. Axonal transection in the lesions of multiple sclerosis. N Engl J Med 1998;338:278.
3. Bermel RA, Bakshi R. The measurement and clinical relevance of brain atrophy in multiple sclerosis. Lancet Neurol 2006;5:158.
4. Fisher E, Rudick RA, Simon JH, et al. Eight-year follow-up study of brain atrophy in patients with MS. Neurology 2002;59:1412.
5. Kappos L, Radue EW, O'Connor P, et al. A placebo-controlled trial of oral fingolimod in relapsing multiple sclerosis. N Engl J Med 2010;362:387.
6. Miller DH, Soon D, Fernando KT, et al. MRI outcomes in a placebo-controlled trial of natalizumab in relapsing MS. Neurology 2007;68:1390.
7. Rudick RA, Fisher E, Lee JC, et al. Use of the brain parenchymal fraction to measure whole brain atrophy in relapsing-remitting MS. Multiple Sclerosis Collaborative Research Group. Neurology 1999;53:1698.
8. Zivadinov R, Reder AT, Filippi M, et al. Mechanisms of action of disease-modifying agents and brain volume changes in multiple sclerosis. Neurology 2008;71:136.
9. Duning T, Kloska S, Steinstrater O, et al. Dehydration confounds the assessment of brain atrophy. Neurology 2005;64:548.
10. Altmann DR, Jasperse B, Barkhof F, et al. Sample sizes for brain atrophy outcomes in trials for secondary progressive multiple sclerosis. Neurology 2009;72:595.
11. Fisher E, Barkhof F, van den Elskamp I, et al. Comparion of brain atrophy measurement methods in the context of a clinical trial. Mult Scler 2009;15:S217.
12. Schmierer K, Tozer DJ, Scaravilli F, et al. Quantitative magnetization transfer imaging in postmortem multiple sclerosis brain. J Magn Reson Imaging 2007; 26:41.
13. Cercignani M, Basile B, Spano B, et al. Investigation of quantitative magnetisation transfer parameters of lesions and normal appearing white matter in multiple sclerosis. NMR Biomed 2009;22:646.
14. Tozer D, Ramani A, Barker GJ, et al. Quantitative magnetization transfer mapping of bound protons in multiple sclerosis. Magn Reson Med 2003;50:83.
15. Barkhof F, Bruck W, De Groot CJ, et al. Remyelinated lesions in multiple sclerosis: magnetic resonance image appearance. Arch Neurol 2003;60(8):1073.
16. Schmierer K, Scaravilli F, Altmann DR, et al. Magnetization transfer ratio and myelin in postmortem multiple sclerosis brain. Ann Neurol 2004;56:407.
17. Chen JT, Kuhlmann T, Jansen GH, et al. Voxel-based analysis of the evolution of magnetization transfer ratio to quantify remyelination and demyelination with histopathological validation in a multiple sclerosis lesion. Neuroimage 2007; 36:1152.
18. Giacomini PS, Levesque IR, Ribeiro L, et al. Measuring demyelination and remyelination in acute multiple sclerosis lesion voxels. Arch Neurol 2009;66:375.
19. Filippi M, Rocca MA, Comi G. Magnetization transfer ratios of multiple sclerosis lesions with variable durations of enhancement. J Neurol Sci 1998;159(2):162.

20. Pike GB, De Stefano N, Narayanan S, et al. Multiple sclerosis: magnetization transfer MR imaging of white matter before lesion appearance on T2-weighted images. Radiology 2000;215(3):824.
21. Richert ND, Ostuni JL, Bash CN, et al. Interferon beta-1b and intravenous methylprednisolone promote lesion recovery in multiple sclerosis. Mult Scler 2001; 7(1):49.
22. Filippi M, Rocca MA, Sormani MP, et al. Short-term evolution of individual enhancing MS lesions studied with magnetization transfer imaging. Magn Reson Imaging 1999;17:979.
23. Lai HM, Davie CA, Gass A, et al. Serial magnetisation transfer ratios in gadolinium-enhancing lesions in multiple sclerosis. J Neurol 1997;244(5):308.
24. Silver N, Lai M, Symms M, et al. Serial gadolinium-enhanced and magnetization transfer imaging to investigate the relationship between the duration of blood-brain barrier disruption and extent of demyelination in new multiple sclerosis lesions. J Neurol 1999;246:728.
25. van Waesberghe JH, van Walderveen MA, Castelijns JA, et al. Patterns of lesion development in multiple sclerosis: longitudinal observations with T1-weighted spin-echo and magnetization transfer MR. AJNR Am J Neuroradiol 1998;19:675.
26. Dousset V, Gayou A, Brochet B, et al. Early structural changes in acute MS lesions assessed by serial magnetization transfer studies. Neurology 1998;51: 1150.
27. Bruck W, Schmied M, Suchanek G, et al. Oligodendrocytes in the early course of multiple sclerosis. Ann Neurol 1994;35:65.
28. Chen JT, Collins DL, Atkins HL, et al. Magnetization transfer ratio evolution with demyelination and remyelination in multiple sclerosis lesions. Ann Neurol 2008; 63:254.
29. Prineas JW, Connell F. Remyelination in multiple sclerosis. Ann Neurol 1979;5:22.
30. De Stefano N, Battaglini M, Stromillo ML, et al. Brain damage as detected by magnetization transfer imaging is less pronounced in benign than in early relapsing multiple sclerosis. Brain 2006;129:2008.
31. Ramio-Torrenta L, Sastre-Garriga J, Ingle GT, et al. Abnormalities in normal appearing tissues in early primary progressive multiple sclerosis and their relation to disability: a tissue specific magnetisation transfer study. J Neurol Neurosurg Psychiatry 2006;77:40.
32. Filippi M, Tortorella C, Rovaris M, et al. Changes in the normal appearing brain tissue and cognitive impairment in multiple sclerosis. J Neurol Neurosurg Psychiatry 2000;68:157.
33. Khaleeli Z, Cercignani M, Audoin B, et al. Localized grey matter damage in early primary progressive multiple sclerosis contributes to disability. Neuroimage 2007;37:253.
34. Amato MP, Portaccio E, Stromillo ML, et al. Cognitive assessment and quantitative magnetic resonance metrics can help to identify benign multiple sclerosis. Neurology 2008;71:632.
35. Santos AC, Narayanan S, de Stefano N, et al. Magnetization transfer can predict clinical evolution in patients with multiple sclerosis. J Neurol 2002;249:662.
36. Khaleeli Z, Altmann DR, Cercignani M, et al. Magnetization transfer ratio in gray matter: a potential surrogate marker for progression in early primary progressive multiple sclerosis. Arch Neurol 2008;65:1454.
37. Bozzali M, Rocca MA, Iannucci G, et al. Magnetization-transfer histogram analysis of the cervical cord in patients with multiple sclerosis. AJNR Am J Neuroradiol 1999;20:1803.

38. Zackowski KM, Smith SA, Reich DS, et al. Sensorimotor dysfunction in multiple sclerosis and column-specific magnetization transfer-imaging abnormalities in the spinal cord. Brain 2009;132:1200.

39. Dwyer M, Bergsland N, Hussein S, et al. A sensitive, noise-resistant method for identifying focal demyelination and remyelination in patients with multiple sclerosis via voxel-wise changes in magnetization transfer ratio. J Neurol Sci 2009;282:86.

40. Arnold DL, Dalton CM, Narayanan S, et al. Magnetization transfer ratio imaging is feasible in large multicenter MS trials. Neurology 2010;74:A118.

41. Calabrese M, Rocca MA, Atzori M, et al. A 3-year magnetic resonance imaging study of cortical lesions in relapse-onset multiple sclerosis. Ann Neurol 2010; 67:376.

42. Geurts JJ, Pouwels PJ, Uitdehaag BM, et al. Intracortical lesions in multiple sclerosis: improved detection with 3D double inversion-recovery MR imaging. Radiology 2005;236:254.

43. Simon B, Schmidt S, Lukas C, et al. Improved in vivo detection of cortical lesions in multiple sclerosis using double inversion recovery MR imaging at 3 Tesla. Eur Radiol 2010;20(7):1675–83.

44. Bagnato F, Butman JA, Gupta S, et al. In vivo detection of cortical plaques by MR imaging in patients with multiple sclerosis. AJNR Am J Neuroradiol 2006; 27:2161.

45. Nelson F, Poonawalla AH, Hou P, et al. Improved identification of intracortical lesions in multiple sclerosis with phase-sensitive inversion recovery in combination with fast double inversion recovery MR imaging. AJNR Am J Neuroradiol 2007;28:1645.

46. Nelson F, Poonawalla A, Hou P, et al. 3D MPRAGE improves classification of cortical lesions in multiple sclerosis. Mult Scler 2008;14:1214.

47. Bagnato F, Yao B, Cantor F, et al. Multisequence-imaging protocols to detect cortical lesions of patients with multiple sclerosis: observations from a postmortem 3 Tesla imaging study. J Neurol Sci 2009;282:80.

48. Stejskal E, Tanner J. Spin diffusion measurements: spin echoes in the presence of a time-dependent field gradient. J Chem Phys 1965;42:288.

49. Moseley ME, Cohen Y, Mintorovitch J, et al. Early detection of regional cerebral ischemia in cats: comparison of diffusion- and T2-weighted MRI and spectroscopy. Magn Reson Med 1990;14:330.

50. Jones DK. The effect of gradient sampling schemes on measures derived from diffusion tensor MRI: a Monte Carlo study. Magn Reson Med 2004;51:807.

51. Feng S, Hong Y, Zhou Z, et al. Monitoring of acute axonal injury in the swine spinal cord with EAE by diffusion tensor imaging. J Magn Reson Imaging 2009;30:277.

52. Kim JH, Budde MD, Liang HF, et al. Detecting axon damage in spinal cord from a mouse model of multiple sclerosis. Neurobiol Dis 2006;21:626.

53. Budde MD, Kim JH, Liang HF, et al. Toward accurate diagnosis of white matter pathology using diffusion tensor imaging. Magn Reson Med 2007; 57:688.

54. DeBoy CA, Zhang J, Dike S, et al. High resolution diffusion tensor imaging of axonal damage in focal inflammatory and demyelinating lesions in rat spinal cord. Brain 2007;130:2199.

55. Ciccarelli O, Werring DJ, Barker GJ, et al. A study of the mechanisms of normal-appearing white matter damage in multiple sclerosis using diffusion tensor imaging–evidence of Wallerian degeneration. J Neurol 2003;250:287.

56. Yu CS, Lin FC, Li KC, et al. Diffusion tensor imaging in the assessment of normal-appearing brain tissue damage in relapsing neuromyelitis optica. AJNR Am J Neuroradiol 2006;27:1009.
57. Song SK, Yoshino J, Le TQ, et al. Demyelination increases radial diffusivity in corpus callosum of mouse brain. Neuroimage 2005;26:132.
58. Simon JH, Zhang S, Laidlaw DH, et al. Identification of fibers at risk for degeneration by diffusion tractography in patients at high risk for MS after a clinically isolated syndrome. J Magn Reson Imaging 2006;24:983.
59. Basser PJ, Pajevic S, Pierpaoli C, et al. In vivo fiber tractography using DT-MRI data. Magn Reson Med 2000;44(4):625.
60. Mori S, Crain B, Chacko V, et al. Three-dimensional tracking of axonal projections in the brain by magnetic resonance imaging. Ann Neurol 1999;45:265.
61. Behrens TE, Berg HJ, Jbabdi S, et al. Probabilistic diffusion tractography with multiple fibre orientations: what can we gain? Neuroimage 2007;34:144.
62. Jian B, Vemuri BC. Multi-fiber reconstruction from diffusion MRI using mixture of Wisharts and sparse deconvolution. Inf Process Med Imaging 2007;20:384.
63. Ozarslan E, Shepherd TM, Vemuri BC, et al. Resolution of complex tissue microarchitecture using the diffusion orientation transform (DOT). Neuroimage 2006; 31:1086.
64. Tuch DS. Q-ball imaging. Magn Reson Med 2004;52:1358.
65. Kreher BW, Mader I, Kiselev VG. Gibbs tracking: a novel approach for the reconstruction of neuronal pathways. Magn Reson Med 2008;60:953.
66. Staempfli P, Jaermann T, Crelier GR, et al. Resolving fiber crossing using advanced fast marching tractography based on diffusion tensor imaging. Neuroimage 2006;30:110.
67. Lowe MJ, Horenstein C, Hirsch JG, et al. Functional pathway-defined MRI diffusion measures reveal increased transverse diffusivity of water in multiple sclerosis. Neuroimage 2006;32:1127.
68. Heiervang E, Behrens TE, Mackay CE, et al. Between session reproducibility and between subject variability of diffusion MR and tractography measures. Neuroimage 2006;33:867.
69. Smith SM, Jenkinson M, Johansen-Berg H, et al. Tract-based spatial statistics: voxelwise analysis of multi-subject diffusion data. Neuroimage 2006;31:1487.
70. Dineen RA, Vilisaar J, Hlinka J, et al. Disconnection as a mechanism for cognitive dysfunction in multiple sclerosis. Brain 2009;132:239.
71. Giorgio A, Palace J, Johansen-Berg H, et al. Relationships of brain white matter microstructure with clinical and MR measures in relapsing-remitting multiple sclerosis. J Magn Reson Imaging 2010;31:309.
72. Filippi M, Cercignani M, Inglese M, et al. Diffusion tensor magnetic resonance imaging in multiple sclerosis. Neurology 2001;56:304.
73. Ge Y, Law M, Johnson G, et al. Preferential occult injury of corpus callosum in multiple sclerosis measured by diffusion tensor imaging. J Magn Reson Imaging 2004;20:1.
74. Naismith RT, Xu J, Tutlam NT, et al. Increased diffusivity in acute multiple sclerosis lesions predicts risk of black hole. Neurology 2010;74:1694.
75. Werring DJ, Clark CA, Barker GJ, et al. Diffusion tensor imaging of lesions and normal-appearing white matter in multiple sclerosis. Neurology 1999;52(8): 1626.
76. Shukla DK, Kaiser CC, Stebbins GT, et al. Effects of pioglitazone on diffusion tensor imaging indices in multiple sclerosis patients. Neurosci Lett 2010;472:153.

77. Sijens PE, Mostert JP, Irwan R, et al. Impact of fluoxetine on the human brain in multiple sclerosis as quantified by proton magnetic resonance spectroscopy and diffusion tensor imaging. Psychiatry Res 2008;164:274.

78. Fox RJ, McColl RW, Lee JC, et al. A preliminary validation study of diffusion tensor imaging as a measure of functional brain injury. Arch Neurol 2008;65: 1179.

79. Reich DS, Zackowski KM, Gordon-Lipkin EM, et al. Corticospinal tract abnormalities are associated with weakness in multiple sclerosis. AJNR Am J Neuroradiol 2008;29:333.

80. Wedeen VJ, Hagmann P, Tseng WY, et al. Mapping complex tissue architecture with diffusion spectrum magnetic resonance imaging. Magn Reson Med 2005; 54:1377.

81. Assaf Y, Ben-Bashat D, Chapman J, et al. High b-value q-space analyzed diffusion-weighted MRI: application to multiple sclerosis. Magn Reson Med 2002;47:115.

82. Mulkern RV, Gudbjartsson H, Westin CF, et al. Multi-component apparent diffusion coefficients in human brain. NMR Biomed 1999;12:51.

83. Jensen JH, Helpern JA, Ramani A, et al. Diffusional kurtosis imaging: the quantification of non-gaussian water diffusion by means of magnetic resonance imaging. Magn Reson Med 2005;53:1432.

84. Fox RJ. Picturing multiple sclerosis: conventional and diffusion tensor imaging. Semin Neurol 2008;28:453.

85. de Graaf RA. In vivo NMR spectroscopy Principles and techniques. New York: John Wiley & Sons; 1998.

86. Govindaraju V, Young K, Maudsley AA. Proton NMR chemical shifts and coupling constants for brain metabolites. NMR Biomed 2000;13:129.

87. Sajja BR, Wolinsky JS, Narayana PA. Proton magnetic resonance spectroscopy in multiple sclerosis. Neuroimaging Clin N Am 2009;19:45.

88. Davie CA, Barker GJ, Thompson AJ, et al. 1H magnetic resonance spectroscopy of chronic cerebral white matter lesions and normal appearing white matter in multiple sclerosis. J Neurol Neurosurg Psychiatry 1997;63:736.

89. Arnold DL, Matthews PM, Francis G, et al. Proton magnetic resonance spectroscopy of human brain in vivo in the evaluation of multiple sclerosis: assessment of the load of disease. Magn Reson Med 1990;14:154.

90. Narayana PA, Doyle TJ, Lai D, et al. Serial proton magnetic resonance spectroscopic imaging, contrast-enhanced magnetic resonance imaging, and quantitative lesion volumetry in multiple sclerosis. Ann Neurol 1998;43:56.

91. Kapeller P, McLean MA, Griffin CM, et al. Preliminary evidence for neuronal damage in cortical grey matter and normal appearing white matter in short duration relapsing-remitting multiple sclerosis: a quantitative MR spectroscopic imaging study. J Neurol 2001;248:131.

92. Chard DT, Griffin CM, McLean MA, et al. Brain metabolite changes in cortical grey and normal-appearing white matter in clinically early relapsing-remitting multiple sclerosis. Brain 2002;125:2342.

93. Gonen O, Catalaa I, Babb JS, et al. Total brain N-acetylaspartate: a new measure of disease load in MS. Neurology 2000;54:15.

94. Tiberio M, Chard DT, Altmann DR, et al. Metabolite changes in early relapsing-remitting multiple sclerosis. A two year follow-up study. J Neurol 2006;253:224.

95. Leary SM, Davie CA, Parker GJ, et al. 1H magnetic resonance spectroscopy of normal appearing white matter in primary progressive multiple sclerosis. J Neurol 1999;246:1023.

96. He J, Inglese M, Li BS, et al. Relapsing-remitting multiple sclerosis: metabolic abnormality in nonenhancing lesions and normal-appearing white matter at MR imaging: initial experience. Radiology 2005;234:211.

97. Inglese M, Li BS, Rusinek H, et al. Diffusely elevated cerebral choline and creatine in relapsing-remitting multiple sclerosis. Magn Reson Med 2003;50:190.

98. Larsson HB, Christiansen P, Jensen M, et al. Localized in vivo proton spectroscopy in the brain of patients with multiple sclerosis. Magn Reson Med 1991;22:23.

99. Arnold DL, Matthews PM, Francis GS, et al. Proton magnetic resonance spectroscopic imaging for metabolic characterization of demyelinating plaques. Ann Neurol 1992;31:235.

100. Tartaglia MC, Narayanan S, De Stefano N, et al. Choline is increased in prelesional normal appearing white matter in multiple sclerosis. J Neurol 2002; 249:1382.

101. Srinivasan R, Sailasuta N, Hurd R, et al. Evidence of elevated glutamate in multiple sclerosis using magnetic resonance spectroscopy at 3 T. Brain 2005; 128:1016.

102. De Stefano N, Matthews PM, Antel JP, et al. Chemical pathology of acute demyelinating lesions and its correlation with disability. Ann Neurol 1995;38:901.

103. Fernando KT, McLean MA, Chard DT, et al. Elevated white matter myo-inositol in clinically isolated syndromes suggestive of multiple sclerosis. Brain 2004;127: 1361.

104. Mader I, Seeger U, Weissert R, et al. Proton MR spectroscopy with metabolite-nulling reveals elevated macromolecules in acute multiple sclerosis. Brain 2001; 124:953.

105. Davie CA, Hawkins CP, Barker GJ, et al. Serial proton magnetic resonance spectroscopy in acute multiple sclerosis lesions. Brain 1994;117(Pt 1):49.

106. Narayana PA, Wolinsky JS, Rao SB, et al. Multicentre proton magnetic resonance spectroscopy imaging of primary progressive multiple sclerosis. Mult Scler 2004;10(Suppl 1):S73.

107. Bastianello S, Paolillo A, Giugni E, et al. MRI of spinal cord in MS. J Neurovirol 2000;6(Suppl 2):S130.

108. Tartaglino LM, Friedman DP, Flanders AE, et al. Multiple sclerosis in the spinal cord: MR appearance and correlation with clinical parameters. Radiology 1995;195:725.

109. Marliani AF, Clementi V, Albini-Riccioli L, et al. Quantitative proton magnetic resonance spectroscopy of the human cervical spinal cord at 3 Tesla. Magn Reson Med 2007;57:160.

110. Kendi AT, Tan FU, Kendi M, et al. MR spectroscopy of cervical spinal cord in patients with multiple sclerosis. Neuroradiology 2004;46:764.

111. Ciccarelli O, Wheeler-Kingshott CA, McLean MA, et al. Spinal cord spectroscopy and diffusion-based tractography to assess acute disability in multiple sclerosis. Brain 2007;130:2220.

112. Brownell B, Hughes JT. The distribution of plaques in the cerebrum in multiple sclerosis. J Neurol Neurosurg Psychiatry 1962;25:315.

113. Kidd D, Barkhof F, McConnell R, et al. Cortical lesions in multiple sclerosis. Brain 1999;122(Pt 1):17.

114. Choi IY, Lee SP, Merkle H, et al. In vivo detection of gray and white matter differences in GABA concentration in the human brain. Neuroimage 2006;33:85.

115. Petroff OA, Pleban LA, Spencer DD. Symbiosis between in vivo and in vitro NMR spectroscopy: the creatine, N-acetylaspartate, glutamate, and GABA content of the epileptic human brain. Magn Reson Imaging 1995;13:1197.

116. Dutta R, McDonough J, Yin X, et al. Mitochondrial dysfunction as a cause of axonal degeneration in multiple sclerosis patients. Ann Neurol 2006;59:478.

117. Bhattacharyya P, Phillips M, Bermel R, et al. Impaired motor performance in MS is associated with increased GABA level in sensorimotor cortex. Proc Int Soc Magn Reson Med 2010;18:390.

118. Kreis R. Issues of spectral quality in clinical 1H-magnetic resonance spectroscopy and a gallery of artifacts. NMR Biomed 2004;17:361.

119. Bhattacharyya PK, Lowe MJ, Phillips MD. Spectral quality control in motion-corrupted single-voxel J-difference editing scans: an interleaved navigator approach. Magn Reson Med 2007;58:808.

120. Felblinger J, Kreis R, Boesch C. Effects of physiologic motion of the human brain upon quantitative 1H-MRS: analysis and correction by retro-gating. NMR Biomed 1998;11:107.

121. Posse S, Cuenod CA, Le Bihan D. Human brain: proton diffusion MR spectroscopy. Radiology 1993;188:719.

122. Ziegler A, Decorp M. Signal-to-noise improvement in in-vivo spin-echo spectroscopy in the presence of motion. J Magn Reson 1993;102:26.

123. Buxton RB, Uludag K, Dubowitz DJ, et al. Modeling the hemodynamic response to brain activation. Neuroimage 2004;23(Suppl 1):S220.

124. Logothetis NK, Pauls J, Augath M, et al. Neurophysiological investigation of the basis of the fMRI signal. Nature 2001;412:150.

125. Kwong KK, Belliveau JW, Chesler DA, et al. Dynamic magnetic resonance imaging of human brain activity during primary sensory stimulation. Proc Natl Acad Sci U S A 1992;89:5675.

126. Ogawa S, Lee TM, Kay AR, et al. Brain magnetic resonance imaging with contrast dependent on blood oxygenation. Proc Natl Acad Sci U S A 1990;87:9868.

127. Biswal B, Yetkin FZ, Haughton VM, et al. Functional connectivity in the motor cortex of resting human brain using echo-planar MRI. Magn Reson Med 1995;34:537.

128. Lowe MJ, Mock BJ, Sorenson JA. Functional connectivity in single and multislice echoplanar imaging using resting-state fluctuations. Neuroimage 1998;7:119.

129. Miki A, Nakajima T, Fujita M, et al. Functional magnetic resonance imaging of the primary visual cortex: evaluation of human afferent visual system. Jpn J Ophthalmol 1995;39:302.

130. Yousry TA, Berry I, Filippi M. Functional magnetic resonance imaging in multiple sclerosis. J Neurol Neurosurg Psychiatry 1998;64(Suppl 1):S85.

131. Gareau PJ, Gati JS, Menon RS, et al. Reduced visual evoked responses in multiple sclerosis patients with optic neuritis: comparison of functional magnetic resonance imaging and visual evoked potentials. Mult Scler 1999;5:161.

132. Audoin B, Ibarrola D, Ranjeva JP, et al. Compensatory cortical activation observed by fMRI during a cognitive task at the earliest stage of MS. Hum Brain Mapp 2003;20:51.

133. Staffen W, Mair A, Zauner H, et al. Cognitive function and fMRI in patients with multiple sclerosis: evidence for compensatory cortical activation during an attention task. Brain 2002;125:1275.

134. Hillary FG, Chiaravalloti ND, Ricker JH, et al. An investigation of working memory rehearsal in multiple sclerosis using fMRI. J Clin Exp Neuropsychol 2003;25:965.

135. Parry AM, Scott RB, Palace J, et al. Potentially adaptive functional changes in cognitive processing for patients with multiple sclerosis and their acute modulation by rivastigmine. Brain 2003;126:2750.

136. Penner IK, Rausch M, Kappos L, et al. Analysis of impairment related functional architecture in MS patients during performance of different attention tasks. J Neurol 2003;250:461.

137. Sweet LH, Rao SM, Primeau M, et al. Functional magnetic resonance imaging of working memory among multiple sclerosis patients. J Neuroimaging 2004;14:150.

138. Lee M, Reddy H, Johansen-Berg H, et al. The motor cortex shows adaptive functional changes to brain injury from multiple sclerosis. Ann Neurol 2000;47:606.

139. Reddy H, Narayanan S, Arnoutelis R, et al. Evidence for adaptive functional changes in the cerebral cortex with axonal injury from multiple sclerosis. Brain 2000;123(Pt 11):2314.

140. Reddy H, Narayanan S, Woolrich M, et al. Functional brain reorganization for hand movement in patients with multiple sclerosis: defining distinct effects of injury and disability. Brain 2002;125:2646.

141. Rocca MA, Matthews PM, Caputo D, et al. Evidence for widespread movement-associated functional MRI changes in patients with PPMS. Neurology 2002; 58:866.

142. Filippi M, Rocca MA, Mezzapesa DM, et al. A functional MRI study of cortical activations associated with object manipulation in patients with MS. Neuroimage 2004;21:1147.

143. Ciccarelli O, Toosy AT, Marsden JF, et al. Functional response to active and passive ankle movements with clinical correlations in patients with primary progressive multiple sclerosis. J Neurol 2006;253:882.

144. Rocca MA, Filippi M. Functional MRI in multiple sclerosis. J Neuroimaging 2007; 17(Suppl 1):36S.

145. Buckle GJ. Functional magnetic resonance imaging and multiple sclerosis: the evidence for neuronal plasticity. J Neuroimaging 2005;15:82S.

146. Pantano P, Mainero C, Lenzi D, et al. A longitudinal fMRI study on motor activity in patients with multiple sclerosis. Brain 2005;128:2146.

147. Korsholm K, Madsen KH, Frederiksen JL, et al. Recovery from optic neuritis: an ROI-based analysis of LGN and visual cortical areas. Brain 2007;130:1244.

148. Audoin B, Reuter F, Duong MV, et al. Efficiency of cognitive control recruitment in the very early stage of multiple sclerosis: a one-year fMRI follow-up study. Mult Scler 2008;14:786.

149. Cardinal KS, Wilson SM, Giesser BS, et al. A longitudinal fMRI study of the paced auditory serial addition task. Mult Scler 2008;14:465.

150. Morgen K, Kadom N, Sawaki L, et al. Training-dependent plasticity in patients with multiple sclerosis. Brain 2004;127:2506.

151. Cader S, Palace J, Matthews PM. Cholinergic agonism alters cognitive processing and enhances brain functional connectivity in patients with multiple sclerosis. J Psychopharmacol 2009;23:686.

152. Pelletier J, Audoin B, Reuter F, et al. Plasticity in MS: from functional imaging to rehabilitation. Int MS J 2009;16:26.

153. Filippi M, Rocca MA, Colombo B, et al. Functional magnetic resonance imaging correlates of fatigue in multiple sclerosis. Neuroimage 2002;15:559.

154. DeLuca J, Genova HM, Hillary FG, et al. Neural correlates of cognitive fatigue in multiple sclerosis using functional MRI. J Neurol Sci 2008;270:28.

155. Tartaglia MC, Narayanan S, Arnold DL. Mental fatigue alters the pattern and increases the volume of cerebral activation required for a motor task in multiple sclerosis patients with fatigue. Eur J Neurol 2008;15:413.

156. White AT, Lee JN, Light AR, et al. Brain activation in multiple sclerosis: a BOLD fMRI study of the effects of fatiguing hand exercise. Mult Scler 2009;15:580.

157. Mainero C, Caramia F, Pozzilli C, et al. fMRI evidence of brain reorganization during attention and memory tasks in multiple sclerosis. Neuroimage 2004;21:858.

158. Rocca MA, Gallo A, Colombo B, et al. Pyramidal tract lesions and movement-associated cortical recruitment in patients with MS. Neuroimage 2004;23:141.

159. Lenzi D, Conte A, Mainero C, et al. Effect of corpus callosum damage on ipsilateral motor activation in patients with multiple sclerosis: a functional and anatomical study. Hum Brain Mapp 2007;28:636.

160. Bonzano L, Pardini M, Mancardi GL, et al. Structural connectivity influences brain activation during PVSAT in Multiple Sclerosis. Neuroimage 2009;44:9.

161. Lowe MJ, Beall EB, Sakaie KE, et al. Resting state sensorimotor functional connectivity in multiple sclerosis inversely correlates with transcallosal motor pathway transverse diffusivity. Hum Brain Mapp 2008;29:818.

162. Mainero C, Pantano P, Caramia F, et al. Brain reorganization during attention and memory tasks in multiple sclerosis: insights from functional MRI studies. J Neurol Sci 2006;245:93.

163. Ingle GT, Thompson AJ, Miller DH. Magnetic resonance imaging in primary progressive multiple sclerosis. J Rehabil Res Dev 2002;39:261.

164. Iannetti GD, Wise RG. BOLD functional MRI in disease and pharmacological studies: room for improvement? Magn Reson Imaging 2007;25:978.

165. Bullmore ET, Brammer MJ, Rabe-Hesketh S, et al. Methods for diagnosis and treatment of stimulus-correlated motion in generic brain activation studies using fMRI. Hum Brain Mapp 1999;7:38.

166. Bhattacharyya PK, Lowe MJ. Cardiac-induced physiologic noise in tissue is a direct observation of cardiac-induced fluctuations. Magn Reson Imaging 2004;22:9.

167. Lund TE, Madsen KH, Sidaros K, et al. Non-white noise in fMRI: does modelling have an impact? Neuroimage 2006;29:54.

Diagnosis of Multiple Sclerosis

Barbara S. Giesser, MD

KEYWORDS

• Multiple sclerosis • Cerebrospinal fluid • MRI
• Evoked potential

There is no pathognomonic symptom, sign, or paraclinical result that provides an unfailingly accurate diagnosis of multiple sclerosis (MS), and hence, MS remains largely a clinical diagnosis. However, being a clinical diagnosis does not mean that the diagnosis of MS is one of exclusion. Increasingly sophisticated guidelines and objective paraclinical findings are generally sufficient to allow the clinician to confirm or rule out the diagnosis with confidence. This article presents the most recent guidelines for using clinical, radiological, and other paraclinical information and the red flags that should alert the clinician to investigate other diagnostic possibilities.

With the advent of disease-modifying therapy in 1993, it became more important to establish (or rule out) a definitive diagnosis of MS as early as possible. This early definitive diagnosis allows the patient not only to begin disease-modifying therapy early, and possibly reduce or delay long-term central nervous system (CNS) damage, but also to begin the process of education, lifestyle modifications as needed, and planning for the future.

DIAGNOSTIC CRITERIA

The clinical criteria published by Schumacher and colleagues[1] still remain the sine qua non for invoking a diagnosis of MS. To reduce these criteria to their quintessential form, the investigators stated that the diagnosis of MS rests on the demonstration of objective CNS white matter lesions separated in space and time, with the exclusion of other conditions that could mimic the clinical and paraclinical findings (**Box 1**).

In 1983, in an attempt to refine the diagnostic criteria so that inclusion of subjects into clinical trials would be more uniform, Poser and colleagues[2] published the first set of diagnostic criteria that included paraclinical (radiological, evoked potentials [EPs]) data, although most of the information remained clinical. This schema also generated a category called laboratory-supported MS that applies to individuals who do not meet the criteria for diagnosis on clinical grounds alone and requires

Department of Neurology, David Geffen University of California, Los Angeles School of Medicine, 710 Westwood Plaza, Los Angeles, CA 90095, USA
E-mail address: bgiesser@mednet.ucla.edu

Neurol Clin 29 (2011) 381–388
doi:10.1016/j.ncl.2010.12.001   neurologic.theclinics.com
0733-8619/11/$ – see front matter © 2011 Elsevier Inc. All rights reserved.

> **Box 1**
> **Criteria for the diagnosis of clinically definite MS by Schumacher and colleagues**
>
> 1. Age of onset of symptoms between 10 and 50 years
>
> 2. Objective abnormalities on neurologic examination
>
> 3. Signs and symptoms localize to CNS (brain, spinal cord, and optic nerve) white matter
>
> 4. Lesions are disseminated in space (2 or more separate lesions)
>
> 5. Lesions are disseminated in time (2 attacks lasting at least 24 hours at least 1 month apart) or insidious progression of lesions over at least 6 months
>
> 6. No other diagnosis
>
> *From* Schumacher G, Beebe G, Kibler R, et al. Problems of experimental trials of therapy in multiple sclerosis. Ann N Y Acad Sci 1965;122:552–68; with permission.

the presence of 2 or more oligoclonal bands (OCBs) in the cerebrospinal fluid (CSF) or evidence of increased intrathecal IgG levels.

An important refinement was introduced in 2001, when an international panel headed by Dr W. Ian McDonald produced what have come to be known as the McDonald criteria, which allow the use of magnetic resonance imaging (MRI) findings to provide evidence of spatiotemporal dissemination.[3] The criteria also specified parameters for the diagnosis of primary progressive MS (**Table 1**).

The most recent modifications of these criteria were published in 2005 by Polman and colleagues[4] and have basically eliminated the requirement of a positive CSF finding to establish a diagnosis of primary progressive MS. The modifications have

Table 1
McDonald criteria

Clinical Episode	Objective Finding	Additional Data Needed to Confirm Diagnosis
2	2	None
2	1	Dissemination in space on MRI OR 2 MRI lesions typical of MS plus presence of OCBs in CSF or elevated CSF IgG levels OR second clinical episode
1	2	Dissemination in time on MRI[a] OR second clinical episode
1	1	Dissemination in space on MRI OR positive CSF finding with 2 MRI lesions typical of MS AND dissemination in time on MRI or second clinical episode
Progressive	1	Positive CSF finding AND dissemination in space on MRI[b] AND dissemination in time on MRI OR continued progression over at least 1 y

[a] Dissemination in time on MRI requires the appearance of a new T2- or gadolinium-enhancing lesion on a scan obtained at least 3 mo after the initial MRI.
[b] MRI criteria: at least 9 T2 cerebral lesions and at least 2 spinal cord lesions OR abnormal VEP with 4 to 8 cerebral MRI lesions OR abnormal VEP with less than 4 cerebral lesions plus 1 spinal cord lesion.
Adapted from Miller AE, Coyle PK. Clinical features of multiple sclerosis. Continuum 2004; 10(6):55; with permission.

simplified the requirement for dissemination in time on MRI in that a new T2 lesion on a follow-up MRI in comparison with a reference scan is sufficient if the reference scan was done at least 30 days after the initial clinical event. The modifications also clarify the use of spinal cord lesions in fulfilling MRI criteria in that a spinal cord lesion may count as an infratentorial lesion, may contribute to the overall total of T2 lesions, and if enhancing, may substitute for a brain-enhancing lesion.

MRI CRITERIA

The criteria for lesions consistent with MS that demonstrate dissemination in space as stated in the McDonald criteria are adapted from the studies by Barkhof and colleagues[5] and Tintore and colleagues.[6] Any 3 of the following criteria are required for the diagnosis:

1. Nine T2 hyperintense or 1 gadolinium-enhancing cerebral lesion
2. At least 1 infratentorial lesion
3. At least 1 juxtacortical lesion
4. At least 3 periventricular lesions.

A spinal cord lesion may substitute for a cerebral lesion with the caveats stated earlier.

In addition to location, which includes the areas listed earlier and in and around the corpus callosum, white matter lesions due to MS may typically be ovoid or irregularly shaped. When the lesions are oriented perpendicularly to the lateral ventricles, they have the eponym Dawson fingers.

A new MRI entity that has been described is radiologically isolated syndrome (RIS).[7] RIS refers to a cerebral MRI finding with lesions characteristic of MS in asymptomatic individuals. In 2 studies that followed up a cohort of patients with RIS for several years, about one-third subsequently developed a clinical event consistent with MS.[8,9] More studies are needed to identify those factors that predict conversion to clinically definite MS in persons with RIS.

CSF

CSF analysis may be performed to help establish a diagnosis of MS when there is a paucity of clinical or radiological findings. The most common abnormalities reflect the presence of intrathecal immunoglobulin synthesis (presence of OCBs, increased IgG synthesis rate and index). However, not all persons with MS have abnormal spinal fluid, and thus, although the presence of normal spinal fluid may raise doubt about the diagnosis, it does not rule out the diagnosis if other diagnostic criteria are met.

OCBs are made of a group of proteins that can be electrophoretically separated from CSF IgG. The antigens eliciting the production of OCBs have not yet been identified. Up to 95% of persons with MS show OCBs in their CSF, and in order to indicate a diagnosis of MS, there have to be at least 2 bands present in the CSF, which are not present in the serum.[10] Other entities can produce OCBs in the CSF,[11–14] and their presence should be interpreted in the appropriate clinical context (**Box 2**).

Another marker of intrathecal IgG production is the IgG index relative to serum IgG. A CSF IgG index greater than 0.7 is abnormal and may be elevated in about 75% of persons with MS.[11] The level of myelin basic protein may be normal in persons with MS and even if elevated, it is a very nonspecific marker and thus is less useful for diagnosis.

Box 2
Diseases that can produce OCBs in the CSF

Inflammatory

    Systemic lupus erythematosus

    Behçet syndrome

    Sarcoid

    Anticardiolipin syndrome

    Sjögren syndrome

Infectious

    Neuroborreliosis

    Neurotuberculosis

    Human immunodeficiency virus infection

    Herpes simplex virus infection

    Neurosyphillis

Neoplastic

    CNS lymphoma

    Paraneoplastic syndromes

    Primary brain tumor

Routine parameters in the CSF, that is, cell count and chemistries are usually normal or only slightly elevated in persons with MS. If the white blood cell count is more than 50 cells/µL or the protein level is greater than 110 mg/dL, alternative diagnoses should be considered.[13] A notable exception is the CSF in neuromyelitis optica (NMO), which may often have elevated white blood cell counts and protein levels and may less commonly show the presence of OCBs.[11,15]

EPs

EP testing assesses the CNS response to specific sensory stimuli and is a sensitive, harmless, noninvasive testing modality. This test is particularly useful for providing evidence of a clinically silent second lesion and can thus often help to establish a diagnosis if there are insufficient clinical findings. The most commonly used EPs are visual (VEP), somatosensory (SSEP), and brainstem auditory (BAEP). VEP can contribute in some specific instances to the diagnosis of MS according to the McDonald criteria.

To record VEP, the subject has recording electrodes placed over the occipital cortex and is then asked to look at an alternating checkerboard pattern on a screen.

A major positive wave, P100, is recorded approximately 100 milliseconds after presentation of the stimulus. Where there is impaired conduction along optic pathways, for example, because of optic neuritis, the latency of the wave is slowed, although morphology and amplitude may be degraded as well. In patients with a history of optic neuritis, the VEP is abnormal about 90% of the time, but VEP may be abnormal on average in more than 50% of patients who have no history of optic neuritis.[16]

BAEPs are recorded while the subject hears a series of auditory stimuli and records 5 waves generated by structures along auditory pathways from the auditory nerve through the brainstem pathways to the auditory cortex. Studies indicate that about 20% to 55% of the time the BAEP is abnormal in patients without clinical brainstem findings.[16]

The SSEPs record responses from peripheral nerve stimulation through dorsal column, medial lemniscus, and thalamic pathways to the somatosensory cortex and can be elicited by upper and/or lower limb stimulation. Reported rates of abnormal SSEPs for persons with possible or suspected MS are around 50%,[16] with abnormalities being found somewhat more frequently with lower limb testing.

As stated earlier, the primary utility of EP testing is to help discern clinically silent evidence of CNS lesions. The American Academy of Neurology guidelines for EPs state that VEPs are recommended as "probably useful" to identify patients at risk for developing clinically definite MS, SSEPs are "possibly useful," and there is "insufficient evidence" to recommend BAEP for this purpose.[17] In patients with a first event or clinically isolated syndrome (CIS) (eg, optic neuritis, brainstem/cerebellar syndrome, or transverse myelitis), the presence of abnormal EPs and/or abnormal CSF findings is associated with a higher risk of converting to clinically definite MS.

PRESENTING SYMPTOMS OF MS
Sensory Symptoms

The most common presenting symptom of MS is sensory, usually numbness and paresthesias. Lightninglike, burning, prickling, or stabbing dysesthesias are not uncommon. Patients may also complain of an unpleasant sensation as though a tight band or girdle is around their thorax, sometimes referred to by patients as the "MS hug." Often, patients describe an electric or vibrating sensation that travels down their limbs or back with neck flexion. This sensation is the Lhermitte sign and indicates a cervical spinal cord lesion.

Motor weakness, especially in the lower limbs, is a common presenting symptom of MS. Patients may also present with gait disturbances due to ataxia. Other cerebellar problems include appendicular ataxia and kinetic tremor.

Other Symptoms

Optic neuritis is a presenting symptom of MS about 15% of the time. Other visual complaints may include diplopia, nystagmus, or oscillopsia. Brainstem symptoms may include trigeminal neuralgia, Bell palsy, vertigo, orofacial numbness, and, uncommonly, tinnitus or hearing loss. Genitourinary symptoms are very common in the population with MS but occur as a presenting symptom in only a few percent of cases.

Unusual or debilitating fatigue may be the very first symptom of MS, but is often ascribed to other causes. Pain occurs in more than 50% of the population diagnosed with MS and has been reported as an initial symptom in up to 11% of patients.[18] Other characteristics that suggest a diagnosis of MS are intermittent nature of symptoms and worsening of symptoms with heat.

RED FLAGS

Some clinical clues that should raise suspicion about the diagnosis include the following: prominent family history (about 80% of persons with MS do not have another affected family member); relentlessly progressive course, particularly in younger individuals; prominent or persistent headache; prominent cortical features (seizures, aphasia, neglect syndromes); abrupt and/or transient (few minutes to hours) duration of symptoms; presence of peripheral neuropathy; and involvement of other organ systems, such as cardiac, hematologic, or rheumatologic. In addition, sensory and genitourinary complaints are so common that their absence should prompt a question about the diagnosis.

As suggested earlier, the differential diagnosis of MS is extensive. Generally, the major categories of disease to consider include vasculitic, infectious, metabolic, neoplastic, and neurodegenerative. A conservative screening evaluation for other causes include metabolic panel and complete blood cell count, erythrocyte sedimentation rate, vitamin B_{12} level, double-stranded DNA test, rheumatoid factor concentration, thyroid-stimulating hormone level, and if suggested by the history, human immunodeficiency virus and *Borrelia* titers. To cite a few other specific examples, a history of clotting disorders or recurrent miscarriage may prompt determination of the presence of anticardiolipin and antiphospholipid antibodies. In African American individuals, it may be appropriate to assay angiotensin-converting enzyme levels to screen for sarcoid. On occasion, there are patients who might best be described as "MS wannabes," that is, patients with a multitude of symptoms and who are very invested in having a diagnosis of MS but have no objective findings on examination or paraclinical testing.

In patients who present with optic neuritis and/or transverse myelitis, the diagnosis of NMO must be considered. The diagnostic criteria state that in addition to optic neuritis and/or transverse myelitis, the diagnosis of NMO requires at least 2 of the following: nondiagnostic cerebral MRI, presence of a spinal cord lesion spanning at least 3 longitudinal vertebral segments, and seropositivity to the NMO antibody, that is, antibody to the water channel aquaporin 4.[19] Brain MRI in persons with NMO may show lesions, but the results are frequently normal. In addition, presence of OCBs in the CSF is much less common in persons with NMO than in those with MS, occurring in only about 20% of cases.[20]

Patients who present with a first neurologic episode and objective evidence of CNS white matter lesions, particularly optic neuritis, transverse myelitis, or brainstem and cerebellar findings, are said to have CIS. These individuals do not fulfill the criteria for the diagnosis of MS because there is no dissemination in time. In a longitudinal study of patients who presented with CIS, O'Riordan and colleagues[21] found that the presence of 2 or more lesions on initial MRI was associated with more than 80% conversion rate to clinically definite MS.

Acute disseminated encephalomyelitis (ADEM) may sometimes be confused with an initial episode of MS. Typically, ADEM tends to occur more commonly in children after a viral illness or vaccination, is monophasic, does not show a female predominance as does MS, and is characterized by diffuse brain lesions with variable gadolinium enhancement. In addition, CSF is more likely to show a pleocytosis and elevated total white cell counts and protein levels and OCBs are less likely to be present in ADEM than in MS.[11] Miller and colleagues[20] propose that the presence of encephalopathy is required for the diagnosis of ADEM and that recurrence of symptoms may occur within a 3-month period but cannot occur after a period of complete remission.

SUMMARY

The diagnosis of MS requires objective clinical and paraclinical documentation of CNS white matter lesions that cannot be ascribed to other causes. Clinical context dictates which other processes may need to be considered, for example, increased suspicion of NMO in a non-White population, ADEM in a child or adolescent, vasculitis if there is evidence of systemic disease, or infection if the history indicates risk factors for an infectious cause. As more knowledge is gained about the pathophysiology of MS, it is hoped that the identification of specific biomarkers will make the diagnosis more timely and specific.

REFERENCES

1. Schumacher G, Beebe G, Kibler R, et al. Problems of experimental trials of therapy in multiple sclerosis. Ann N Y Acad Sci 1965;122:552–68.
2. Poser C, Paty D, Scheinberg L, et al. New diagnostic criteria for multiple sclerosis: guidelines for research protocols. Ann Neurol 1983;13:227–31.
3. McDonald WI, Compston A, Edan G, et al. Recommended diagnostic criteria for multiple sclerosis: guidelines from the international panel on the diagnosis of multiple sclerosis. Ann Neurol 2001;50:121–7.
4. Polman C, Reingold S, Edan G, et al. Diagnostic criteria for multiple sclerosis: 2005 revisions to the "McDonald criteria". Ann Neurol 2005;58:840–6.
5. Barkhof F, Rocca M, Francis G, et al. Validation of diagnostic magnetic resonance imaging criteria for multiple sclerosis and response to interferon beta1a. Ann Neurol 2003;53:718–24.
6. Tintore M, Rovira A, Rio J, et al. New diagnostic criteria for multiple sclerosis: application in first demyelinating episode. Neurology 2003;60:27–30.
7. Okuda DT, Mowry EM, Beheshtian A, et al. Incidental MRI anomalies suggestive of multiple sclerosis: the radiologically isolated syndrome. Neurology 2009;72(9): 800–5.
8. Lebrun C, Bensa C, Debouverie M, et al. Association between clinical conversion to multiple sclerosis in radiologically isolated syndrome and magnetic resonance imaging, cerebrospinal fluid, and visual evoked potential: follow up of 70 patients. Arch Neurol 2009;66(7):841–6.
9. Siva S, Saip S, Altintas A, et al. Multiple sclerosis risk in radiologically uncovered asymptomatic possible inflammatory demyelinating disease. Mult Scler 2009; 15(8):918–27.
10. Link H, Huang YM. Oligoclonal bands in multiple sclerosis cerebrospinal fluid: an update on methodology and clinical usefulness. J Neuroimmunol 2006;180(1): 17–28.
11. Mehling M, Kuhle J, Regeniter A. 10 most commonly asked questions about cerebrospinal fluid characteristics in demyelinating disorders of the central nervous system. Neurologist 2008;14(1):60–5.
12. Franciotta D, Columba-Cabezas S, Andreoni L, et al. Oligoclonal IgG band patterns in inflammatory demyelinating human and mouse diseases. J Neuroimmunol 2008;200(1):125–8.
13. Bourahoui A, de Seze J, Guttierez R, et al. CSF isoelectrofocusing in a large cohort of MS and other neurological diseases. Eur J Neurol 2004;11:525–9.
14. Tourtellotte WW, Tumani H. Multiple sclerosis cerebrospinal fluid. In: Raine CS, Mc Farland H, Tourtellotte WW, editors. Multiple sclerosis: clinical and pathological basis. London, Weinheim, Toyko, New York, Melbourne, Madras: Chapman & Hall Medical; 1997. p. 58–9.
15. Zaffaroni M. Cerebrospinal fluid findings in Devic's neuromyelitis optica. Neurol Sci 2004;24(Suppl 4):S368–70.
16. Chiappa K. Pattern shift visual, brainstem auditory, and short latency somatosensory evoked potentials in MS. Ann N Y Acad Sci 1984;436:315–27.
17. Gronseth G, Ashman E. Practice parameter: the usefulness of evoked potentials in identifying clinically silent lesions in patients with suspected MS (an evidence based review). Neurology 2000;54:1720–5.

18. Paty D, Noseworthy J, Ebers G. Diagnosis of multiple sclerosis. In: Paty D, Ebers G, editors. Multiple sclerosis. Philadelphia: F.A. Davis Co; 1998. p. 73.
19. WIngerchuk D. Diagnosis and treatment of neuromyelitis optica. Neurologist 2007;13(1):2–11.
20. Miller D, Weinshenker B, Fillipi M, et al. Differential diagnosis of suspected multiple sclerosis: a consensus approach. Mult Scler 2008;14:1157–74.
21. O'Riordan J, Thompson A, Kingsley D, et al. The prognostic value of brain MRI in clinically isolated syndromes of the CNS. A 10-year follow-up. Brain 1998; 121(Pt 3):495–503.

Treatment of Multiple Sclerosis Exacerbations

Pavle Repovic, MD, PhD[a], Fred D. Lublin, MD[b],*

KEYWORDS

- Multiple sclerosis • Exacerbation • Relapse
- Steroid • Treatment

For most patients with multiple sclerosis (MS), exacerbations are a powerful reminder of the unpredictability of their disease. Variously referred to as *exacerbations*, *flares*, *bouts*, *relapses*, or *attacks*, they are a hallmark of the disease for about 85% of the patients with MS. For these patients, no other feature of MS is as frightening as a prospect of an acute neurologic deficit that strikes at random and in such protean ways. The understanding of what constitutes an exacerbation has evolved along with the advances in the knowledge of MS in general. Most often, an exacerbation is thought of as a new neurologic deficit lasting 24 hours or more, in the absence of fever or infection.[1] There are, however, exceptions to this rule. Exacerbation may present as a paroxysmal symptom that recurs in a stereotypical fashion over the course of a day, lasting no more than a few seconds or minutes at a time. Worsening of a preexisting symptom may also be an exacerbation if no alternative explanation can be found. Most exacerbations evolve in severity over hours to days, although sudden onset has been described. Neurologic symptoms evolving over months, in contrast, are more typical of progressive MS.

An exacerbation can present as any symptom of a central nervous system lesion, from a typical optic neuritis to coma and pulmonary edema.[2,3] However, random exacerbations may appear, and there may be a pattern of recurrence such that a previously affected neuroanatomic site is more likely to be a target of subsequent exacerbation. For example, if the initial demyelinating event affected the optic nerve or spinal cord, the odds of a subsequent exacerbation affecting the same site are about 6-fold for the optic nerve and 3-fold for the spinal cord.[4]

This work was supported by Sylvia Lawry Fellowship Grant no. FP 1764-A-1 awarded to P.R. from the National Multiple Sclerosis Society.

[a] Multiple Sclerosis Center, Swedish Neuroscience Institute, 1600 East Jefferson Street, Suite 205, Seattle, WA 98122, USA
[b] Corinne Goldsmith Dickinson Center for Multiple Sclerosis, Department of Neurology, Mount Sinai Medical Center, 5 East 98th Street, Box 1138, New York, NY 10029, USA
* Corresponding author.
E-mail address: fred.lublin@exchange.mssm.edu

Neurol Clin 29 (2011) 389–400
doi:10.1016/j.ncl.2010.12.012
0733-8619/11/$ – see front matter © 2011 Elsevier Inc. All rights reserved.

neurologic.theclinics.com

It has long been recognized that heat, fever, and infection may lead to reemergence of symptoms from a prior exacerbation. This reemergence is known as a pseudoexacerbation and is thought to arise from a temperature-dependent conduction block across demyelinated segments of axons.[5] More recently, N-methyl-D-aspartate (NMDA) antagonist memantine has joined the list of pseudoexacerbation triggers, suggesting a role for NMDA in this process.[6] Pseudoexacerbations are expected to resolve once the offending agent is removed. However, some infections may lead to a bona fide exacerbation.[7]

An exacerbation is usually followed by a variable period of self-repair that manifests clinically as remission of symptoms. Although a complete recovery can occur, usually early in the disease process, the residual deficit may persist and contribute to the stepwise progression of disability across the course of MS.[8–11] Minimizing the risk of an exacerbation has been the mainstay of current MS treatment. Nevertheless, none of the available therapies have been able to entirely prevent exacerbations. For this reason, appropriate management of MS exacerbations remains a cornerstone of MS care. This article reviews the current body of knowledge regarding the treatment of MS exacerbations.

STEROIDS

Corticosteroids have been used for the treatment of MS exacerbations since the 1950s. Their use was first reported by Jonsson and colleagues[12] and Glaser and Merritt[13] in 1951, but it was not until 1970 that the first large randomized control trial established firm evidence in support of corticosteroid use in this setting.[14] In this landmark study, the largest to date specifically addressing the treatment of MS exacerbations, Rose and colleagues[14] randomized 197 patients in a double-blind fashion to receive placebo (94 patients) or intramuscular adrenocorticotropic hormone (ACTH) (103 patients; 40 U twice a day for 7 days, 20 U twice a day for 4 days, 20 U daily for 3 days). Only patients with diagnosed MS who were within 8 weeks of an exacerbation and showed no or minimal spontaneous improvement were enrolled. Patients were evaluated a day before treatment and weekly thereafter up to 1 month. Patients treated with ACTH were found to be more likely to improve than those treated with placebo, and to do so sooner. There was no evidence that ACTH-treated patients improved to a greater extent than the placebo arm.

A major contribution of this study was that it provided a roadmap for subsequent studies in the treatment of MS exacerbations. No fewer than 7 rating scales were used: Disability Status Scale (DSS), clinical estimate of overall condition, standard neurologic examination, functional systems, 7-day symptom scoring, worsening of existing symptoms, and quantitative examination of neurologic function. Comparing various rating scales, the investigators concluded that the "disability status scale, together with the functional systems, comprises an adequate system of evaluating change in a therapeutic trial of MS and, of all the measures used in this study, apparently is the most consistent indicator of change."[14]

In 1985, Durelli and colleagues[15] published the first randomized controlled trial of intravenous (IV) steroids. This randomized double-blind trial was conducted on 23 patients and compared IV methylprednisolone (MP) with placebo. A total of 13 patients received a tapering dose of IV MP totaling 100.5 mg/kg over 15 days; thereafter, both placebo and treatment arms received a lengthy taper of oral prednisone over 120 days. Recipients of IV MP were more likely to improve on day 5, 10, and 15 compared with placebo-treated patients, with improvement defined as a decrease of 1.0 or more on the Expanded DSS (EDSS). The investigators concluded that the IV MP shortened the duration of exacerbations and increased the odds of improvement over 15 days. However, the extent of recovery was not reported. Furthermore, although IV MP was relatively well tolerated, most patients developed significant side effects on the long prednisone taper.

Milligan and colleagues[16] eliminated the oral steroid taper and treated 50 patients, 22 with acute exacerbation and 28 in the progressive phase, with 500 mg IV MP or saline placebo for 5 days (total dose, 2500 mg). Following an exacerbation, the residual deficits measured by DSS were significantly lower in the IV MP-treated group at 1 and 4 weeks of treatment.

The utility of steroids in the treatment of MS exacerbations was further supported by meta-analyses. Including all of the studies mentioned earlier, Filippini and colleagues[17] found that treatment with ACTH or MP minimizes the risk of worsening or no improvement by 5 weeks from exacerbation (Peto odds ratio, 0.37). This result implies that, for every 1000 patients treated with ACTH or MP, 247 more patients will have improved within 5 weeks compared with placebo. The effect was greater, but not significantly so, for MP than for ACTH. Miller and colleagues,[18] in their meta-analysis, also found a positive effect of MP in lowering the EDSS score by a mean of 0.76 compared with placebo at 1 or 3 to 4 weeks.

Steroid Route

Parenteral administration of steroids has been recognized as not only cumbersome for the patient but also expensive and not without inherent risks associated with venipuncture. Oral steroids, depending on the type, can be dosed to achieve a bioavailability similar to that of steroids administered parenterally. A small but helpful study by Morrow and colleagues[19] found that, over 24 hours, both 1250 mg oral prednisone and 1000 mg IV MP achieved the same mean area under the concentration-time curve, a major component of bioavailability. The 2 routes, however, were different with respect to the time-to-peak concentration (1 hour for IV MP vs 2 hours for prednisone) and peak concentrations (about 12 mg/mL for IV MP vs 4 mg/mL for prednisone).

In 1998, Sellebjerg and colleagues[20] reported on the use of oral MP in the treatment of MS exacerbations. A total of 25 patients were randomized to placebo or 500 mg oral MP for 5 days, with a 10-day taper in a double-blind fashion (total steroid dose, 3676 mg). Significantly more patients administered oral MP than placebo improved by at least 1 EDSS unit at 1, 3, and 8 weeks. A similar study demonstrated benefit of the same oral steroid regimen in optic neuritis.[21]

Sellebjerg and colleagues'[20] findings on oral steroids, however, came against a backdrop of a much larger and influential Optic Neuritis Treatment Trial (ONTT), published in 1992.[22] The ONTT recruited 457 patients with acute unilateral optic neuritis and randomized patients to 1 of 3 arms: oral placebo, oral prednisone (1 mg/kg/d for 14 days), or IV MP (250 mg every 6 hours for 3 days, followed by oral prednisone 1 mg/kg/d for 11 days). Each group received a brief oral prednisone taper on days 15 (20 mg), 16 (10 mg), and 18 (10 mg). The trial was blinded only between the non-IV arms (prednisone and placebo) but not with respect to the IV treatment. Although most patients across all treatment groups experienced vision recovery within 2 weeks, the recovery was significantly more rapid in the IV MP group than in the placebo group, with the greatest difference noted on days 4 and 15. Thereafter, the difference between the groups decreased, and by 1 year, was negligible. Recovery in the low-dose oral prednisone group did not differ from that in the placebo group at any point. Among various theories put forth to explain the difference in outcomes between prednisone and IV MP, it was suggested that the oral route may have been inferior to the IV route. Others have implicated the difference in dose, rather than the route, as responsible for different outcomes.

Several trials have addressed the question of whether oral and IV routes are equivalent. Alam and colleagues[23] conducted a double-blind placebo-controlled trial of MP (500 mg daily) administered either IV or orally for 5 days to 35 patients, without detecting any significant difference in the EDSS score among the groups 5 and 28 days after administration of the steroids. This study, however, may have been underpowered (98 patients per group would have detected a 10% difference in the outcome).

Barnes and colleagues[24] reported a double-blind trial of 80 patients randomized to IV MP (1 g/d for 3 days) or oral MP (48 mg/d for 7 days, 24 mg/d for 7 days, 12 mg/d for 7 days). There was no difference between the groups in terms of the EDSS score, Hauser Ambulation Index, and arm-function index at any point during the study (1–24 weeks). The study had more than 90% power to detect a change in 1 EDSS unit at 4 weeks (primary outcome measure) but did not use a noninferiority design.

A noninferiority trial of IV and oral MP (both 1 g/d for 5 days) was performed by Martinelli and colleagues[25] on 40 patients. The primary end point of this trial was a reduction in the number of gadolinium-enhancing lesions on magnetic resonance imaging (MRI) at 1 week. Oral MP was noninferior to IV MP on this outcome, even though there were more enhancing lesions in the oral MP group at baseline. The groups also did not differ significantly in their EDSS scores.

A meta-analysis comparing oral and IV steroids for the treatment of MS exacerbations found no evidence that the 2 routes were significantly different in terms of improvement of their EDSS scores by week 4.[26] However, because of the small number of patients studied and trial methodologies used, the investigators concluded that it may be premature to declare equivalence of oral and IV steroids in terms of their efficacy and safety.

In addition to the oral route, intrathecal administration of steroids has also been investigated in MS exacerbation treatment. The intrathecal route was no more effective in MS exacerbation treatment than the IV route and, for obvious reasons, did not garner much additional testing.[27]

Steroid Dose and Type

The earliest attempt at comparing different types of corticosteroids was reported by Abruzzese and colleagues,[28] but the study was open label. Barnes and colleagues[29] compared IV MP with IM ACTH (**Table 1**) in a randomized examiner-blinded study and found that IV MP led to faster recovery than ACTH at 7 and 28 days, although at 3 months the groups did not differ. Subsequent trials have not confirmed the superiority of MP. Thompson and colleagues'[30] randomized double-blind study of IV MP and ACTH in 61 patients, although at doses somewhat different from those in the study by Barnes and colleagues, found no difference in the EDSS response at any time between 3 days and 3 months. In another study by Milanese and colleagues,[31] 30 patients were assigned to ACTH, dexamethasone (78 mg), and low-dose MP (390 mg), all administered by the IV route in a double-blinded fashion (see **Table 1**). Both the ACTH and dexamethasone groups performed better than the low-dose MP group as measured by the change in the EDSS score at 7 and 30 days posttreatment. However, the groups were not well matched in terms of mean disease duration (43 months for ACTH vs 75–85 months for others) and preexacerbation EDSS scores (2.7 in MP group vs 0.75–1 in others). There were more patients with progressive MS in the MP group as well. A similar study by La Mantia and colleagues[32] compared dexamethasone with 2 doses of MP (high and low), administered IV. Dexamethasone and

Table 1
Studies comparing various types and routes of steroids for treatment of MS exacerbations

Study	Group 1 (Total Dose [mg]); n	Group 2 (Total Dose); n	Group 3 (Total Dose [mg]); n	Definition of Relapse	EDSS Measurement
Barnes et al,[29] 1985	IV MP (7000); 14 1000 mg × 7 d	IM ACTH (1120 U); 11 80 U × 7 d 60 U × 7 d 20 U × 7 d		CDMS, within 4 wk without improvement in EDSS: 3.9–4.4	0, 3, 7, 30, 90 d
Thompson et al,[30] 1989	IV MP (3000); 29 1000 mg × 3 d + IM placebo	IM ACTH (750 U); 32 80 U × 7 d 40 U × 4 d 20 U × 3 d + IV placebo		CDMS within 4 wk, not improving, EDSS<5 prerelapse EDSS 4.3–4.6	3, 7, 14, 30, 90 d
La Mantia et al,[32] 1994	IV MP (390); 10 40 mg × 7 d 20 mg × 4 d 10 mg × 3 d	IV MP (5750 mg); 10 1000 mg × 3 d 500 mg × 3 d 250 mg × 3 d 125 mg × 3 d 62.5 mg × 2 d	Dexamethasone (78); 11 8 mg × 7 d 4 mg × 4 d 2 mg × 3 d	RRMS, at least 1 EDSS, <4 wk, >6 d, not improving EDSS 4.36–4.77	–1, 2, 4, 7, 14, 30, 60, 120, 180, 365 d
Milanese et al,[31] 1989	IV MP (390); 10 40 mg × 7 d 20 mg × 4 d 10 mg × 3 d	IM ACTH (437.5 U); 10 50 U × 7 d 25 U × 4 d 12.5 U × 3 d	Dexamethasone (78); 10 8 mg × 7 d 4 mg × 4 d 2 mg × 3 d	>1 d, <4 wk EDSS: 0.75–2.7	–1, 2, 4, 7, 14, 15, 60, 120, 180 d
Oliveri et al,[33] 1998	IV MP (2500); 15 500 mg × 5 d	IV MP (10,000 mg); 14 2000 mg × 5 d		<2 wk with at least 1 Gd enhancing lesion, not improving	0, 7, 15, 30, 60 d
Barnes et al,[24] 1997	IV MP (3000); 38 1000 mg × 3 d	Oral MP (588 mg); 42 48 mg × 7 d 24 mg × 7 d 12 mg × 7 d		<4 wk	

Abbreviations: CDMS, clinically definite multiple sclerosis; Gd, gadolinium; RRMS, relapsing-remitting multiple sclerosis.

high-dose MP were similarly beneficial in terms of the number of patients who improved at 1 month (10 of 11 and 8 of 10, respectively), even though the high-dose MP group had a significantly longer disease duration compared with the dexamethasone group (117 vs 30 months). In contrast, only 4 of 10 patients improved in the low-dose MP group.

Exactly what dose of MP constitutes a high dose is not clear, although some have suggested any cumulative dose greater than 500 mg to be high.[18] By this criterion, Oliveri and colleagues[33] compared ultrahigh (10,000 mg total) and high (2500 mg) doses of IV MP administered over 5 days to 31 patients with MS exacerbation. Using the change in the EDSS score and the number of MRI contrast-enhancing lesions as coprimary outcome measures, they found that both doses were equally effective in improving the EDSS score and decreasing the number of MRI contrast-enhancing lesions over the first 2 weeks. However, at 30 and 60 days, the ultrahigh dose of IV MP was more effective in reducing the number of MRI contrast-enhancing lesions, but not the EDSS score, compared with high-dose IV MP.

Adverse Events Associated with Steroid Use

Susceptibility to steroid side effects varies from patient to patient and depends not only on the individual patient's comorbidities but also on the dose, duration, and possibly type and route of steroid administration. The trials reviewed earlier report no serious adverse events associated with steroid use, but virtually all trials tended to exclude patients prone to complications from steroid use.

Steroids often have gastrointestinal side effects.[20] Dysgeusia, described as metallic taste, has been associated with oral steroids more so than parenteral steroids in one study,[25] but not in another.[23] Pyrosis appears to be equally common with IV or oral MP.[23,25,34] Prophylactic sucralfate use may explain no reports of pyrosis in 1 study.[15] Peptic ulcer or gastrointestinal bleeding was reported with IM ACTH in 1% of treated patients and 3% of controls.[14]

Psychiatric side effects of steroids can manifest as insomnia,[14,20,25] elevated mood,[15] anxiety,[20] or frank psychosis,[30] whereas some patients experience dysphoria after steroid cessation. Hyperglycemia is not uncommon during steroid treatment, and latent or overtly diabetic patients may necessitate inpatient monitoring. Increased appetite may lead to unwanted weight gain, a side effect that may also result from fluid retention and ankle edema related to the effects of corticosteroids on the kidney, because all synthetic corticosteroids have some mineralocorticoid activity. Renal sodium retention can lead to frank hypertension, whereas potassium excretion can result in hypokalemia. Short-term steroid treatment is not expected to suppress the endogenous hypothalamic-pituitary-adrenal axis,[35] obviating oral taper,[36] although some investigators have found the oral taper helpful in alleviating "let-down" after steroid treatment.[29] A longer steroid regimen, such as with IM ACTH, is often associated with acne, moon facies, and hypertrichosis (30%, 6.8%, and 6.8%, respectively).[14] Long-term corticosteroid use is also associated with osteoporosis, a problem to which disabled patients with MS may be predisposed owing to their decreased physical activity. An algorithm was recently proposed to streamline osteoporosis management in patients with MS.[37] Less-common side effects of steroids include hiccups,[25] elevated levels of liver enzymes,[33] pancreatitis,[38] and, improbably, anaphylactoid reactions.[39] Patients should be educated about the more-common side effects before steroids are administered. A useful rule of thumb is that the first-time steroid infusions are best performed under supervision, either in a clinic or in an inpatient setting.

TREATMENT OF STEROID-UNRESPONSIVE EXACERBATIONS

It has long been recognized that some MS exacerbations do not improve even after repeated courses of steroids. Among the alternative treatments in this setting, the evidence is strongest in support of plasmapheresis. In a landmark study, Weinshenker and colleagues[40] conducted a randomized, double-blind, sham-controlled trial of plasma exchange in patients who did not improve when given steroids alone (at least 5 days of 7 mg/kg/d of IV MP). A total of 22 patients (12 with MS, 10 with other acute inflammatory demyelinating diseases) were randomized to either plasma exchange or sham treatment (7 exchanges every other day) for 14 days. On day 14, the patients were examined by 2 blinded evaluators. Those who did not have at least moderate improvement crossed over to the opposite treatment arm for another 14 days. In total, 19 courses of plasma exchange were performed, resulting in 8 moderate or marked improvements, as determined by a change in mean power score, a metric developed specifically for this study to evaluate the targeted neurologic deficit. Change in the EDSS score was also noted, but it did not meet statistical significance, possibly because the EDSS did not reflect improvements in upper extremity strength among responders. In contrast, only 1 moderate improvement was noted across 17 courses of sham treatment. The order of treatment (sham or exchange first), age, sex, and diagnosis (MS or non-MS) were not significantly related to the response to plasma exchange, although a tendency to respond was noted among patients who were male and younger.

In a subsequent retrospective review of 59 steroid-unresponsive demyelinating events treated by plasmapheresis, Keegan and colleagues[41] found that male sex, preserved or brisk reflexes, and early initiation of treatment (<60 days) were associated with a moderate or marked improvement. Conversely, patient age and white blood cell count, protein level, and presence of oligoclonal bands in the cerebrospinal fluid were not significantly associated with the response. Technical factors related to exchange, that is, the type of replacement solution and total volume or number of exchanges, were also not significantly related to the response. These findings were partly confirmed in another retrospective review of 41 patients by Llufriu and colleagues,[42] who found that early initiation of plasma exchange (<60 days), but not age or male sex, was associated with a greater likelihood of response. However, in their series, 43% of patients treated after 60 days also showed improvement, suggesting that plasma exchange should not be overlooked as a treatment modality for steroid-unresponsive exacerbations beyond 60 days. This result was corroborated by a recent report of the response among patients more than 90 days after the exacerbation.[43]

More recently, Keegan and colleagues[44] correlated the pathologic features of demyelination with responsiveness to plasma exchange. All the patients with MS who responded to plasma exchange in their series (10 of 19) had a particular pattern of demyelination, characterized by the presence of antibodies and complement (pattern II),[45] whereas nonresponders had pathologic characteristics of T-cell/macrophage-associated demyelination (pattern I) or distal oligodendrogliopathy (pattern III).

The response to plasma exchange was initially thought to occur rapidly or not at all.[40] However, Llufriu and colleagues[42] documented a delayed effect of plasma exchange. At discharge 39% of patients had achieved improvement (as compared with 41% in the Weinshenker series), but at 6 months the response rate reached 63%. Delayed response to plasma exchange was also noted by Trebst and colleagues[46] in a review of 12 steroid-unresponsive optic neuritis cases treated with plasma exchange. Although most of their patients (80%) experienced some improvement by the end of plasmapheresis, all 12 cases had improved by 90 days. Although optic neuritis by natural history tends to improve by 2 to 4 weeks, the patients in this study underwent plasma exchange at 19 to 180 days (median, 44), with acuities mostly below 20/50, that is, having features associated with poor recovery.[47] Thus, their recovery on account of natural history or steroids alone would be unexpected and likely reflects the effects of plasma exchange.

Across the reported series, plasma exchanges were relatively well tolerated. Treatments were performed every other day to minimize the risk of hypotension, but it nevertheless occurred in 6% to 24% of the exchanges.[42,46] Most exchanges were performed via peripheral access, but some necessitated placement of a central catheter. Less commonly reported were anemia,[40,41] heparin-induced thrombocytopenia,[41] and paresthesias.[40,46] Only 1 series reported 5% bacterial infections related to line placement.[42]

Therapeutic alternatives to plasma exchange as a second-line treatment of steroid-unresponsive exacerbations are not established. Immunoadsorption, in which instead of all plasma proteins only immunoglobulins, immune complexes, and complement are removed, has been tried but seems no more effective than plasma exchange.[48,49] Kerr and colleagues[50] retrospectively reviewed a series of 122 patients with idiopathic transverse myelitis, caused in some by systemic autoimmune disease but none clearly identified as having MS at the time of treatment. They found that patients with American Spinal Injury Association (ASIA) level A (complete loss of motor and sensory function) benefited from IV cyclophosphamide (1000 mg/m^2), but not plasma exchange, following 3 to 5 days of IV MP. In contrast, non-ASIA A patients had more improvement with plasma exchange after steroid administration, with no benefit from IV cyclophosphamide. Because most of the responders to cyclophosphamide were patients with systemic autoimmune diseases who generally tend to respond better to this medication,[51] the role of IV cyclophosphamide in acute MS exacerbation remains to be validated.

Trials of monoclonal antibodies for treatment of MS exacerbations, including natalizumab[52] and anti-CD11/CD18 monoclonal antibody,[53] demonstrated no clinical benefit over placebo. IV immunoglobulin (IVIG) has anecdotally been reported as beneficial in MS exacerbations, but most studies to date provide no evidence of IVIG benefit when used concurrently with, or immediately following, IV MP.[54,55] However, an open-label study by Tselis and colleagues[56] suggested that some patients with steroid-unresponsive optic neuritis may respond to IVIG. A total of 23 patients whose visual acuity remained worse than 20/400 three months after the attack in spite of IV MP treatment were treated with IVIG (0.4 mg/kg/d for 5 days, followed by monthly 400 mg/kg infusion for 5 months). Compared with 24 controls, who received only IV MP, the treatment group showed a remarkable response rate (78% vs 12.5%) in terms of improving visual acuity to 20/30 or better 1 year later. This is in marked contrast with a failed trial of IVIG alone in acute optic neuritis[57] and a large, double-blind, placebo-controlled trial by Noseworthy and colleagues,[58] who found that delayed IVIG administration had no effect on recovery from optic neuritis. The latter trial, however, enrolled only patients whose optic neuritis occurred more than 6 months before (mean, 4.3 years), because the objective was to test the utility of IVIG in promoting recovery from irreversible damage to the optic nerve.

SUMMARY AND FUTURE DIRECTIONS

The understanding of the mechanisms that lead to MS exacerbations continues to produce novel treatments for patients with relapsing forms of MS. Even with the most potent agents available, the exacerbations remain a distinct possibility and a source of concern for patients and clinicians. Therefore, the treatment of acute MS exacerbations remains an indispensable element of MS care. The research outlined in this review highlights the central role of corticosteroids in speeding up recovery from exacerbations. It is worth emphasizing, however, that not all exacerbations require steroid treatment. Mild exacerbations may be left to their natural course, which entails a certain degree of recovery. The authors reserve steroids for the treatment of exacerbations that result in symptoms that a patient perceives as disabling.

As with any work spanning decades, the methodologies across different trials of steroids in MS have changed over time, making individual studies difficult to compare, even with meta-analyses. The question of the optimal timing of steroid administration illustrates this point. Early studies enrolled patients within 8 weeks of exacerbation,[14–16] whereas later studies narrowed this window to 4 weeks[20,24,30] or even 2 weeks.[33] There are reasons to believe that earlier administration of steroids should result in greater recovery, but there exists a lack of evidence. A current study of oral steroids, OMEGA (Oral Megadose Corticosteroid Therapy of Acute Exacerbations of Multiple Sclerosis), may answer the question of optimal timing and route of steroid administration. In this study, 140 patients aged 18 to 50 years with relapsing forms of MS who are experiencing an acute exacerbation are randomized to receive, within 7 days of exacerbation onset, 1000 mg/d IV MP or 1400 mg/d oral MP for 5 days. The primary objective of the trial is to determine whether the 2 groups (oral and IV) have equivalent recovery from day 0 to day 28, as assessed by the EDSS. Secondary outcome measures include change in the multiple sclerosis functional score, improvement of specific neurologic deficit, and relapse rate up to 1 year following treatment.

For those patients whose exacerbation symptoms fail to respond to steroids, therapeutic plasma exchange may provide a chance for recovery. Physical and occupational therapy, although not as rigorously studied as corticosteroids or plasma exchange, probably facilitate the recovery from MS exacerbations,[59] and should be part of a comprehensive rehabilitation treatment plan. Beyond that, there is little to offer, underscoring a need for alternative treatments. The roles of IVIG and IV cyclophosphamide in this setting remain uncertain and require additional confirmation. On the other hand, looking beyond antiinflammatory therapies, MS exacerbations present a unique opportunity to explore and harness the neuroprotective and regenerative potential of novel therapeutic agents.

REFERENCES

1. Schumacher GA. Critique of experimental trials of therapy in multiple sclerosis. Neurology 1974;24(11):1010–4.
2. Yetimalar Y, Seçil Y, Inceoglu AK, et al. Unusual primary manifestations of multiple sclerosis. N Z Med J 2008;121(1277):47–59.
3. Crawley F, Saddeh I, Barker S, et al. Acute pulmonary oedema: presenting symptom of multiple sclerosis. Mult Scler 2001;7(1):71–2.
4. Mowry EM, Deen S, Malikova I, et al. The onset location of multiple sclerosis predicts the location of subsequent relapses. J Neurol Neurosurg Psychiatry 2009;80(4):400–3.
5. Smith KJ, McDonald WI. The pathophysiology of multiple sclerosis: the mechanisms underlying the production of symptoms and the natural history of the disease. Philos Trans R Soc Lond B Biol Sci 1999;354(1390):1649–73.
6. Villoslada P, Arrondo G, Sepulcre J, et al. Memantine induces reversible neurologic impairment in patients with MS. Neurology 2009;72(19):1630–3.

7. Sibley WA, Bamford CR, Clark K. Clinical viral infections and multiple sclerosis. Lancet 1985;1(8441):1313–5.

8. Bosca I, Coret F, Valero C, et al. Effect of relapses over early progression of disability in multiple sclerosis patients treated with beta-interferon. Mult Scler 2008;14(5):636–9.

9. Lublin FD, Baier M, Cutter G. Effect of relapses on development of residual deficit in multiple sclerosis. Neurology 2003;61(11):1528–32.

10. Vercellino M, Romagnolo A, Mattioda A, et al. Multiple sclerosis relapses: a multivariable analysis of residual disability determinants. Acta Neurol Scand 2009; 119(2):126–30.

11. Leray E, Yaouanq J, Le Page E, et al. Evidence for a two-stage disability progression in multiple sclerosis. Brain 2010;133(Pt 7):1900–13.

12. Jonsson B, von Reis G, Sahlgren E. Treatment of sclerosis disseminata with ACTH. Nord Med 1950;43(9):380–1 [in Undetermined Language].

13. Glaser GH, Merritt HH. Effects of ACTH and cortisone in multiple sclerosis. Trans Am Neurol Assoc 1951;56:130–3.

14. Rose AS, Kuzma JW, Kurtzke JF, et al. Cooperative study in the evaluation of therapy in multiple sclerosis. ACTH vs. placebo–final report. Neurology 1970; 20(5):1–59.

15. Durelli L, Cocito D, Riccio A, et al. High-dose intravenous methylprednisolone in the treatment of multiple sclerosis: clinical-immunologic correlations. Neurology 1986;36(2):238–43.

16. Milligan NM, Newcombe R, Compston DA. A double-blind controlled trial of high dose methylprednisolone in patients with multiple sclerosis: 1. Clinical effects. J Neurol Neurosurg Psychiatry 1987;50(5):511–6.

17. Filippini G, Brusaferri F, Sibley WA, et al. Corticosteroids or ACTH for acute exacerbations in multiple sclerosis. Cochrane Database Syst Rev 2000;4: CD001331.

18. Miller DM, Weinstock-Guttman B, Béthoux F, et al. A meta-analysis of methylprednisolone in recovery from multiple sclerosis exacerbations. Mult Scler 2000;6(4): 267–73.

19. Morrow SA, Stoian CA, Dmitrovic J, et al. The bioavailability of IV methylprednisolone and oral prednisone in multiple sclerosis. Neurology 2004;63(6):1079–80.

20. Sellebjerg F, Frederiksen JL, Nielsen PM, et al. Double-blind, randomized, placebo-controlled study of oral, high-dose methylprednisolone in attacks of MS. Neurology 1998;51(2):529–34.

21. Sellebjerg F, Nielsen HS, Frederiksen JL, et al. A randomized, controlled trial of oral high-dose methylprednisolone in acute optic neuritis. Neurology 1999; 52(7):1479–84.

22. Beck RW, Cleary PA, Anderson MM, et al. A randomized, controlled trial of corticosteroids in the treatment of acute optic neuritis. The Optic Neuritis Study Group. J Neurol Neurosurg Psychiatry 1992;326(9):581–8.

23. Alam SM, Kyriakides T, Lawden M, et al. Methylprednisolone in multiple sclerosis: a comparison of oral with intravenous therapy at equivalent high dose. J Neurol Neurosurg Psychiatry 1993;56(11):1219–20.

24. Barnes D, Hughes RA, Morris RW, et al. Randomised trial of oral and intravenous methylprednisolone in acute relapses of multiple sclerosis. Lancet 1997; 349(9056):902–6.

25. Martinelli V, Rocca MA, Annovazzi P, et al. A short-term randomized MRI study of high-dose oral vs intravenous methylprednisolone in MS. Neurology 2009;73(22): 1842–8.

26. Burton JM, O'Connor PW, Hohol M, et al. Oral versus intravenous steroids for treatment of relapses in multiple sclerosis. Cochrane Database Syst Rev 2009; 3:CD006921.
27. Heun R, Sliwka U, Rüttinger H, et al. Intrathecal versus systemic corticosteroids in the treatment of multiple sclerosis: results of a pilot study. J Neurol 1992;239(1): 31–5.
28. Abbruzzese G, Gandolfo C, Loeb C. "Bolus" methylprednisolone versus ACTH in the treatment of multiple sclerosis. Ital J Neurol Sci 1983;4(2):169–72.
29. Barnes MP, Bateman DE, Cleland PG, et al. Intravenous methylprednisolone for multiple sclerosis in relapse. J Neurol Neurosurg Psychiatry 1985;48(2):157–9.
30. Thompson AJ, Kennard C, Swash M, et al. Relative efficacy of intravenous methylprednisolone and ACTH in the treatment of acute relapse in MS. Neurology 1989;39(7):969–71.
31. Milanese C, La Mantia L, Salmaggi A, et al. Double-blind randomized trial of ACTH versus dexamethasone versus methylprednisolone in multiple sclerosis bouts. Clinical, cerebrospinal fluid and neurophysiological results. Eur Neurol 1989;29(1):10–4.
32. La Mantia L, Eoli M, Milanese C, et al. Double-blind trial of dexamethasone versus methylprednisolone in multiple sclerosis acute relapses. Eur Neurol 1994;34(4): 199–203.
33. Oliveri RL, Valentino P, Russo C, et al. Randomized trial comparing two different high doses of methylprednisolone in MS: a clinical and MRI study. Neurology 1998;50(6):1833–6.
34. Metz LM, Sabuda D, Hilsden RJ, et al. Gastric tolerance of high-dose pulse oral prednisone in multiple sclerosis. Neurology 1999;53(9):2093–6.
35. Lević Z, Micić D, Nikolić J, et al. Short-term high dose steroid therapy does not affect the hypothalamic-pituitary-adrenal axis In relapsing multiple sclerosis patients. Clinical assessment by the insulin tolerance test. J Endocrinol Invest 1996;19(1):30–4.
36. Perumal JS, Caon C, Hreha S, et al. Oral prednisone taper following intravenous steroids fails to improve disability or recovery from relapses in multiple sclerosis. Eur J Neurol 2008;15(7):677–80.
37. Hearn AP, Silber E. Osteoporosis in multiple sclerosis. Mult Scler 2010;16(9): 1031–43.
38. Sellebjerg F, Barnes D, Filippini G, et al. EFNS guideline on treatment of multiple sclerosis relapses: report of an EFNS Task Force on treatment of multiple sclerosis relapses. Eur J Neurol 2005;12(12):939–46.
39. van den Berg JS, van Eikema Hommes OR, Wuis EW, et al. Anaphylactoid reaction to intravenous methylprednisolone in a patient with multiple sclerosis. J Neurol Neurosurg Psychiatry 1997;63(6):813–4.
40. Weinshenker BG, O'Brien PC, Petterson TM, et al. A randomized trial of plasma exchange in acute central nervous system inflammatory demyelinating disease. Ann Neurol 1999;46(6):878–86.
41. Keegan M, Pineda AA, McClelland RL, et al. Plasma exchange for severe attacks of CNS demyelination: predictors of response. Neurology 2002;58(1):143–6.
42. Llufriu S, Castillo J, Blanco Y, et al. Plasma exchange for acute attacks of CNS demyelination: predictors of improvement at 6 months. Neurology 2009;73(12): 949–53.
43. Magana S, Weigand S, Thomsen K, et al. Duration following severe attacks of CNS demyelinating disease to plasma exchange initiation: how long is too long? In: Annual Meeting Program. Toronto: American Academy of Neurology; 2010. p. A370.

44. Keegan M, Konig F, Mcclelland R, et al. Relation between humoral pathological changes in multiple sclerosis and response to therapeutic plasma exchange. Lancet 2005;366(9485):579–82.
45. Lucchinetti C, Brück W, Parisi J, et al. Heterogeneity of multiple sclerosis lesions: implications for the pathogenesis of demyelination. Ann Neurol 2000;47(6): 707–17.
46. Trebst C, Reising A, Kielstein JT, et al. Plasma exchange therapy in steroid-unresponsive relapses in patients with multiple sclerosis. Blood Purif 2009; 28(2):108–15.
47. Kupersmith MJ, Gal RL, Beck RW, et al. Visual function at baseline and 1 month in acute optic neuritis: predictors of visual outcome. Neurology 2007;69(6):508–14.
48. Palm M, Behm E, Schmitt E, et al. Immunoadsorption and plasma exchange in multiple sclerosis: complement and plasma protein behaviour. Biomater Artif Cells Immobilization Biotechnol 1991;19(1):283–96.
49. Schmitt E, Behm E, Buddenhagen F, et al. Immunoadsorption (IA) versus plasma exchange (PE) in multiple sclerosis–first results of a double blind controlled trial. Prog Clin Biol Res 1990;337:289–92.
50. Greenberg BM, Thomas KP, Krishnan C, et al. Idiopathic transverse myelitis: corticosteroids, plasma exchange, or cyclophosphamide. Neurology 2007; 68(19):1614–7.
51. Barile-Fabris L, Ariza-Andraca R, Olguín-Ortega L, et al. Controlled clinical trial of IV cyclophosphamide versus IV methylprednisolone in severe neurological manifestations in systemic lupus erythematosus. Ann Rheum Dis 2005;64(4):620–5.
52. O'Connor PW, Goodman A, Willmer-Hulme AJ, et al. Randomized multicenter trial of natalizumab in acute MS relapses: clinical and MRI effects. Neurology 2004; 62(11):2038–43.
53. Lublin F. A phase II trial of anti-CD11/CD18 monoclonal antibody in acute exacerbations of multiple sclerosis. In: Annual Meeting Program. Toronto: American Academy of Neurology; 1999. p. A290–1.
54. Sorensen PS, Haas J, Sellebjerg F, et al. IV immunoglobulins as add-on treatment to methylprednisolone for acute relapses in MS. Neurology 2004;63(11):2028–33.
55. Visser LH, Beekman R, Tijssen CC, et al. A randomized, double-blind, placebo-controlled pilot study of i.v. immune globulins in combination with i.v. methylprednisolone in the treatment of relapses in patients with MS. Mult Scler 2004;10(1): 89–91.
56. Tselis A, Perumal J, Caon C, et al. Treatment of corticosteroid refractory optic neuritis in multiple sclerosis patients with intravenous immunoglobulin. Eur J Neurol 2008;15(11):1163–7.
57. Roed HG, Langkilde A, Sellebjerg F, et al. A double-blind, randomized trial of IV immunoglobulin treatment in acute optic neuritis. Neurology 2005;64(5):804–10.
58. Noseworthy JH, O'Brien PC, Petterson TM, et al. A randomized trial of intravenous immunoglobulin in inflammatory demyelinating optic neuritis. Neurology 2001; 56(11):1514–22.
59. Craig J, Young CA, Ennis M, et al. A randomised controlled trial comparing rehabilitation against standard therapy in multiple sclerosis patients receiving intravenous steroid treatment. J Neurol Neurosurg Psychiatry 2003;74(9):1225–30.

FDA-Approved Preventative Therapies for MS: First-line Agents

Mariko Kita, MD[a,b]

KEYWORDS

- Relapsing-remitting multiple sclerosis • Preventative therapy
- First-line agents • Clinically isolated syndrome

The focus of this article is the first-line disease-modifying treatments for relapsing forms of multiple sclerosis (MS). At the time of this writing in 2010, 7 therapies for the treatment of multiple sclerosis are approved by the Food and Drug Administration (FDA) in the United States (Betaseron, Avonex, Copaxone, Rebif, Novantrone, Tysabri, and Extavia). Although all may be used in patients who are treatment naïve, the self-injectable therapies (Betaseron, Avonex, Copaxone, Rebif, Extavia) are considered to be the standard first-line agents, with the infused therapies (Novantrone, Tysabri) generally being reserved for more aggressive disease. With newer therapies quickly on the horizon, it is worthwhile to revisit these standard therapies and how they are used at this time as this is the backdrop on which the newer agents will emerge.

Class I studies have been performed for the interferon (IFN) beta formulations[1-4] and glatiramer acetate[5] using what we have come to expect as standard primary and secondary outcome measures for MS: measures of clinical relapse (relapse rate, percent relapse-free, time to next relapse, and so forth), measures of clinical disability (time to sustained Expandable Disability Status Scale [EDSS] progression, percent of patients progressing, and so forth), and measures of MRI activity (new/enlarging T2 lesions, gadolinium-enhancing lesions, combined unique lesions, T2 or T1 lesion volume, and so forth). These studies, which are summarized briefly, have shown efficacy of all of these agents compared with placebo in reducing measures of clinical relapse, impacting clinical disability, and limiting new MRI activity.

INTERFERONS

Interferon beta-1b was the first disease-modifying therapy (DMT) to be FDA-approved for the treatment of relapsing-remitting multiple sclerosis (RRMS) in the United States.

[a] Virginia Mason Multiple Sclerosis Center, PO Box 900, Seattle, WA 98101, USA
[b] Department of Neurology, University of Washington School of Medicine, Seattle, WA 98195, USA
E-mail address: Mariko.Kita@vmmc.org

Neurol Clin 29 (2011) 401–409
doi:10.1016/j.ncl.2011.01.007
0733-8619/11/$ – see front matter © 2011 Elsevier Inc. All rights reserved.

The pivotal study,[1] in 372 subjects, showed significantly lower relapse rates in subjects treated with 8 mIU every other day compared with placebo (annualized relapse rate [ARR] 1.27 vs 0.84; $P = .0001$) at 2 years. A low dose of IFN (1.6 mIU every other day) was also studied in this clinical trial demonstrating superiority to placebo (ARR 1.27 vs 1.17; $P = .0101$). Exacerbation rates between low-dose and high-dose arms were statistically significantly different ($P = .0086$) suggesting a dose effect. In an extension study to 5 years,[2] the proportion of subjects experiencing confirmed disability progression was lower in the group treated with 8 mIU every other day than placebo (35% vs 46%; $P = .096$). Furthermore, the treated group had no significant increase in MRI lesion burden ($P = .917$) compared with baseline; whereas, the placebo group experienced a 30% increase in MRI lesions ($P = .0001$).

After being reconstituted by patients in 1 mL saline, IFN beta-1b is administered subcutaneously every other day, with the option of using an autoinjector. Lyophilized, IFN beta-1b may remain at room temperature until it is ready to be used. The full listing of side effects can be found in the package insert,[6] but in the author's experience the side effects most commonly encountered in clinical practice include redness at the injection site that can last several days to weeks, flu-like symptoms, and, less commonly, burning at the injection site. Because there is a possibility for hepatic transaminitis and leukopenia, routine liver function tests (LFTs) and cell blood counts (CBCs) should be done every 3 to 6 months.

There are 2 formulations of IFN beta-1a: once weekly intramuscular IFN and 3 times weekly subcutaneous IFN. Weekly intramuscular IFN beta-1a at a dose of 30 mcg was shown in a phase III study of 301 subjects with RRMS to delay time to progression of disability when compared with placebo with fewer treated subjects experiencing disability progression (21.9% vs 34.9%; $P = .02$).[3] Relapse rates over a 2-year period were also lower compared with placebo (ARR 0.61 vs 0.90 $P = .03$), as was accumulation of gadolinium-enhancing (Gd+) MRI lesion burden. The weekly administered injection is available in a lyophilized form, which may remain at room temperature for 30 days and needs to be reconstituted by patients. It is also available in a premixed form (0.5 mL), which must be refrigerated but can remain at room temperature for up to 7 days. For a complete listing of side effects the reader is directed to the package insert.[7] In the experience of the author, flu-like symptoms can occur and may be more commonly experienced in patients who take the premixed formulation. Injection-site redness is uncommon with the intramuscular formulation. CBC and LFTs should be performed every 6 months.

Subcutaneous IFN beta-1a was studied in 560 subjects against placebo at a 22 mcg dose versus a 44 mcg dose 3 times per week over a 2-year period.[4] Both doses proved effective against placebo as measured by annualized relapse rate (ARR 1.82, 22 mcg; ARR 1.73, 44 mcg; and ARR 2.56 placebo [PLC]; $P<.005$), reducing risk of relapse by 27% (22 mcg) to 33% (44 mcg). Subjects on active treatment accumulated less T2 lesion burden (22 mcg: -1.2%; 44 mcg: -3.8%; PLC +10.9%; $P<.001$ for both vs PLC) and experienced a delay in the progression of sustained disability ($P<.05$). A subset of subjects with EDSS greater than 3.5 was analyzed and had a reduction in the probability of disability progression only when treated with the higher dose. Similarly, the higher dose was favored when looking at the outcome of the number of T2 active lesions on biannual scans.

After the first 2 years, the placebo recipients were randomized to the 22-mcg or 44-mcg dosing groups and followed for an additional 2 years.[8] Making the switch to treatment improved measures of disease activity, but the subjects who had been maintained on the 44-mcg dose during the entire 4 years had the best disability outcome at the end of the study prolonging time to disability progression by 18 months (P = .047) when compared with those who had been on placebo for 2 years.

Subcutaneous IFN beta-1a is available in a premixed formulation (0.5 mL) and may be administered with an autoinjector. When refrigeration is not available, it can remain at room temperature for up to 30 days. Both 22-mcg and 44-mcg premixed doses are available. For a complete list of side effects, the reader is directed to the package insert.[9] In the author's clinical experience, side effects include flu-like symptoms, redness at the injection site that can last several days to weeks, and burning at the injection site. CBC and LFTs should be monitored every 3 to 6 months. The provider should be aware of the possible emergence or worsening of clinical depression with the initiation of interferon therapy so as not to lose an opportunity to be recognized and appropriately treated. Premorbid depression is not a contraindication to use of interferons in the treatment of MS.

Neutralizing antibodies (NAbs) may develop with use of the IFNs and have the potential to interfere with efficacy as measured by clinical and imaging outcomes.[10–14] Furthermore, NAbs to IFN beta-1a and IFN beta-1b appear to cross react with one another.[15] The use of routine NAb testing in clinical practice varies widely between practitioners and reflects the lack of consensus regarding its utility. In 2005, the European Federation of Neurologic Societies (EFNS) published guidelines regarding the routine use of Nab testing. It was recommended that all interferon recipients be tested for NAbs at 12 and 24 months.[16] If patients were NAb negative at these time points, it was suggested that testing was no longer necessary because the likelihood of conversion to NAb-positive status was low after 24 months.[17] However, if patients tested NAb positive, repeat testing was recommended at 3 and 6 months. If high titers persisted, the EFNS recommended discontinuation of interferon. In contrast, the American Academy of Neurology issued an expert consensus report in 2007 that concluded that there were insufficient data to make specific recommendations "regarding when to test, which test to use, how many tests are necessary, or which cutoff titer to apply".[18] Commercially available testing in the United States uses the viral cytopathic effect assay; the Myxovirus A induction assay is not commercially available. Given that NAbs can interfere with IFN efficacy and that antibodies can cross-react, it would seem reasonable to use antibody testing when considering a change in therapy between the IFNs for reasons of breakthrough activity. Nabs testing should not be performed immediately an IFN injection because IFN may saturate the antibodies and impact the result of the assay.

GLATIRAMER ACETATE

In the pivotal trial of glatiramer acetate (GA), 251 subjects with RRMS were randomized to receive a daily dose of 20 mg subcutaneously versus placebo.[5] Over 2 years treatment with GA reduced relapses by 29% (ARR 0.59 vs 0.84; P = .007). Fewer recipients of glatiramer acetate experienced a worsening in their disability score. In a separate study of 239 subjects with RRMS randomized to GA versus placebo, active treatment resulted in reduction in new Gd+ MRI lesions over 9 months.[19] GA is available premixed (1 mL) and can be administered with an autoinjector. For a full listing of side effects, the reader is directed to the package insert.[20] In the author's clinical experience, commonly encountered side effects include injection-site redness, itching, and induration. Patients may also experience lipoatrophy over time. So-called postinjection reactions, including systemic flushing, chest tightness, and so forth, rarely occur with injections and are self-limited.

INITIATING TREATMENT

Because all of the aforementioned DMTs have been shown to be effective in treating RRMS when compared with placebo, it would be reasonable to treat patients with RRMS with any of these agents. A unified algorithm for how to choose the first therapy, as well as how and when to move on to the next, would imply that all patients with MS can be treated exactly the same way, with predictable, similar degrees of disease activity off treatment, identical anticipated responses to therapy, with universal experience of side effects. Clearly this is not the case. In an effort to better guide therapy choices, head-to-head studies have been performed.

IFN beta-1b (250 mcg subcutaneously every other day) was compared with once-weekly intramuscular interferon beta-1a (30 mcg) in the INCOMIN study. In this 2-year, single-blind, randomized study in 188 subjects with RRMS, significantly more subjects on IFN beta-1b were relapse free and had accumulated fewer new T2 and Gd+ lesions.[21] A second study, the ABOVE study, comparing these two agents was performed in a randomized, double-blind fashion over 2 years and was completed in 2008, but results have not been reported.[22]

In the BEYOND study, double-dose IFN beta-1b (500 mcg) was compared with standard IFN-1b (250 mcg). There was no difference between the doses with regard to reduction in relapse risk, EDSS progression, T1-hypointense lesion volume, or change in normalized brain volume.[23]

When 3-times weekly subcutaneous interferon beta-1a was compared with once-weekly intramuscular interferon beta-1a (EVIDENCE)[24] in 677 subjects with RRMS in a single-blind fashion, over 48 weeks the high-dose recipients had fewer relapses and T2 lesions (combined unique lesions) with differences between the doses seen primarily in the first 24 weeks. Progression of disability, however, was not different between the two doses.

Based on the available evidence, there appears to be a dose effect with the IFN preparations. How this translates in clinical practice is not straightforward because not all patients require the highest dose to control their disease, and some patients appear resistant to IFN. Further, the frequency of NAbs to IFN is different according to the agent used. There are practitioners who choose to limit the use of IFNs to only the highest-dosing regimen. Others choose to start with the lower-dose regimen, leaving open the opportunity for dose escalation, if necessary. The apparent dose effect must be balanced by the issue of tolerability and schedule of administration, and involving patients in this decision process is highly important.

Head-to-head trials have also been performed comparing IFNs to GA.[23,25] In the REGARD trial, GA was compared with 3-times weekly subcutaneous IFN beta-1a in 764 subjects with RRMS over 96 weeks. There was no difference seen in relapse measure, time to EDSS progression, or multiple MRI outcomes (T2 lesion number and volume, Gd+ volume). Subjects randomized to IFN had fewer numbers of Gd+ lesions per scan.

In the BEYOND study, GA was compared with standard-dose IFN beta-1b and double-dose IFN beta-1b. In addition to there being no significant differences between the two IFN dosing regimens, treatment effect was similar between IFN beta-1b and GA with respect to relapse measures, EDSS progression, and several MRI outcomes. Differences were seen in new T2 lesions, T2 lesions volume, and Gd+ lesion volume, but not Gd+ number.

The available MS therapies are effective. However, it appears from clinical practice and from clinical trial results that not every therapy is equally effective in every individual. Predictors of response remain aggressively under study. In the absence of reliable markers and a consensus on how to define treatment response, it seems that the key message to our patients is to encourage initiation of treatment for RRMS, rather than promoting any specific treatment: treat first, tweak later. It is the author's practice to engage patients in a careful discussion of the details of drug administration and side-effect profile and anticipated outcome. Based on these factors, after a decision is made on which therapy to start, it falls on the provider to continue to make ongoing assessments of adequate efficacy. Throughout this process efforts need to be directed at minimizing side effects to maximize compliance. Patients may often expect to feel poorly on MS medications and therefore do not always express the difficulties that they are experiencing. Often times the side-effect profile may dictate whether a drug is tolerable enough for patients to remain compliant. Side effects, such as flu-like symptoms and site reactions, should be targeted to be minimal.

CLINICALLY ISOLATED SYNDROME

The first opportunity to initiate DMT in an individual with MS is at the time of their first attack. Often referred to as the *clinically isolated syndrome* (CIS), it bears mentioning that the emergence of this entity has proven to be problematic at times for patients and providers alike. There are individuals for whom a demyelinating event may represent a manifestation of a systemic disorder or a truly isolated phenomenon with little future risk of experiencing a second attack. For others, the initial demyelinating event heralds the onset of multiple sclerosis. CIS is a term that in and of itself does not distinguish the former from the latter, which can lead to much confusion. Therefore, it is important to rule out disorders that can mimic MS at the time of this attack.

Entry criteria for CIS trials required that other causes for the demyelinating event were ruled out and that there was subclinical evidence for dissemination of the demyelinating process in space (at least 2 clinically silent lesions on cranial MRI scans). Given sufficient certainty that these individuals ought to experience another clinical attack,[26–29] the studies focused on the potential of the DMTs to prevent or delay a second attack (thus confirming MS by Poser criteria) and to impact other measures of MS (MRI activity, disability progression).

All of the first-line, disease-modifying therapies have been tested in patients with abnormal MRI scans of the brain after their first demyelinating attack.[30–33] All have been found to be effective in delaying the second attack of MS and in reducing new MRI lesions. The first of the IFNs to be tested in CIS was intramuscular IFN beta-1a. In the CHAMPS study, 383 subjects with CIS were randomized to 30-mcg once weekly intramuscular IFN beta-1a versus placebo. Treatment significantly reduced the proportion of subjects experiencing a second attack (50% vs 35%; $P = .002$) over 3 years [30] when compared with placebo. The Early Treatment of MS (ETOMS) study examined a similar regimen of once-weekly IFN. Subcutaneous interferon beta-1a at a once-weekly 22-mcg subcutaneous dose was tested in 308 subjects with CIS against placebo with similar results (34% vs 45%; $P = .046$).[31] Higher-dose, higher-frequency IFN beta-1a in CIS is currently under investigation exploring effectiveness of 44 mcg administered subcutaneously 1 or 3 times weekly compared with placebo,[34] but high-dose, high-frequency IFN beta-1b has already been tested in CIS and shown to be effective.[32] In the BENEFIT study, IFN beta-1b at a dose of 250 mcg every other day in 292 subjects with CIS significantly reduced the proportion of subjects experiencing a second attack over 2 years compared with placebo (44% vs 26%; $P<.0001$). Significant reductions in MRI activity were also noted in all of these studies.[30–32] A meta-analysis of all 3 of these studies in 1160 subjects with CIS confirmed the efficacy of interferon treatment in reducing the probability of experiencing a second relapse, thus converting to MS at both 1 year (pooled odds ratio [OR] 0.53; 95% confidence interval [CI], 0.40 to 0.71; $P<.0001$) and 2 years (pooled OR 0.52; 95% CI, 0.38 to 0.70; $P<.0001$) when compared with placebo.[35]

In open-label extension studies, early initiation of treatment has shown long-term benefit. Subjects enrolled in CHAMPS were offered treatment with weekly intramuscular IFN beta-1a and were followed in the CHAMPIONS study.[36] At 5 years, the group who had been treated from onset remained less likely to have a second attack compared with the group with delayed treatment. Similar results were seen with extension of the BENEFIT study[37,38] at 3 and 5 years. In both extension studies, disability progression was similar between groups that were treated immediately and those whose treatment was delayed. This result may be caused in part by the fact that even the delayed groups were being treated early in their disease course, and also by the impact of subject dropouts.

When GA was tested in 481 subjects presenting with unifocal CIS for up to 3 years, the proportion of subjects experiencing a second attack was reduced compared with placebo (25% vs 43%; $P<.0001$).[33] MRI lesion burden was also significantly reduced in the active arm. This cohort is being followed in an on-going 5-year extension study.[39]

Given the data, it appears that there is compelling evidence to support the treatment of CIS. Reluctance to treat should not stem from uncertainty about the diagnosis. For that reason, it is the author's preference to avoid the term CIS once other causes are ruled out and to stipulate that this individual has had their first attack of MS. Reluctance to treat may stem more from uncertainty about a particular patient's prognosis, driven by a desire not to overtreat. Because of this uncertainty, some patients and providers may choose not to initiate therapy at the first demyelinating event, instead waiting for formal criteria to be met. In this instance, one could consider close clinical follow-up with MRI scans to be done on a serial basis, looking for subclinical disease activity. According to revised McDonald criteria,[40] a new T2 lesion as soon as 1 month after the first event and scan would qualify as dissemination in time, thus establishing a diagnosis of MS. Practical issues, such as insurance coverage and out-of-pocket patient costs, may limit the frequency with which such follow-up scans can be performed. A 3- to 6-month interval might prove more feasible. A detailed discussion of early prognostic indicators is covered elsewhere, but such factors (degree of abnormality of MRI, degree of dissemination in space, cerebrospinal fluid abnormality, recovery from event) may provide helpful information to identify those patients who have a higher propensity for a more active disease course at the time of their first event.

SUMMARY

RRMS is highly variable in its presentation and disease course. The approach to initiating first-line preventative therapies must focus on individualizing treatment strategies. Careful discussion of available treatment options and appropriate expectations regarding outcomes is important to ensure a successful start. Early treatment is recommended, as is on-going monitoring of patients who may choose to forego therapy.

REFERENCES

1. The IFNB Multiple Sclerosis Study Group. Interferon beta-1b is effective in relapsing-remitting multiple sclerosis. I. Clinical results of a multicenter, randomized, double-blind, placebo-controlled trial. The IFNB Multiple Sclerosis Study Group. Neurology 1993;43:655–61.

2. Interferon beta-1b in the treatment of multiple sclerosis: final outcome of the randomized controlled trial. The IFNB Multiple Sclerosis Study Group and The University of British Columbia MS/MRI Analysis Group. Neurology 1995;45(7): 1277–85.

3. Jacobs LD, Cookfair DL, Rudick RA, et al. Intramuscular interferon beta-1a for disease progression in relapsing multiple sclerosis. The Multiple Sclerosis Collaborative Research Group (MSCRG). Ann Neurol 1996;39(3):285–94.

4. Randomised double-blind placebo-controlled study of interferon beta-1a in relapsing/remitting multiple sclerosis. PRISMS (Prevention of Relapses and Disability by Interferon beta-1a Subcutaneously in Multiple Sclerosis) Study Group. Lancet 1998;352(9139):1498–504.

5. Johnson KP, Brooks BR, Cohen JA, et al. Copolymer 1 reduces relapse rate and improves disability in relapsing-remitting multiple sclerosis: results of a phase III multicenter, double-blind placebo-controlled trial. The Copolymer 1 Multiple Sclerosis Study Group. Neurology 1995;45(7):1268–76.

6. Betaseron [package insert]. Montville (MJ): Berlex; 2007.

7. Avonex [package insert]. Cambridge (MA): BiogenIdec Inc; 2006.

8. PRISMS Study Group and the University of British Columbia MS/MRI Analysis Group. PRISMS-4: long-term efficacy of interferon-beta-1a in relapsing MS. Neurology 2001;56(12):1628–36.

9. Rebif [package insert]. Rocklan (MA): Serono Inc; 2005.

10. Sorensen PS, Ross C, Clemmesen KM, et al. Clinical importance of neutralising antibodies against interferon beta in patients with relapsing-remitting multiple sclerosis. Lancet 2003;362(9391):1184–91.

11. Malucchi S, Sala A, Gilli F, et al. A Neutralizing antibodies reduce the efficacy of Beta IFN during treatment of multiple sclerosis. Neurology 2004;62(11):2031–7.

12. Kappos L, Clanet M, Sandberg-Wollheim M, et al. Neutralizing antibodies and efficacy of interferon beta-1a: a 4-year controlled study. Neurology 2005;65(1): 40–7.

13. Francis GS, Rice GP, Alsop JC. Interferon beta-1a in MS: results following development of neutralizing antibodies in PRISMS. Neurology 2005;65(1):48–55.

14. Bertolotto A, Gilli F, Sala A, et al. Persistent neutralizing antibodies abolish the interferon beta bioavailability in MS patients. Neurology 2003;60(4):634–9.

15. Khan OA, Dhib-Jalbut SS. Neutralizing antibodies to interferon beta-1a and interferon beta-1b in MS patients are cross-reactive. Neurology 1998;51:1698–702.

16. Sorensen PS, Deisenhammer F, Duda P, et al. Guidelines on use of anti-IFN-beta antibody measurements in multiple sclerosis: report of an EFNS Task Force on IFN-beta antibodies in multiple sclerosis. Eur J Neurol 2005;12(11):817–27.

17. Sorensen PS, Koch-Henriksen N, Ross C, et al. Appearance and disappearance of neutralizing antibodies during interferon-beta therapy. Neurology 2005;65(1): 33–9.

18. Goodin DS, Frohman EM, Hurwitz B, et al. Neutralizing antibodies to interferon beta: assessment of their clinical and radiographic impact: an evidence report: report of the Therapeutics and Technology Assessment Subcommittee of the American Academy of Neurology. Neurology 2007;68(13):977–84.

19. Comi G, Filippi M, Wolinsky JS. European/Canadian multicenter, double-blind, randomized, placebo-controlled study of the effects of glatiramer acetate on magnetic resonance imaging–measured disease activity and burden in patients with relapsing multiple sclerosis. European/Canadian Glatiramer Acetate Study Group. Ann Neurol 2001;49(3):290–7.

20. Copaxone [package insert]. Kansas City (MO): Teva Neuroscience Inc; 2007.

21. Durelli L, Verdun E, Barbero P, et al. Every-other-day interferon beta-1b versus once-weekly interferon beta-1a for multiple sclerosis: results of a 2-year prospective randomised multicentre study (INCOMIN). Lancet 2002;359(9316): 1453–60.

22. Available at: http://www.clinicaltrial.gov/. Accessed January 24, 2011.

23. O'Connor P, Filippi M, Arnason B, et al. 250 microg or 500 microg interferon beta-1b versus 20 mg glatiramer acetate in relapsing-remitting multiple sclerosis: a prospective, randomised, multicentre study. Lancet Neurol 2009;8(10): 889–97.

24. Panitch H, Goodin DS, Francis G, et al. Randomized, comparative study of interferon beta-1a treatment regimens in MS: The EVIDENCE Trial. Neurology 2002; 59(10):1496–506.

25. Mikol DD, Barkhof F, Chang P, et al. Comparison of subcutaneous interferon beta-1a with glatiramer acetate in patients with relapsing multiple sclerosis (the Rebif vs Glatiramer Acetate in Relapsing MS Disease [REGARD]study): a multicentre, randomised, parallel, open-label trial. Lancet Neurol 2008;7(10):903–14.

26. Beck RW, Trobe JD, Moke PS, et al. High- and low-risk profiles for the development of multiple sclerosis within 10 years after optic neuritis: experience of the optic neuritis treatment trial. Arch Ophthalmol 2003;121(7):944–9.

27. Brex PA, Ciccarelli O, O'Riordan JI, et al. A longitudinal study of abnormalities on MRI and disability from multiple sclerosis. N Engl J Med 2002;346(3): 158–64.

28. Miller D, Barkhof F, Montalban X, et al. Clinically isolated syndromes suggestive of multiple sclerosis, part I: natural history, pathogenesis, diagnosis, and prognosis. Lancet Neurol 2005;4(5):281–8.

29. Montalban X, Tintore M, Swanton J, et al. MRI criteria for MS in patients with clinically isolated syndromes. Neurology 2010;74(5):427–34.

30. Jacobs LD, Beck RW, Simon JH, et al. Intramuscular interferon beta-1a therapy initiated during a first demyelinating event in multiple sclerosis. CHAMPS Study Group. N Engl J Med 2000;343(13):898–904.

31. Comi G, Filippi M, Barkhof F, et al. Effect of early interferon treatment on conversion to definite multiple sclerosis: a randomised study. Lancet 2001;357(9268): 1576–82.

32. Kappos L, Polman CH, Freedman MS, et al. Treatment with interferon beta-1b delays conversion to clinically definite and McDonald MS in patients with clinically isolated syndromes. Neurology 2006;67(7):1242–9.

33. Comi G, Martinelli V, Rodegher M, et al. Effect of glatiramer acetate on conversion to clinically definite multiple sclerosis in patients with clinically isolated syndrome (PreCISe study): a randomised, double-blind, placebo-controlled trial. Lancet 2009;374(9700):1503–11.

34. Available at: http://www.clinicaltrial.gov/. Accessed January 24, 2011.

35. Clerico M, Faggiano F, Palace J, et al. Recombinant interferon beta or glatiramer acetate for delaying conversion of the first demyelinating event to multiple sclerosis. Cochrane Database Syst Rev 2008;2:CD005278.

36. Kinkel RP, Kollman C, O'Connor P, et al. IM interferon beta-1a delays definite multiple sclerosis 5 years after a first demyelinating event. Neurology 2006; 66(5):678–84.

37. Kappos L, Freedman MS, Polman CH, et al. Effect of early versus delayed interferon beta-1b treatment on disability after a first clinical event suggestive of multiple sclerosis: a 3-year follow-up analysis of the BENEFIT study. Lancet 2007;370(9585):389–97.

38. Kappos L, Freedman MS, Polman, et al. Long-term effect of early treatment with interferon beta-1b after a first clinical event suggestive of multiple sclerosis: 5-year active treatment extension of the phase 3 BENEFIT trial. Lancet Neurol 2009;8(11):987–97.
39. Available at: http://www.clinicaltrial.gov/. Accessed January 24, 2011.
40. Polman CH, Reingold SC, Edan G, et al. Diagnostic criteria for multiple sclerosis; 2005 revisions to the "McDonald Criteria." Ann Neurol 2005;58(6):840–6.

Definitions of Breakthrough Disease and Second-Line Agents

James J. Marriott, MD, FRCPC[a],
Paul W. O'Connor, MD, MSc, FRCPC[b,c],*

KEYWORDS

- Multiple sclerosis • Breakthrough disease • Natalizumab
- Mitoxantrone • Cyclophosphamide • Management

Frequently, patients with relapsing-remitting multiple sclerosis (RRMS) on the standard injectable immunomodulating agents, interferon (IFN)-β1a/b or glatiramer acetate (GA), continue to have some level of disease activity. This disease activity has been called suboptimal response, treatment nonresponse, treatment failure, or break-through disease, with the last term being preferred by Rudick and Polman,[1] as it does not carry the connotations of failure. This article reviews the second-line therapy options available at present and other potential future therapies discussed in greater length elsewhere (**Table 1**). It then discusses the various tools and guidelines developed to help guide the clinician and patient who are considering second-line therapies before finally reviewing the available literature on treatment outcomes in patients with RRMS who have switched therapies.

SECOND-LINE AGENTS

Approved Therapies

Of the 3 main second-line agents used in RRMS, the best quality evidence exists for the most recent agent, natalizumab, which has been studied in 2 phase 3 trials as both monotherapy AFFIRM[2] and in combination with intramuscular IFN-β1a SENTINEL.[3] Natalizumab is a monoclonal antibody directed against the α4 subunit

[a] Section of Neurology, University of Manitoba, GF-543 Health Sciences Centre, 820 Sherbrook Street, Winnipeg, MB, Canada, R3A 1R9
[b] Division of Neurology, University of Toronto, St Michael's Hospital, Shuter 3-007, 30 Bond Street, Toronto, Ontario, Canada
[c] Department of Neurology, MS Clinic and MS Research, St Michael's Hospital, Shuter 3-007, 30 Bond Street, Toronto, Ontario, Canada M5B 1W8
* Corresponding author. MS Clinic and MS Research, Department of Neurology, St Michael's Hospital, Shuter 3-007, 30 Bond Street, Toronto, Ontario, Canada M5B 1W8.
E-mail address: oconnorp@smh.ca

Neurol Clin 29 (2011) 411–422
doi:10.1016/j.ncl.2010.12.005
0733-8619/11/$ – see front matter © 2011 Elsevier Inc. All rights reserved.

neurologic.theclinics.com

Table 1
Approved, off-label, and emerging second-line MS therapies

Therapy	Trial Characteristics	Trial Results	Breakthrough Disease Patients Enrolled
Approved			
Natalizumab[2,3]	Double-blind RCTs	Effective alone or in combination with IFN-β	No
Mitoxantrone[12,63-67]	Double-blind RCTs, unblinded cohort studies	Effective (clinical ± MRI end points)	No (RCT); yes (cohort)
Off label			
Cyclophosphamide[24-26,68-75]	Unblinded RCTs and cohort studies	Variable results; induction and booster effective in active inflammatory MS	No (RCT); yes (cohort)
AHSCT[28-31]	Unblinded cohort studies	Effective (may not be sustained)	Yes
Corticosteroids[32-34]	Double-blind RCTs	Benefit as add-on to IFN-β,[32] not replicated[33,34]	Yes,[32,33] no[34]
Rituximab[40]	Double-blind RCT	Effective	No
Awaiting approval/ongoing trials			
Fingolimod[35,36]	Double-blind RCT	Effective	No
Cladribine[37]	Double-blind RCT	Effective	No
Alemtuzumab[38,39]	Rater-blinded RCTs	Effective,[38] ongoing[39]	No,[30] yes[31]
Ocrelizumab[41]	Rater-blinded RCT	Ongoing	No

Abbreviations: AHSCT, autologous hematopoietic stem cell transplantation; RCT, randomized controlled trial.

of α4β1-integrin expressed on circulating T lymphocytes.[4] Binding of natalizumab prevents α4β1-integrin from interacting with endothelial vascular cell adhesion molecule 1 (VCAM-1), a necessary step in lymphocyte transmigration.

In the AFFIRM monotherapy trial, 942 patients with RRMS with a relapse in the preceding year were randomized 2:1 to receive either natalizumab 300 mg, or placebo intravenously (IV) monthly.[2] Patients with recent immunosuppressant or immunomodulator exposure were excluded, as were patients who had been administered IFN or GA for longer than 6 months at any time in the past. After 1 year of treatment, the annualized relapse rate (ARR) in the placebo-treated patients was 0.81 compared with 0.26 in the natalizumab-treated patients (relative risk reduction [RRR], 68%; $P<.001$). After 2 years, disability progression, as defined by the Expanded Disability Status Scale (EDSS) change sustained for 12 weeks, had occurred in 29% of patients in the placebo arm compared with only 17% in the natalizumab arm (RRR, 42%; $P<.001$). Significant reductions in both T1 gadolinium (Gd^+)-enhancing lesions and T2 hyperintense lesions were also seen.

In the SENTINEL trial, almost 1171 patients with RRMS who had been administered intramuscular IFN-β1a for at least 1 year with at least 1 relapse in the year preceding study entry were randomized in a 1:1 ratio to either add-on natalizumab (at the same dose and frequency as in AFFIRM) or add-on placebo.[3] At 1 year, the ARR in the combination IFN/natalizumab arm was 0.38 compared with 0.82 in the IFN-β1a alone arm (RRR, 54%; $P<.001$). At 2 years, sustained disability progression in the combination arm was also significantly lower at 23% relative to 29% in the control arm (RRR, 24%; $P = .02$). A subsequent post hoc analysis of those patients with highly active disease (defined as ≥2 relapses in the previous year or ≥1 Gd^+ lesion at study entry) showed that combination therapy reduced the ARR by 76% and disability progression by 66% over 2 years (both $P<.001$).[5]

Because enrolled patients had to have had a relapse when administered Intramuscular IFN-β1a, SENTINEL can be considered a study of "breakthrough disease." However, given that there was no natalizumab-only arm in this trial, it does not answer the key clinical question of whether patients with breakthrough disease do better after switching to natalizumab monotherapy. An ongoing trial, SURPASS, will better examine this question, as it is recruiting patients with breakthrough clinical or magnetic resonance imaging (MRI) disease activity while being administered either GA or subcutaneous IFN-β1a.[6] Patients will be randomized to continue their current therapy, switch to the other first-line agent (ie, GA to IFN-β1a or vice versa), or switch to natalizumab.

Natalizumab can cause both immediate and delayed hypersensitivity reactions in approximately 4% of patients, the former occurring most commonly during a patient's second infusion.[7,8] The main concern with natalizumab treatment is the risk of progressive multifocal leukoencephalopathy (PML) caused by the presumed reactivation of latent JC virus in the central nervous system. Older patient age, previous immunosuppressant use, and prolonged natalizumab exposure increase the risk of PML. To date, in the postmarketing setting, the approximate rates of PML are 0.01, 0.37, and 1.49 per 1000 patients in the first, second, and third years of therapy, respectively (Biogen-Idec, personal communication, 2010).[9,10]

Mitoxantrone hydrochloride (MX) is an anthracenedione that prevents lymphocyte proliferation through the dual mechanisms of intercalation into DNA strands, causing strand breakage, and inhibiting topoisomerase II, a DNA repair enzyme.[11] The pivotal Mitoxantrone in Multiple Sclerosis Group (MIMS) phase 3 trial compared the administration of MX (at doses of both 5 and 12 mg/m^2) every 3 months for 2 years with placebo.[12] A total of 194 patients with either worsening RRMS or secondary progressive multiple sclerosis (SPMS) were enrolled. Patients previously treated with IFN, GA, and MX were excluded. The primary end point (a composite of disability progression and unblinded relapse outcomes without any MRI measures) was significantly lower in both the high-dose MX arm ($P<.0001$) and the low-dose MX arm ($P = .005$) relative to placebo. MRI outcomes in a nonrandomized subset of 110 patients from the MIMS cohort seen at specific sites were subsequently reported.[13] A trend toward a decreased number of scans showing Gd+ lesions at 24 months was seen in the high-dose MX arm relative to placebo ($P = .065$). Patients previously treated with IFN or GA were excluded, so as with the natalizumab trials, MIMS does not provide any direct evidence to support the use of MX as a second-line disease-modifying therapy (DMT).

Use of MX in cancer chemotherapy has been known to be associated with ventricular dysfunction and therapy-related acute leukemia (TRAL). These risks initially seemed smaller in MX-treated patients with multiple sclerosis (MS);[14,15] however, since licensing of this agent as a second-line DMT, an increasing number of reports have resulted in mandated "black box" product monograph changes.[16] The risk of ventricular dysfunction has been estimated to be as high as 12%, including a 0.4% risk of congestive heart failure and the risk of TRAL as high as 0.8%.[17]

Off-Label Therapies

Trials of the alkylating agent cyclophosphamide in MS date back to the 1960s. Through alkylating guanosine residues, cyclophosphamide creates cross-links in both DNA and RNA strands, preventing DNA synthesis and protein production, respectively.[18] In modern practice, cyclophosphamide is typically used either as a high-dose induction therapy for fulminant MS or as booster administered every 1 to 3 months.[18,19] There has been great debate in the literature about the merits of cyclophosphamide administration in MS, with the main North American trials producing divergent results, likely related to the clinical characteristics of the enrolled patients.[18–23]

An early unblinded randomized controlled trial (RCT) of 60 patients with chronic progressive MS (CPMS) compared cyclophosphamide induction and adrenocorticotropic hormone (ACTH); oral cyclophosphamide, plasma exchange, and ACTH; and ACTH alone.[24] Compared with ACTH alone, cyclophosphamide induction resulted in a higher likelihood of disease stabilization ($P = .002$), with the plasma exchange/oral cyclophosphamide group showing an intermediate favorable trend.

The Northeast Cooperative Treatment Group also demonstrated beneficial effects of cyclophosphamide administration in a 4-arm rater-blinded trial comparing 2 different induction protocols, with or without follow-up monthly cyclophosphamide boosters for 2 years.[25] Enrolled patients were followed up for an additional year off-treatment. The 2 induction protocols produced equivalent results. However, at the 1-year mark, a separation was seen in the survival curves of the patients who did and did not receive boosters. The patients who received the booster had less EDSS progression during the second year of treatment and in the subsequent year of follow-up ($P = .03$). Subgroup analyses showed that patients with primary progressive multiple sclerosis fared worse than patients with SPMS regardless of the treatment protocol used ($P = .04$) and that the benefits of boosters seemed to be confined to younger patients ($P = .003$), with similar progression rates seen in those older than 40 years regardless of whether or not boosters were used ($P = .97$).

In contrast, the rater-blinded Canadian Cooperative Multiple Sclerosis Study Group results did not show a benefit of cyclophosphamide induction in patients with CPMS.[26] The reasons for these divergent results have been debated, but the general consensus is that cyclophosphamide administration is likely to be of benefit only in younger patients with an active inflammatory component as manifested clinically by continued relapses or radiologically by an increasing T2 and/or T1 Gd$^+$ burden of disease.[18]

Cyclophosphamide therapy is generally well tolerated at the doses used in patients with MS, although nausea, alopecia, and fatigue are common.[18,19] Patients need be counseled about the high likelihood of menstrual irregularities and fertility issues with high cumulative doses, the need to monitor for febrile neutropenia and hemorrhagic cystitis, and the possibility of bladder cancer and other secondary malignancies.

The most aggressive second-line therapy is autologous hematopoietic stem cell transplantation.[27] Several small nonrandomized, uncontrolled studies have reported generally positive outcomes with this approach in severely affected patients with MS,[28] although there is still a significant up-front mortality risk. However, recent reports suggest that, although there can be a dramatic early improvement/stabilization,[29,30] disease progression occurs with longer patient follow-up, especially in older patients with SPMS.[31]

At the other end of the spectrum of "aggressiveness," the combination of pulse steroid and IFN therapy has been explored.[32–34] In the NORMIMS RCT, the addition of monthly oral methylprednisolone courses to standard subcutaneous IFN-β1a therapy in a cohort of 66 patients with breakthrough disease resulted in a mean annual relapse rate of 0.22 compared with 0.59 in the IFN-β1a-alone arm (RRR, 62%; $P<.0001$); however, this trial was compromised by a high drop-out rate.[32] This positive benefit of the steroid/IFN-β combination therapy was not replicated in 2 other RCTs. The Avonex Combination Trial (ACT) was a 2 × 2 factorial-design trial evaluating add-on monthly IV methylprednisolone boosters and weekly oral methotrexate (either alone or in combination) in patients with breakthrough clinical or MRI disease activity when administered intramuscular IFN-β1a.[33] The investigators did not find any reduction in the number of new or enlarged T2 lesions at 12 months when either methylprednisolone (OR, 0.74; $P = .18$) or methotrexate (OR, 0.98; $P = .93$) was added to IFN-β1a. In the MECOMBIN study of treatment-naive patients, monthly pulse oral methylprednisolone or placebo was added to intramuscular IFN-β1a therapy.[34] No effect was seen on the primary end point of EDSS progression sustained for 6 months (hazard ratio, 0.88; $P = .57$).

Therapies awaiting the US Food and Drug Administration approval

Several novel therapies are in various stages of clinical development, including the probable licensing of the first oral DMTs, fingolimod and cladribine, in the next 1 to 2 years. Because of the impressive efficacy results coupled with concerns about the potential toxicities of these oral agents identified in the pivotal phase 3 trials,[35–37] the initial use of these therapies in clinical practice might be as second-line agents, given the relative safety of the current first-line injectable DMTs. However, the phase 3 trials of fingolimod and cladribine were not designed to specifically focus on patients with breakthrough disease. Indeed, the pivotal cladribine trial (CLARITY)[37] specifically excluded patients who had failed therapy with 2 or more DMTs. The active-comparator fingolimod trial (TRANSFORMS) demonstrated that this agent was more effective than intramuscular IFN-β1a, indirectly suggesting that it might be useful as a second-line agent.[36]

The monoclonal antibodies alemtuzumab and ocrelizumab/rituximab may also be available as second-line therapies in the next few years. The phase 2 alemtuzumab trial comparing this agent with subcutaneous IFN-β1a specifically enrolled early, treatment-naive patients.[38] However, the benefit observed relative to the active-comparator indirectly suggests that it would be useful as a second-line therapy. This question is being addressed in 1 of the 2 ongoing phase 3 alemtuzumab trials, which is specifically recruiting patients who have had breakthrough disease when administered either IFN or GA.[39] Similarly, although the completed phase 2 trial of the anti-CD20 monoclonal antibody rituximab did not focus on breakthrough disease,[40] the recently completed trial of the related molecule ocrelizumab has both placebo and active-comparator arms.[41] If the final results favor ocrelizumab, the trial may provide some indirect evidence to support the use of ocrelizumab as a second-line therapy despite not specifically enrolling patients who have failed first-line therapy.

DEFINITIONS OF BREAKTHROUGH DISEASE

There is neither a standard definition for breakthrough disease in MS nor a clear consensus on how to manage such patients, given that this particular group has not been the primary population enrolled in class I, assessor-blinded RCTs. Furthermore, as Rudick and Polman[1] have noted, given that approximately two-thirds of patients randomized to DMTs in the pivotal IFN and GA trials had further relapses and/or evidence of MRI activity, breakthrough disease has to be considered "the rule and not the exception." Therefore, the important issue becomes what degree of break-through disease is felt to be acceptable by the patient and/or the treating clinician and what represents treatment failure. Implicit in this formulation is that this threshold of treatment failure is inherently subjective and may be defined differently by the patient and clinician and between different patients and clinicians.

Rudick and Polman[1] concisely summarize the extensive literature examining specific clinical and MRI parameters used to define the presence of breakthrough disease or to predict who will subsequently develop breakthrough disease.[1] Although study results are by no means uniform, the development of T2 hyperintensities, Gd[+] lesions, T1 hypointensities, and brain atrophy while patients are administered IFN or GA therapy are all either associated with or predictive of breakthrough disease as measured by future disability progression or relapse rates. Neutralizing antibodies to IFN[42,43] and natalizumab[44] block the biologic effect of these agents and are associated with a loss of clinical and MRI effectiveness. In contrast, antibodies to GA are not physiologically significant and are not associated with an increased risk of break-through disease.[45]

In the absence of RCT data to indicate when second-line therapies should be used, a variety of expert opinion statements and guidelines have been published.[46–52] Specifically focusing on the use of natalizumab, Ransohoff[46] suggested that this drug should be considered in any patient given a first-line DMT with 1 or more relapses over a 12-month period with or without Gd[+] lesional activity or in patients unable to tolerate first-line therapy. Canadian consensus guidelines developed by an expert panel also highlight that the main indication for natalizumab at present is in patients with a suboptimal response to a minimum of 1 year of IFN or GA treatment.[47] The panel felt that this inadequate response had to be clinical; MRI worsening in isolation would not mandate a change in therapy. In addition, treatment-naive patients with rapid disability progression or any relapsing patient unable to tolerate the conventional injectable agents could be considered for natalizumab treatment. Similarly, natalizumab and MX have been recommended for use in breakthrough disease and rapidly progressive, highly inflammatory MS by various researchers.[48–50]

Bashir and colleagues[51] proposed an analog model to assess treatment response and decide if alternative therapy is warranted. The model used gauges for relapse activity, disease progression, and MRI activity, with each gauge having "no concern," "notable," "worrisome," and "actionable" regions. If the dial reads "notable" on all gauges, "worrisome" on 2, or "actionable" on 1, the investigators suggested that an alternative medication be considered. This approach was subsequently adapted by the Canadian Multiple Sclerosis Working Group's Treatment Optimization Recommendations (CANTOR),[52] with the caveat that this group felt that changes in the MRI gauge could not be used in isolation to support a change in therapy. To assess the utility of the CANTOR approach, the relapse and progression gauge criteria were retrospectively applied to the active-treatment-arm patients enrolled in the pivotal subcutaneous IFN-β1a trial.[53] Patients with a medium or high level of concern in the first year of therapy had an 89% chance of developing breakthrough disease in the next 3 years compared with a 67% chance in the group with a low level of concern (P = .01). A computerized version of CANTOR applied retrospectively over 1 year to intramuscular IFN-β1a-treated patients at a single center in Spain also suggested that these criteria could predict future relapse rates and disability progression.[54] The CANTOR model has been incorporated into a study of subcutaneous IFN-β1a in clinically isolated syndrome patients.[55]

STUDIES OF SWITCHING/ESCALATING THERAPY

Several published retrospective observational studies have examined the utility of switching between different classes of licensed DMTs.[56–60] Gajofatto and colleagues[56] assessed the utility of switching between the 4 first-line DMTs among non-responders (as judged by the treating neurologist) and found that the global median ARR decreased from 0.67 on the first DMT to zero on the second DMT (P<.0001). Although this decrease in ARR was observed for all combinations of first- and second-line DMTs (IFN to GA, GA to IFN, IFN to different IFN), it was not statistically significant in the IFN to GA subgroup, but this subgroup was small. Whereas drawing definite conclusions from such an observational study is limited by the lack of randomization and possible phenomenon of regression-to-the-mean, the ARR did not change between the baseline and first-DMT periods, suggesting that the observed drop with switching was a real effect of the treatment change. This study is also intriguing in the context of the 2 recent RCTs comparing subcutaneous IFN-β1a and IFN-β1b with GA, neither of which demonstrated any significant differences between these agents.[61,62] The report of Gajofatto and colleagues suggests that although these first-line DMTs are essentially equivalent at the population level, individual patients who do not respond to one DMT may respond to another without the need to switch to so-called second-line treatments such as natalizumab.

Various groups have reported significant benefits of switching from IFN or GA to natalizumab in postmarketing studies.[57–60] Putzki and colleagues[57] initially assessed the real-world utility of switching from IFN or GA to natalizumab in patients who failed therapy on the first-line agents (defined as ≥1 relapse or Gd+ lesion over the course of a year on therapy) at a single center. The overall ARR decreased from 2.1 on IFN/GA to 0.2 on natalizumab, an RRR of 91%. This analysis was subsequently extended in 2 other studies of the experiences of MS clinics in Germany and Switzerland[58,59] (one clinic is discussed in both studies). In these populations, approximately 90% to 95% of natalizumab-treated patients had previously been administered IFN or GA. The ARR declined from 2.0–2.3 to 0.2–0.3 after initiating natalizumab in these 2 cohorts (P<.001). Similar results were obtained in a single-center Canadian study, in which the on-treatment ARR mirrored that found in the pivotal trials.[60]

In addition to the large main RCTs discussed in the article, numerous small, open-label, unblinded studies of both MX[63–67] and cyclophosphamide[68–75] have suggested that these agents are effective in patients with aggressive breakthrough disease on conventional DMTs.

SUMMARY

Breakthrough disease, if defined broadly as any ongoing clinical or MRI activity while on conventional injectable DMTs, is common. However, the degree of breakthrough disease that can be considered as treatment failure is not standardized and inherently is a subjective decision involving both the patient and physician. Several approved and off-label agents are suitable options for treating breakthrough disease; however, the risk-benefit ratios of these agents need to be individualized.

REFERENCES

1. Rudick RA, Polman CH. Current approaches to the identification and management of breakthrough disease in patients with multiple sclerosis. Lancet Neurol 2009;8:545–59.
2. Polman CH, O'Connor PW, Havrdova E, et al. A randomized, placebo-controlled trial of natalizumab for relapsing multiple sclerosis. N Engl J Med 2006;354:899–910.
3. Rudick RA, Stuart WH, Calabresi PA, et al. Natalizumab plus interferon beta-1a for relapsing multiple sclerosis. N Engl J Med 2006;354:911–23.
4. Niino M, Bodner C, Simard ML, et al. Natalizumab effects on immune cell responses in multiple sclerosis. Ann Neurol 2006;59:748–54.
5. Hutchinson M, Kappos L, Calabresi PA, et al. The efficacy of natalizumab in patients with relapsing multiple sclerosis: subgroup analyses of AFFIRM and SENTINEL. J Neurol 2009;256:405–15.
6. Biogen Idec. Study evaluating Rebif, Copaxone, and Tysabri for active multiple sclerosis (SURPASS). ClinicalTrials.gov [Internet]. Bethesda (MD): National Library of Medicine (US); 2000. Available at: http://clinicaltrials.gov/ct2/show/NCT01058005. NLM Identifier: NCT01058005. Accessed June 15, 2010.
7. Phillips JT, O'Connor PW, Havrdova E, et al. Infusion-related hypersensitivity reactions during natalizumab treatment. Neurology 2006;67:1717–8.
8. Hellwig K, Schimrigk S, Fischer M, et al. Allergic and nonallergic delayed infusion reactions during natalizumab therapy. Arch Neurol 2008;65:656–8.
9. Yousry TA, Major EO, Ryschkewitsch C, et al. Evaluation of patients treated with natalizumab for progressive multifocal leukoencephalopathy. N Engl J Med 2006;354:924–33.
10. Food and Drug Administration. FDA drug safety communication: risk of progressive multifocal leukoencephalopathy (PML) with the use of Tysabri (natalizumab) [updated 02/05/2010] In: FDA.gov [Internet]. Silver Springs (MD): U.S. Food and Drug Administration. Available at: http://www.fda.gov/Drugs/DrugSafety/PostmarketDrugSafetyInformationforPatientsandProviders/ucm199872.htm. Accessed June 15, 2010.
11. Crespi MD, Ivanier SE, Genovese J, et al. Mitoxantrone affects topoisomerase activities in human breast cancer cells. Biochem Biophys Res Commun 1986;136:521–8.
12. Hartung HP, Gonsette R, Konig N, et al. Mitoxantrone in progressive multiple sclerosis: a placebo-controlled, double-blind, randomized, multicentre trial. Lancet 2002;360:2018–25.

13. Krapf H, Morrissey SP, Zenker O, et al. Effect of mitoxantrone on MRI in progressive MS: results of the MIMS trial. Neurology 2005;65:690–5.
14. Ghalie RG, Edan G, Laurent M, et al. Cardiac adverse effects associated with mitoxantrone (Novantrone) therapy in patients with MS. Neurology 2002;59:909–13.
15. Ghalie RG, Mauch E, Edan G, et al. A study of therapy-related leukemia after mitoxantrone therapy for multiple sclerosis. Mult Scler 2002;8:441–5.
16. EMD Serono, Inc. Novantrone (mitoxantrone) for injection concentrate. [Product Monograph]. 2009. Available at: http://www.novantrone.com/assets/pdf/novantrone_prescribing_info.pdf. Accessed June 1, 2010.
17. Marriott JJ, Miyasaki JM, Gronseth G, et al. Evidence report: the efficacy and safety of mitoxantrone (Novantrone) in the treatment of multiple sclerosis. Report of the Therapeutics and Technology Assessment Subcommittee of the American Academy of Neurology. Neurology 2010;74:1463–70.
18. Weiner HL, Cohen JA. Treatment of multiple sclerosis with cyclophosphamide: critical review of clinical and immunologic effects. Mult Scler 2002;8:142–54.
19. Perini P, Calabrese M, Rinaldi L, et al. The safety profile of cyclophosphamide in multiple sclerosis therapy. Expert Opin Drug Saf 2007;62:183–90.
20. Weiner HL, Hauser SL, Dawson DM, et al. Cyclophosphamide and plasma exchange in multiple sclerosis [letter]. Lancet 1991;337:1033–4.
21. Noseworthy JH, Vandervoort MK, Penman M, et al. Cyclophosphamide and plasma exchange in multiple sclerosis [letter]. Lancet 1991;337:1540–1.
22. Noseworthy JH, Ebers GC, Roberts R. Cyclophosphamide and MS [letter]. Neurology 1994;44:579.
23. Weiner HL, Orav EJ, Hafler DA, et al. Cyclophosphamide and MS [letter]. Neurology 1994;44:580–1.
24. Hauser SL, Dawson DM, Lehrich JR, et al. Intensive immunosuppression in progressive multiple sclerosis. A randomized, three-arm study of high-dose intravenous cyclophosphamide, plasma exchange and ACTH. N Engl J Med 1983; 308:173–80.
25. Weiner HL, Mackin GA, Orav EJ, et al. Intermittent cyclophosphamide pulse therapy in progressive multiple sclerosis: final report of the Northeast Cooperative Multiple Sclerosis Treatment Group. Neurology 1993;43:910–8.
26. The Canadian Cooperative Multiple Sclerosis Study Group. The Canadian cooperative trial of cyclophosphamide and plasma exchange in progressive multiple sclerosis. Lancet 1991;337:441–6.
27. Atkins H, Freedman M. Immunoablative therapy as a treatment for aggressive multiple sclerosis. Neurol Clin 2005;23:273–300.
28. Mancardi G, Saccardi R. Autologous haematopoietic stem-cell transplantation in multiple sclerosis. Lancet Neurol 2008;7:626–36.
29. Burt RK, Loh Y, Cohen B. Autologous non-myeloablative haemopoietic stem cell transplantation in relapsing-remitting multiple sclerosis: a phase I/II study. Lancet Neurol 2009;8:244–53.
30. Fagius J, Lundgren J, Oberg G. Early highly aggressive MS successfully treated by hematopoietic stem cell transplantation. Mult Scler 2009;15:229–37.
31. Krasulová E, Trneny M, Kozák T. High-dose immunoablation with autologous haematopoietic stem cell transplantation in aggressive multiple sclerosis: a single centre 10-year experience. Mult Scler 2010;16:685–93.
32. Sorensen PS, Mellgren SI, Svenningsson, et al. NORdic trial of oral Methylprednisolone as add-on therapy to Interferon beta-1a for treatment of relapsing-remitting Multiple Sclerosis (NORMIMS study): a randomised, placebo-controlled trial. Lancet Neurol 2009;8:519–29.

33. Cohen JA, Imrey PB, Calabresi PA, et al. Results of the Avonex Combination Trial (ACT) in relapsing-remitting MS. Neurology 2009;72:535–41.
34. Ravnborg M, Sørensen PS, Andersson M, et al. Methylprednisolone in combination with interferon beta-1a for relapsing-remitting multiple sclerosis (MECOMBIN study): a multicentre, double-blind, randomised, placebo-controlled, parallel-group trial. Lancet Neurol 2010;9:672–80.
35. Kappos L, Radue E-W, O'Connor P, et al. A placebo-controlled trial of oral fingolimod in relapsing multiple sclerosis. N Engl J Med 2010;362:387–401.
36. Cohen J, Barkhof F, Comi G, et al. Oral fingolimod or intramuscular interferon for relapsing multiple sclerosis. N Engl J Med 2010;362:402–15.
37. Giovannoni G, Comi G, Cook S, et al. A placebo-controlled trial of oral cladribine for relapsing multiple sclerosis. N Engl J Med 2010;355:1124–40.
38. The CAMMS223 Trial Investigators. Alemtuzumab vs. interferon beta-1a in early multiple sclerosis. N Engl J Med 2008;359:1786–801.
39. Genzyme. Comparison of alemtuzumab and Rebif® efficacy in multiple sclerosis, study two (CARE-MS II). ClinicalTrials.gov [Internet]. Bethesda (MD): National Library of Medicine (US); 2000. Available at: http://clinicaltrials.gov/ct2/show/NCT00548405. NLM Identifier: NCT00530348. Accessed June 15, 2010.
40. Hauser SL, Waubant E, Arnold DL, et al. B-cell depletion with rituximab in relapsing-remitting multiple sclerosis. N Engl J Med 2008;358:676–88.
41. Genentech A. Study of the efficacy and safety of ocrelizumab in patients with relapsing-remitting multiple sclerosis. ClinicalTrials.gov [Intranet]. Betheseda (MD): National Library of Medicine (US); 2000. Available at: http://clinicaltrials.gov/ct2/show/NCT00676715. NLM Identifier: NCT00676715. Accessed June 15, 2010.
42. Goodin DS, Frohman EM, Hurwitz B, et al. Neutralizing antibodies to interferon beta: assessment of their clinical and radiographic impact: an evidence report: report of the Therapeutics and Technology Assessment Subcommittee of the American Academy of Neurology. Neurology 2007;68:977–84.
43. Polman CH, Bertolotto A, Deisenhammer F, et al. Recommendations for clinical use of data on neutralising antibodies to interferon-beta therapy in multiple sclerosis. Lancet Neurol 2010;9:740–50.
44. Calabresi PA, Giovannoni G, Confavreux C, et al. The incidence and significance of anti-natalizumab antibodies: results from AFFIRM and SENTINEL. Neurology 2007;69:1391–403.
45. Teitelbaum D, Brenner T, Abramsky O, et al. Antibodies to glatiramer acetate do not interfere with its biological functions and therapeutic efficacy. Mult Scler 2003; 9:592–9.
46. Ransohoff RM. Natalizumab for multiple sclerosis. N Engl J Med 2007;356:2622–9.
47. O'Connor PW. Use of natalizumab in multiple sclerosis patients. Can J Neurol Sci 2010;37:98–104.
48. Karussis D, Biermann LD, Bohlega S, et al. A recommended treatment algorithm in relapsing multiple sclerosis: report of an international consensus meeting. Eur J Neurol 2006;13:61–71.
49. Wiendl H, Toyka KV, Rieckmann P, et al. Basic and escalating immunomodulatory treatments in multiple sclerosis: current therapeutic recommendations. J Neurol 2008;255:1449–63.
50. Boster A, Edan G, Frohman E, et al. Intense immunosuppression in patients with rapidly worsening multiple sclerosis: treatment guidelines for the clinician. Lancet Neurol 2008;7:173–83.

51. Bashir K, Buchwald L, Coyle PK, et al. MS patient management: optimizing the benefits of immunomodulatory therapy. Int J MS Care 2002;4:3–7.
52. Freedman MS, Patry DG, Grand'Maison F, et al. Treatment optimization in multiple sclerosis. Can J Neurol Sci 2004;31:157–68.
53. Freedman MS, Forrestal FG. Canadian treatment optimization recommendations (TOR) as a predictor of disease breakthrough in patients with multiple sclerosis treated with interferon beta-1a: analysis of the PRISMS study. Mult Scler 2008; 14:1234–41.
54. Ruiz-Pena JL, Duque P, Izquierdo G. Optimization of treatment with interferon beta in multiple sclerosis. Usefulness of automatic system application criteria. BMC Neurol 2008;8:3.
55. Serono EMD. A prospective study looking at the use of Rebif® in subjects with clinically isolated syndrome (CIS-ON). ClinicalTrials.gov [Internet]. Bethesda (MD): National Library of Medicine (US); 2000. Available at: http://clinicaltrials. gov/ct2/show/NCT00287079. NLM Identifier: NCT00287079. Accessed June 15, 2010.
56. Gajofatto A, Bacchetti P, Grimes B, et al. Switching first-line disease-modifying therapy after failure: impact on the course of relapsing–remitting multiple sclerosis. Mult Scler 2009;15:50–8.
57. Putzki N, Kollia K, Woods S, et al. Natalizumab is effective as second line therapy in the treatment of relapsing remitting multiple sclerosis. Eur J Neurol 2009;16: 424–6.
58. Putzki N, Yaldizli O, Mäurer M, et al. Efficacy of natalizumab in second line therapy of relapsing-remitting multiple sclerosis: results from a multi-center study in German speaking countries. Eur J Neurol 2010;17:31–7.
59. Putzki N, Yaldizli O, Bühler R, et al. Natalizumab reduces clinical and MRI activity in multiple sclerosis patients with high disease activity: results from a multicenter study in Switzerland. Eur Neurol 2010;63:101–6.
60. Krysko KM, O'Connor PW. Comparability of randomized controlled versus observational studies: findings from the Toronto observational study of natalizumab in multiple sclerosis [abstract P05.081]. In the 62nd Annual Meeting of the American Academy of Neurology. Toronto, April 10–17, 2010.
61. Mikol DD, Barkhof F, Chang P, et al. Comparison of subcutaneous interferon beta-1a with glatiramer acetate in patients with relapsing multiple sclerosis (the REbif vs Glatiramer Acetate in Relapsing MS Disease [REGARD] study): a multicentre, randomised, parallel, open-label trial. Lancet Neurol 2008;7:903–14.
62. O'Connor P, Filippi M, Arnason B, et al. 250 microg or 500 microg interferon beta-1b versus 20 mg glatiramer acetate in relapsing-remitting multiple sclerosis: a prospective, randomised, multicentre study. Lancet Neurol 2009;8:889–97.
63. Jeffery DR, Chepuri N, Durden D, et al. A pilot trial of combination therapy with mitoxantrone and interferon beta-1b using monthly gadolinium-enhanced magnetic resonance imaging. Mult Scler 2005;11:296–301.
64. Correale J, Rush C, Amengual A, et al. Mitoxantrone as rescue therapy in worsening relapsing-remitting MS patients receiving IFN-beta. J Neuroimmunol 2005; 162:173–83.
65. Benesova Y, Stourac P, Beranek M, et al. Mitoxantrone therapy in rapidly worsening multiple sclerosis. Bratisl Lek Listy 2005;106:141–3.
66. Cocco E, Marchi P, Sardu C, et al. Mitoxantrone treatment in patients with early relapsing-remitting multiple sclerosis. Mult Scler 2007;13:975–80.
67. Buttinelli C, Clemenzi A, Borriello G, et al. Mitoxantrone treatment in multiple sclerosis: a 5-year clinical and MRI follow-up. Eur J Neurol 2007;14:1281–7.

68. Khan OA, Zvartau-Hind M, Caon C, et al. Effect of monthly intravenous cyclophosphamide in rapidly deteriorating multiple sclerosis patients resistant to conventional therapy. Mult Scler 2001;7:185–8.

69. Perini P, Gallo P. Cyclophosphamide is effective in stabilizing rapidly deteriorating secondary progressive multiple sclerosis. J Neurol 2003;250:834–8.

70. Patti F, Cataldi ML, Nicoletti F, et al. Combination of cyclophosphamide and interferon-beta halts progression in patients with rapidly transitional multiple sclerosis. J Neurol Neurosurg Psychiatry 2001;71:404–7.

71. Reggio E, Nicoletti A, Fiorilla T, et al. The combination of cyclophosphamide plus interferon beta as rescue therapy could be used to treat relapsing-remitting multiple sclerosis patients: twenty-four months follow-up. J Neurol 2005;252: 1255–61.

72. Smith DR, Weinstock-Guttman B, Cohen JA, et al. A randomized blinded trial of combination therapy with cyclophosphamide in patients with active multiple sclerosis on interferon beta. Mult Scler 2005;11:573–82.

73. Gladstone DE, Zamkoff KW, Krupp L, et al. High-dose cyclophosphamide for moderate to severe refractory multiple sclerosis. Arch Neurol 2006;63:1388–93.

74. Krishnan C, Kaplin AI, Brodsky RA, et al. Reduction of disease activity and disability with high-dose cyclophosphamide in patients with aggressive multiple sclerosis. Arch Neurol 2008;65:1044–51.

75. Makhani N, Gorman MP, Branson HM, et al. Cyclophosphamide therapy in pediatric multiple sclerosis. Neurology 2009;72:2076–82.

Progressive Multiple Sclerosis: Characteristics and Management

Kathleen Hawker, MD

KEYWORDS

- Primary and secondary progressive multiple sclerosis
- Treatments • MRI • Relapsing remitting multiple sclerosis

PROGRESSIVE FORMS OF MULTIPLE SCLEROSIS

Multiple sclerosis (MS) is thought to be an autoimmune disease of the central nervous system preferentially affecting women and young people aged 20 to 40 years and is one of the most common causes of disability during this age.[1]

The most common form, relapsing remitting MS (RRMS), is characterized by intermittent attacks and subsequent partial improvement of neurologic symptoms, with stability of symptoms in between attacks, and comprises 85% of all patients at the onset of disease. However, natural history studies show that up to 85% to 90% of untreated patients with RRMS develop secondary progressive MS (SPMS), whereby gradual disability accrues over a variable amount of time, with or without superimposed relapses.[2]

A less common clinical phenotype, primary progressive MS (PPMS), encompasses 10% to 15% of the population with MS. This phenotype is equally common in men and women and tends to occur in a population that is older than that with RRMS (approximately 10 years older on average), and disease progression starts slowly from the onset without any identifiable relapses. Relapsing progressive MS is a rare subtype, occurring in about 1% of patients, and presents as a progressive increase in disability from the onset, superimposed by occasional relapses.[3]

The prevailing opinion has been that PPMS represents a distinct clinical phenotype, although many have questioned the accuracy of this assumption and, in particular, whether PPMS is distinct from SPMS. A second assumption is that progression is caused by neurodegeneration and thus not treatable by drugs that mitigate inflammation. Data from clinical trials in conjunction with information available from magnetic

Funding source: none.
Conflicts of interest: The author has received personal compensation as an employee and holds stock in Eli Lilly.
Eli Lilly and Company, Lilly Corporate Center, Indianapolis, IN 46285, USA
E-mail address: hawkerks@lilly.com

Neurol Clin 29 (2011) 423–434
doi:10.1016/j.ncl.2011.01.002
0733-8619/11/$ – see front matter © 2011 Elsevier Inc. All rights reserved.

resonance imaging (MRI) studies on the differences in age, gender, and genetics have examined this postulate.[4–7]

IMAGING OF PROGRESSIVE DISEASE

On the basis of MRI and autopsy studies, it has been proposed and is generally well accepted that there are 2 pathologic components to MS: inflammation and neurodegeneration. Furthermore, it has been proposed that the former, as evidenced by gadolinium (Gd)-enhancing (reflecting blood-brain barrier disruption) and T2-bright lesions, is the pathophysiologic correlate of relapses, whereas the latter, as measured by brain and spinal cord atrophy, is the correlate of progression. Conventional MRI techniques are primarily used to evaluate inflammation, although they can be used to measure tissue loss, that is, brain and spinal cord atrophy.

In 1990, Thompson's group found that PPMS was associated with fewer T2 brain lesions than SPMS and RRMS. This observation has since been replicated and extended to Gd-enhancing lesions in many studies.[8–14] Despite the quantitative differences between the groups, there is evidence of an early, clinically silent inflammatory component in PPMS. Ingle and colleagues[15] performed an MRI study with a triple dose of Gd in a cohort of 45 patients in the early stages of PPMS (within 5 years of symptom onset) and showed that the Gd enhancing T1 lesion load was seen in 42% of patients on brain MRI as compared with 80% in RRMS and much higher than shown in previous studies. This finding was corroborated in a study by Bieniek and colleagues[16] demonstrating that 49% of patients with PPMS had Gd-enhancing lesions, with an average disease duration of 3.3 years. In addition, patients with enhancing lesions had a greater T2 lesion load, higher brain atrophy, and greater disability compared with patients without enhancement.

Other MRI studies on PPMS have reported much lower numbers of Gd-enhancing lesions, possibly reflecting the longer disease duration of patients in the studies. Not surprisingly, and similar to PPMS, studies on the degree of inflammation in SPMS, as measured by Gd-enhancing lesions, have varied, depending on the cohort imaged.[17]

In a study of 80 patients by Kidd and colleagues,[18] MRI of the brain and spinal cord demonstrated that T2 lesions of the spinal cord are relatively common in patients with progressive MS, occurring in 74% of patients and more predominantly in the cervical than thoracic cord. The frequency of lesions found in patients with PPMS and SPMS was no different.

Atrophy can be evaluated by numerous techniques, has a higher correlation with long-term disability, and has been thought to represent the sum of acute loss of tissue from inflammatory lesions and neurodegeneration. Studies quantifying the degree of gray matter atrophy in PPMS and SPMS on conventional MRI, magnetic transfer imaging, and diffusion tensor imaging have been varied, showing either equal amounts in both forms of the disease or a predominance in SPMS.[19] Equally, in the early phase of RRMS and in clinically isolated syndromes, there are numerous studies documenting the underlying subclinical disease progression, as measured by progressive brain atrophy.[20–22]

Cord atrophy occurs in progressive disease in addition to brain atrophy, although in a study by Losseff and colleagues[23] the degree of spinal cord atrophy seemed to be less extensive in PPMS than in SPMS; however, overall the degree of atrophy seemed to predict disability. A subsequent study with a 5-year follow-up showed no correlation of disability with cord atrophy, with the only predictors being a lower Expanded Disability Status Scale (EDSS) at baseline and gray matter mean diffusivity.[24] The disparity between the 2 studies was thought to reflect the difficulty in measurement of the spinal cord because of its relatively small size. In another 5-year study of progressive disease, no correlation between progression of cord atrophy and brain atrophy was observed, suggesting that independent processes may result in the differential rates of atrophy in the brain and cord.[25]

Advances in MRI technology are also changing the understanding of the pathogenesis of MS subtypes. The nonconventional MRI techniques, magnetization transfer imaging, diffusion tensor imaging, and magnetic resonance spectroscopy, can be used to evaluate more subtle changes in the brain and spinal cord tissue that appear normal on conventional MRI. Numerous studies using these nonconventional techniques have shown that compared with healthy controls, patients with PPMS have widespread changes to the so-called normal-appearing tissues of the brain and spinal cord in the white and especially gray matter (normal-appearing white matter [NAWM] and normal-appearing gray matter [NAGM]).[26–28] These data collectively indicate that there are diffuse abnormalities and axonal loss in the NAWM and NAGM of the brain and spinal cord in patients with PPMS. Some studies have also shown similar abnormalities in SPMS and changes in NAWM (with lesser changes in NAGM) in RRMS.

Consistent with the findings from brain atrophy studies described earlier,[20–22] the results of nonconventional MRI studies indicate that clinically silent neurodegeneration occurs earlier in the disease process of RRMS than originally thought, with changes indicative of axonal loss even when the T2 burden is low.[29]

There are several caveats that may produce conflicting data when comparing the studies; first, the specific patient characteristics or heterogeneity of patients with progressive MS included in the study may skew or limit the conclusions, and second, technical limitations may limit extrapolation between studies. Despite these caveats, there are many MRI similarities between the 2 forms of progressive disease, possibly reflecting relatively similar pathogenic mechanisms driving disability progression.

In addition, although MS is classified by relapsing and progressive clinical phenotypes, the aforementioned studies suggest that progressive tissue loss occurs at an early stage of the disease and is independent of the clinical manifestation.[30]

The data mentioned earlier, together with the results of studies showing that current immunosuppressants and immunomodulators are generally effective for RRMS but not SPMS and PPMS (see section on clinical trials in progressive MS later in the article) have been interpreted as evidence that progressive disease is distinct from relapsing onset disease and that it is a primarily neurodegenerative rather than an inflammatory condition. However, it is now clear that the inflammation/neurodegeneration dichotomy is much too simplistic.

There has been a paucity of treatments for progressive disease (SPMS and PPMS), possibly reflecting the incomplete understanding of the pathogenesis of progression in MS. Both inflammation and degeneration have been implicated; however, there has been debate in the literature as to their relative contributions and the heterogeneity within the 2 populations, and specific cohorts studied likely contributed to the contradictory conclusions. Thus, it is postulated that progression is caused by the interaction of multiple biologic processes, and a deeper understanding of these mechanisms may aid in developing effective treatment protocols.[31]

The controversy of the role of inflammation as a significant component of progression is illustrated in several natural studies that have suggested a lack of correlation between disability progression and relapses. Data from the Lyon Multiple Sclerosis Cohort also show that the clinical phenotype and course of MS are age dependent. Thus, the age at which patients reached specified disability milestones was independent of relapses and the initial course of the disease. Furthermore, in the London, Ontario, cohort, it was also shown that age at onset and age at observation were important determinants of clinical phenotype.[32,33] In a study by Confavreux and colleagues,[34] once SPMS and PPMS patients reached a Disability Status Scale of 4, the rate of disability progression was the same irrespective of relapses.[35]

The same disconnect between relapses and disease progression has been observed in clinical trials. In the European study of interferon beta-1a, disability was slowed in all patients irrespective of previous or ongoing relapses.[36]

However, other studies have shown a treatment effect in those patients with evidence of ongoing inflammation as measured by Gd-enhancing lesions on the MRI scan. It may be that subclinical inflammation mediated by various components of the immune system, in the absence of relapses, initiates irreversible damage–producing progression; however, the clinical manifestations of progression may not be evident until compensatory mechanisms in the central nervous system are overwhelmed.[37,38]

There are several factors that may modify the degree of inflammation and progression in individual patients. Genetic studies have shown that modifiers may influence both the severity of the inflammation (interleukin-7 receptor, interleukin-2 receptor, cadherin 10, neuroligin-1, huntingtin interacting protein 2) and the mediators of repair.[39–41]

Although there is a paucity of large data sets of the hormonal influence on immunity in humans, there are some suggestions from animal data that testosterone may protect against developing the disease; however, estrogens, through effects on multiple steroid receptors, may downmodulate the immune response. However, effects of the modulation of both estrogen and testosterone on various immune cells may be altered or lost with aging. The experimental data raise the possibility that glial cells may be more reactive in older individuals with MS, whereas T and B cells may be less reactive because of hormonal influences.

In combination with genetic and hormonal influences, aging (immunosenescence) modifies the immune responses, and studies suggest that the inflammatory response lessens over time; thus, the relative contribution of specific pathogenic cells causing progression may be altered in older individuals as compared with younger patients. It also has been demonstrated that older neurons are less amenable to recovery after an insult, leading to a greater rate of axonal loss after injury with aging.

The equal predominance of men and women in PPMS as compared with the increased women to men ratio in RRMS and SPMS may partially be explained by an effect of aging and changes in hormonal influences. The protective effect of testosterone is diminished, making men more susceptible to the development of the disease, and the downregulation of T and B cells may predispose to the lesser inflammatory phenotype of PPMS.[42–45]

To target patients with SPMS and PPMS who may respond to antiinflammatory treatments, it is crucial to identify predictive factors. Several cross-sectional and long-term studies of progressive disease have identified some patient and MRI characteristics that may predict a faster progression.

Although there was a marked variation among patients with PPMS, the best predictors of subsequent disability progression included male sex, a slower timed walk at baseline, deterioration of the EDSS score in the first 2 years and reduction in brain volume on the MRI scan of the brain over 2 years, an increase in T2 lesion load, and the development of new lesions and cord atrophy over 2 years.[46] A significant percentage of patients have been shown to have Gd-enhancing lesions early in the course of PPMS (although less numerous than RRMS; 50% vs 80%). In addition, Gd-enhancing lesions may be predictive of a more rapid disability progression in PPMS.[38,46–48]

TREATMENT OF PROGRESSIVE DISEASE

The treatment of progressive disease can be subdivided into 2 categories; the first is prevention of the disease to slow progression, and the second is treatment of symptoms to improve the quality of life.

Disease Prevention

At present, there are only 2 drugs approved for the progressive forms of MS (specifically SPMS), interferon beta-1b in Europe and mitoxantrone (Novantrone) in Europe and the United States for worsening MS (**Table 1**). Despite the paucity of approved treatments for progressive disease, there have been numerous clinical trials for the treatment of SPMS and PPMS. Although the results of most of the studies have been negative, they provide a clearer picture of the pathogenesis of progression and patient cohorts that may be amenable to treatment.

Several drug trials have included both SPMS and PPMS in their cohorts and range from small, open-label observational studies to large, double-blind, placebo-controlled, randomized studies. Specific patient baseline characteristics were not addressed in some studies, making comparisons and conclusions somewhat difficult. Several phase 3 trials have also included patients with SPMS who had superimposed relapses (natalizumab, fingolimod).[49,50] All of the drugs previously tested act to prevent inflammation, mostly targeting either T or B cells. Many of the therapies tested carry concerning risks (particularly infections); thus, it becomes important to be able to select patients with progressive disease that may respond to these drugs so that the benefit outweighs the risk.

There have been several large, randomized, placebo-controlled trials of interferon beta in SPMS and PPMS.

Two trials examined the effect of interferon beta-1b (Betaferon in Europe and Betaseron in North America) on disability progression in SPMS. There were conflicting results: the North American trial showed no effect, whereas the European trial showed a significant effect of slowing of the disease. A meta-analysis that was performed to elucidate the reasons behind the differing outcomes showed a greater percentage of younger patients, lesser duration of disease, and patients with more relapses in the prior 2 years before randomization in the European trial, and patients with a more rapid rate of EDSS progression seemed to benefit the most from therapy, suggesting that signs of ongoing inflammation may predict patients who may respond to this drug.[8,36,51]

The SPECTRIMS (Secondary Progressive Efficacy Clinical Trial of Recombinant Interferon beta-1a in MS) (Rebif, 22 and 44 μg 3 times a week, in SPMS) and the IMPACT (International MS Secondary Progressive Avonex Controlled Trial) trials (Avonex, 60 μg once a week, in SPMS) showed results that were similar to the North American Betaseron trial. Neither trial showed an effect on the time to confirmed disease progression as measured by the EDSS; however, significant effects on MRI parameters (Gd-enhancing and T2 lesions) and relapse rate were seen for both drugs. There was a trend to slowing of disease progression in patients who had a relapse in the previous 2 years before randomization in the SPECTRIMS trial and significant effects on the Multiple Sclerosis Functional Composite (MSFC) Z score in the IMPACT trial.[52,53]

No benefit was seen on slowing of progression in several smaller trials of interferon beta (Avonex 30 and 60 μg once a week vs placebo in 50 patients, and Betaseron 8 million IU vs placebo in 73 patients) in PPMS; however, statistical differences in the MSFC score, T1 and T2 lesion volume, and active lesions were seen with interferon

Table 1
Randomized, class 1, clinical trials in patients with PPMS and SPMS

Drug	Study Design (Duration)	Treatment (Number of Patients)	Primary End Point	Results	References
Interferon beta-1a PPMS	Exploratory, randomized, double-blind, placebo-controlled study (2 y)	Interferon beta-1a, 30 μg; interferon beta-1a, 60 μg; or placebo (n = 50)	Disease progression (increase in EDSS score ≥1 if baseline score ≤5.0 or ≥0.5 if baseline score ≥5.5) sustained for 3 mo	No significant treatment effect on EDSS progression for individual or combined treatment arms vs placebo	Leary et al,[54] 2003
Interferon beta-1b PPMS	Randomized, placebo-controlled pilot study (2 y)	Interferon beta-1b or placebo (n = 73)	As above, but sustained for 6 mo	No significant treatment effect on progression	Montalban et al,[55] 2004
Interferon beta-1b (Europe) SPMS	Randomized, placebo-controlled study (2 y)	Interferon beta-1b or placebo (n = 718)	As above, but sustained for 3 mo	Significant treatment effect on progression (P = .0008)	European Study Group,[36] 1998
Interferon beta-1b (NA) SPMS	Randomized, placebo-controlled study (2 y)	Interferon beta-1b or placebo (n = 939)	Disability sustained for 3 mo	No significant treatment effect	NA Study Group,[51] 2004
Interferon beta-1a SPMS-Avonex	Randomized, placebo-controlled study (2 y)	Interferon beta-1a (60 μg) or placebo (n = 436)	Disability sustained for 3 mo	No effect EDSS; effect of MRI and MSFCS	Cohen et al,[53] 2002
Interferon beta-1a SPMS-Rebif	Randomized, placebo-controlled study (2 y)	Interferon beta-1a 22 or 44 μg (n = 618)	Disability sustained for 3 mo	No significant treatment effect	SPECTRIMS Study Group,[52] 2001
Mitoxantrone PPMS	Randomized, double-blind, placebo-controlled study (2 y)	Mitoxantrone or placebo (n = 61)	Composite end point of EDSS progression (defined as above) or worsening performance (≥20%) on 9-peg hole test, sustained for 3 mo	No significant treatment effect on progression	Kita et al,[58] 2004
Mitoxantrone SPMS/RRMS	Randomized, double-blind, placebo-controlled study (2 y)	Mitoxantrone 12 mg/m^2 or placebo (n = 194)	Sustained disability at 3 mo	Significant effect on disability progression (P = .019)	Hartung et al,[56] 2002
Glatiramer acetate PPMS	Randomized, double-blind, placebo-controlled study (3 y)	Glatiramer acetate or placebo (n = 943)	As for interferon beta-1a study	No significant treatment effect on progression[a]	Wolinsky et al,[59] 2007
Rituximab PPMS	Randomized, double-blind, placebo-controlled study	Rituximab, 1000 mg × 2 every 6 mo (n = 439)	Sustained disability at 3 mo	No significant treatment effect on progression	Hawker et al,[38] 2009

Abbreviations: EDSS, Expanded Disability Status Scale; MSFCS, multiple sclerosis functional composite score; NA, North America.

[a] Data from 2-year interim analysis; study was stopped after this interim analysis.

beta-1b compared with placebo.A decrease in the number of T2 lesions was also seen with interferon beta-1a compared with placebo.[54,55]

A significant slowing of disability progression, as measured by the EDSS and ambulation index, was observed in a mixed cohort of patients with RRMS and SPMS treated with 12 mg/m^2 of mitoxantrone every 3 months. The inclusion criteria selected a group of patients with evidence of change on the EDSS before randomization, somewhat analogous to the patients with a more rapid disease progression seen in the European Betaferon trial. Effects on the relapse rate and MRI parameters were also positive in the mitoxantrone arm compared with placebo. Significant side effects in the trial included nausea, urinary tract infections, menstrual abnormalities, leukopenia, and decreased left ventricular ejection fraction. Although not seen in this study, cases of acute myelogenous leukemia have since been reported with the use of mitoxantrone.[56,57]

Despite the positive outcome in the patients with SPMS, negative results were reported in a smaller and shorter PPMS trial with mitoxantrone. It is unclear whether this discrepancy on treatment outcomes relates to patient selection, as results have not yet been published.[58]

The progressive MS trial was a placebo-controlled trial of 943 patients with PPMS examining the effect of glatiramer acetate (Copaxone) versus placebo. The study was stopped early at 2 years for futility. Although there was no statistical difference in the 2 arms of the study on disease progression, there was a decrease in the number of new T2-bright lesions at year 2 ($P = .0026$) and Gd-enhancing lesions at year 1 but not at year 2 ($P = .0022; P = .07$). There was also a trend to lesser disability progression in men receiving glatiramer acetate compared with placebo, whereas men overall had a more rapid disability progression. A smaller number of patients progressed than was expected, and the early discontinuation of the study may have limited the power to detect a treatment effect.[59]

Rituximab (Rituxan), a B-cell depleting monoclonal antibody, was investigated in 439 patients with PPMS. Although the primary outcome of time to confirmed disease progression was negative, a preplanned subanalysis revealed a significant effect on the slowing of disability in younger patients ($P = .01$), patients who had at least 1 Gd-enhancing lesion on their baseline MRI ($P = .007$), and younger patients with at least 1 Gd-enhancing lesion at baseline ($P = .009$). Although the accumulation of new T2-bright disease burden was lesser in rituximab recipients at 2 years ($P = .001$), no effect was found on brain volume between the 2 groups.[38]

Placebo versus intravenous immunoglobulin at a dose of 0.4 g/kg was infused monthly for 24 months to 197 patients with SPMS and 34 patients with PPMS. A small effect ($P = .03$) on the slowing of sustained disability progression was seen in the PPMS cohort but not in the SPMS cohort. In that study, patients with SPMS and a relapse in the previous year before randomization were excluded and no MRI parameters were reported.[60]

There have been 2 trials of intravenous cladribine for progressive MS. The initial study evaluated cladribine versus placebo in a 2-year crossover study in 48 patients with progressive disease. Analysis of the results showed improvement on the EDSS, the Scripps Neurologic Rating Scale, and MRI findings in the cladribine-treated patients.[61]

This study was in contradistinction to a second study done several years later, in which 159 patients (30% with PPMS, 70% with SPMS) were randomized to placebo or 2 doses of intravenous cladribine for 12 months. About 63% of the patients had no Gd-enhancing lesions on their baseline MRI, and disability levels were high at study entry (the median EDSS score was 6.0). There was no effect on disability progression, but both cladribine doses decreased the proportion of patients having Gd-enhancing lesions as well as the volume and number of Gd-enhancing lesions ($P \leq .003$), starting at 6 months, with a modest decrease in the accumulation of T2-bright lesions. The differences were mainly driven by the SPMS subgroup.[62]

The explanation to the differing outcomes in these 2 trials is somewhat unclear. A direct comparison is difficult because of the different study designs and entry patient characteristics in the studies; however, patients in the initial study had a lower mean EDSS (4.5 vs 6.0), and disability changes were assessed over 2 years, which might be a better time frame to evaluate the effect of the medication tested in the progressive forms of MS.

Goodkin and colleagues[63] reported slowing of progression of upper limb function in 60 patients with SPMS and 18 patients with PPMS administered low-dose (7.5 mg) weekly methotrexate. Serial MRIs were performed in 35 patients for 6 months, and a decrease in new T2 lesions as compared with placebo was demonstrated, correlating with the lesser changes on the 9-hole peg test but not on the EDSS score.

There has been a variety of open-label studies showing both negative and positive effects on slowing disease progression; however, the results are difficult to interpret because of the design and number of patients in the studies.

Monthly pulses of cyclophosphamide (Cytoxan) were used to treat 362 patients with SPMS and 128 patients with PPMS selected because of at least a 1-point worsening on the EDSS during the previous year. Over 70% of the patients either stabilized or improved on the EDSS after 12 months of treatment, but there was no control group.[64]

Intermittent steroids, given by intrathecal injection (triamcinolone acetate) in 1 open-label trial, showed no effect on the progression, whereas monthly intravenous methylprednisolone administered in patients with SPMS and PPMS who had evidence of inflammation on the MRI demonstrated a treatment effect.[65]

Small, open-label, and crossover studies of riluzole, autologous stem cell transplantation, and pirfenidone reported stabilization on various MRI and clinical outcomes.[66–68]

When the results are examined from the class 1 evidence trials and other studies, there seems to be several common themes among all the progressive disease cohorts. First, subsets of patients with progressive forms of MS may still have evidence of ongoing inflammation as evidenced by Gd-enhancing lesions, new T2-bright lesions (SPMS and PPMS), or relapses (SPMS). Second, certain parameters, including Gd-enhancing lesions on the MRI, ongoing relapses, younger age, and possibly gender, might predict a treatment response in progressive disease possibly because some subgroups of patients have a faster disability progression, making the detection of a treatment effect easier. Several meta-analyses of RRMS treatment and natural history studies have also noted a more rapid progression to disability with the same parameters.[69,70]

These data suggest that inflammation and progressive tissue loss are integral components of all clinical subtypes of MS; thus, it may no longer be appropriate to dichotomize patients into relapsing and progressive forms of MS. Multiple factors including genetic, immunologic, environmental, hormonal, and aging (immunosenescence) influences may interact to produce quantitative, rather than qualitative, differences, and further analysis of those factors that influence the clinical subtype may aid in the selection of patients responsive to treatment.

Based on the aforementioned studies, it may be possible to identify patients with progressive disease who may benefit from disease-modifying drugs to suppress inflammation and slow disability progression. Careful selection may prevent exposure of patients to drugs with concerning risks without significant benefit. Thus, it may be feasible to identify patients with certain clinical and MRI characteristics, whose progression is more rapid and not primarily driven by neurodegeneration, where the risk-benefit ratio may warrant treatment with a disease-modifying therapy that targets inflammation.

REFERENCES

1. Hauser S, Oksenberg J. The neurobiology of multiple sclerosis: genes, inflammation, and neurodegeneration. Neuron 2006;52:61–76.
2. Noseworthy JH, Lucchinetti C, Rodriguez M, et al. Multiple sclerosis. N Engl J Med 2000;343:938.
3. Miller DH, Leary SM. Primary-progressive multiple sclerosis. Lancet Neurol 2007; 6:903–12.
4. Ebers GC. Prognostic factors for multiple sclerosis: the importance of natural history studies. J Neurol 2005;252(Suppl 3):iii15–20.
5. McDonnell GV, Hawkins SA. Primary progressive multiple sclerosis: a distinct syndrome? Mult Scler 1996;2:137–41.
6. Rudick R. Mechanisms of disability progression in primary progressive multiple sclerosis: are they different from secondary progressive multiple sclerosis? Mult Scler 2003;9:210–2.
7. Vukusic S, Confavreux C. Primary and secondary progressive multiple sclerosis. J Neurol Sci 2003;206:153–5.
8. Thompson AJ, Kermode AG, MacManus DG, et al. Patterns of disease activity in multiple sclerosis: clinical and magnetic resonance imaging study. BMJ 1990; 300:631–4.
9. Lycklama à Nijeholt GJ, Van Wlderveen MA, Castelijins JA, et al. Brain and spinal cord abnormalities in multiple sclerosis. Correlation between MRI parameters, clinical subtypes and symptoms. Brain 1998;121:687–97.
10. Thompson AJ, Kermode AG, Wicks D, et al. Major differences in the dynamics of primary and secondary progressive multiple sclerosis. Ann Neurol 1991;29: 53–62.
11. Ingle GT, Stevenson VL, Miller DH, et al. Two-year follow-up study of primary and transitional progressive multiple sclerosis. Mult Scler 2002;8:108–14.
12. Kidd D, Thorpe JW, Kendall BE, et al. MRI dynamics of brain and spinal cord in progressive multiple sclerosis. J Neurol Neurosurg Psychiatry 1996;60:15–9.
13. Stevenson VL, Miller DH, Rovaris M, et al. Primary and transitional progressive MS: a clinical and MRI cross-sectional study. Neurology 1999;52:839–45.
14. van Walderveen MA, Lycklama ANG, Ader HJ, et al. Hypointense lesions on T1-weighted spin-echo magnetic resonance imaging: relation to clinical characteristics in subgroups of patients with multiple sclerosis. Arch Neurol 2001;58:76–81.
15. Ingle GT, Sastre-Garriga J, Miller DH, et al. Is inflammation important in early PPMS? a longitudinal MRI study. J Neurol Neurosurg Psychiatry 2005;76:1255–8.
16. Bieniek M, Altmann DR, Davies GR, et al. Cord atrophy separates early primary progressive and relapsing remitting multiple sclerosis. J Neurol Neurosurg Psychiatry 2006;77:1036–9.
17. Zhao Y, Petkau AJ, Traboulsee A, et al. Does MRI lesion activity regress in secondary progressive multiple sclerosis? Mult Scler 2010;16:434–42.
18. Kidd D, Thorpe JW, Thompson AJ, et al. Spinal cord MRI using multi-array coils and fast spin echo. II. Findings in multiple sclerosis. Neurology 1993;43(12): 2632–7.
19. Filippi M, Rocca MA. MR imaging of gray matter involvement in multiple sclerosis: implications for understanding disease pathophysiology and monitoring treatment efficacy. AJNR Am J Neuroradiol 2010;31(7):1171–7.

20. Chard DT, Griffin CM, Parker GJ, et al. Brain atrophy in clinically early relapsing-remitting multiple sclerosis. Brain 2002;125:327–37.
21. Luks TL, Goodkin DE, Nelson SJ, et al. A longitudinal study of ventricular volume in early relapsing-remitting multiple sclerosis. Mult Scler 2000;6:332–7.
22. Rudick RA, Fisher E, Lee JC, et al. Use of the brain parenchymal fraction to measure whole brain atrophy in relapsing-remitting MS. Multiple Sclerosis Collaborative Research Group. Neurology 1999;53:1698–704.
23. Losseff NA, Webb SL, O'Riordan JI, et al. Spinal cord atrophy and disability in multiple sclerosis. A new reproducible and sensitive MRI method with potential to monitor disease progression. Brain 1996;119(Pt 3):701–8.
24. Rovaris M, Judica E, Gallo A, et al. Grey matter damage predicts the evolution of primary progressive multiple sclerosis at 5 years. Brain 2006;129:2628–34.
25. Ingle GT, Stevenson VL, Miller DH, et al. Primary progressive multiple sclerosis: a 5-year clinical and MR study. Brain 2003;126:2528–36.
26. Filippi M, Rovaris M, Rocca MA. Imaging primary progressive multiple sclerosis: the contribution of structural, metabolic, and functional MRI techniques. Mult Scler 2004;10(Suppl 1):S36–44.
27. Filippi M, Agosta F. Magnetization transfer MRI in multiple sclerosis. J Neuroimaging 2007;17(Suppl 1):22S–6S.
28. Rovaris M, Judica E, Sastre-Garriga J, et al. Large-scale, multicentre, quantitative MRI study of brain and cord damage in primary progressive multiple sclerosis. Mult Scler 2008;14:455–64.
29. Lisak RP. Neurodegeneration in multiple sclerosis: defining the problem. Neurology 2007;68(22 Suppl 3):S5–12.
30. DeStephano N, Giorgio A, Battaglini M, et al. Assessing brain atrophy rates in a large population of untreated multiple sclerosis subtypes. Neurology 2010;74:1868–76.
31. Trapp B, Nave KA. Multiple sclerosis: an immune or neurodegenerative disorder? Annu Rev Neurosci 2008;31:247–69.
32. Confavreux C, Vukusic S. Natural history of multiple sclerosis: a unifying concept. Brain 2006;129:606–16.
33. Kremenchutzky M, Rice GP, Baskerville J, et al. The natural history of multiple sclerosis: a geographically based study 9: observations on the progressive phase of the disease. Brain 2006;129:584–94.
34. Confavreux C, Vukusic S, Adeleine P. Early clinical predictors and progression of irreversible disability in multiple sclerosis: an amnesic process. Brain 2003;126:770–82.
35. Scalfari A, Neuhaus A, Degenhardt A. The natural history of multiple sclerosis; a geographically based study 10: relapses and long-term disability. Brain 2010;133(Pt 7):1914–29.
36. European Study Group on Interferon-1b in Secondary Progressive MS. Placebo-controlled multicentre randomised trial of interferon-1b in treatment of secondary progressive multiple sclerosis. Lancet 1998;352:1491–7.
37. Filippi M, Anderson VM, Altmann DR. Brain atrophy and lesion load measures over 1 year relate to clinical status after 6 years in patients with clinically isolated syndromes. J Neurol Neurosurg Psychiatry 2010;81:204–8.
38. Hawker KS, O'Connor P, Freedman MS, et al. Rituximab in patients with primary progressive multiple sclerosis: results of a randomized double-blind placebo-controlled multicenter trial. Ann Neurol 2009;66:460–71.
39. Oksenberg J, Baranzini SE, Sawcer S, et al. The genetics of multiple sclerosis: SNPs to pathways to pathogenesis. Nat Rev Genet 2008;9:516–26.

40. Baranzini SE, Wang J, Gibson RA, et al. Genome-wide association analysis of susceptibility and clinical phenotype in multiple sclerosis. Hum Mol Genet 2009;18:767–78.
41. Matejuk A, Hopke C, Vandenbark A, et al. Middle aged male mice have increased severity of experimental autoimmune encephalomyelitis and are unresponsive to testosterone therapy. J Immunol 2005;174:2387–95.
42. Chen J, Buchanan JB, Sparkman NL, et al. Neuroinflammation and disruption in working memory in aged mice after acute stimulation of the peripheral innate immune system. Brain Behav Immun 2008;22:301–11.
43. Godbout JP, Chen J, Abraham J, et al. Exaggerated neuroinflammation and sickness behavior in aged mice following activation of the peripheral innate immune system. FASEB J 2005;19:1329–31.
44. Hasler P, Zouali M. Immune receptor signaling, aging, and autoimmunity. Cell Immunol 2005;233:102–8.
45. Sawada M, Sawada H, Nagatsu T. Effects of aging on neuroprotective and neurotoxic properties of microglia in neurodegenerative diseases. Neurodegener Dis 2008;5:254–6.
46. Khaleeli Z, Ciccarelli O, Manfredonia F, et al. Predicting progression in primary progressive multiple sclerosis. Ann Neurol 2008;63:790–3.
47. Sastre-Garriga J, Ingle GT, Rovaris M. Long-term clinical outcome of primary progressive MS: predictive value of clinical and MRI data. Neurology 2005;65:633–5.
48. Ingle GT, Sastre-Garriga J, Miller DH, et al. Does inflammation have a role in early PPMS: a longitudinal MRI study. Mult Scler 2003;9:S13.
49. Kappos L, Radue EW, O'Connor P, et al. A placebo-controlled trial of oral fingolimod in relapsing multiple sclerosis. N Engl J Med 2010;362:387–401.
50. Polman C, O'Connor P, Havrdova E, et al. A randomized, placebo-controlled trial of natalizumab for relapsing multiple sclerosis. N Engl J Med 2006;354:899–910.
51. The North American Study Group on Interferon beta-1b in Secondary Progressive MS. Interferon beta-1b in secondary progressive MS: results from a 3-year controlled study. Neurology 2004;63:1788–95.
52. Secondary Progressive Efficacy Clinical Trial of Recombinant Interferon-beta-1a in MS (SPECTRIMS) Study Group. Randomized controlled trial of interferon beta-1a in secondary progressive MS. Neurology 2001;56:1496–504.
53. Cohen J, Cutter G, Fischer JS, et al. Benefit of interferon beta-1a on MSFC progression in secondary progressive MS. Neurology 2002;59:679–87.
54. Leary SM, Miller DH, Stevenson VL, et al. Interferon beta-1a in primary progressive MS. Neurology 2003;60:44–51.
55. Montalban X, Sastre-Garriga J, Tintoré M, et al. A single-center, randomized, double-blind, placebo-controlled study of interferon beta-1b on primary progressive and transitional multiple sclerosis. Mult Scler 2009;15:1195–205.
56. Hartung HP, Gonsette R, König N, et al. Mitoxantrone in progressive multiple sclerosis: a placebo controlled, double-blind, randomised, multicentre trial. Lancet 2002;360:2018–25.
57. Martinelli M, Radaelli L, Straffi H, et al. Mitoxantrone: benefits and risks in multiple sclerosis patients. Neurol Sci 2009;30:1590–874.
58. Kita M, Cohen JA, Fox RJ, et al. A phase II trial of mitoxantrone in patients with progressive forms of multiple sclerosis. Neurology 2004;62(Suppl 5):A99.
59. Wolinsky JS, Narayana PA, O'Connor P, et al. Glatiramer acetate in primary progressive multiple sclerosis: results of a multinational, multicenter, double-blind, placebo-controlled trial. Ann Neurol 2007;61:14–24.

60. Pöhlau D, Przuntek H, Sailer M, et al. Intravenous immunoglobulin in primary and secondary chronic progressive multiple sclerosis: a randomized placebo controlled multicentre study. Mult Scler 2007;13:1007–17.

61. Beutler E, Sipe JC, Romine JS, et al. The treatment of chronic progressive multiple sclerosis with cladrabine. Proc Natl Acad Sci U S A 1996;93:1716–20.

62. Rice G, Filippi M, Comi G, et al. Cladribine and progressive MS: clinical and MRI outcomes of a multicenter controlled trial. Cladribine MRI Study Group. Neurology 2000;54:1145–55.

63. Goodkin DE, Rudick RA, VanderBrug Medendorp S, et al. Low-dose (7.5 mg) oral methotrexate is effective in reducing the rate of progression of neurological impairment in patients with chronic progressive multiple sclerosis. Ann Neurol 1995;37:30–40.

64. Zephir H, de Seze J, Duhamel A, et al. Treatment of progressive forms of multiple sclerosis by cyclophosphamide: a cohort study of 490 patients. J Neurol Sci 2004;218:73–7.

65. Pirko I, Rodriguez M. Pulsed intravenous methylprednisolone therapy in progressive multiple sclerosis: need for a controlled trial. Arch Neurol 2004;61:1148–9.

66. Kalkers N, Barkhof F, Bergers E, et al. The effect of the neuroprotective agent riluzole on MRI parameters in primary progressive multiple sclerosis: a pilot study. Mult Scler 2002;8:532–53.

67. Saccardi R, Kozak T, Bocelli-Tyndall C, et al. Autologous stem cell transplantation for progressive multiple sclerosis: update of the European Group for Blood and Marrow Transplantation autoimmune disease working party database. Mult Scler 2006;12:814–23.

68. Bowen JD, Maravilla K, Margolin SB. Open-label study of pirfenidone in patients with progressive forms of multiple sclerosis. Mult Scler 2003;9:280–3.

69. Mowry EM, Pesic M, Grimes B, et al. Clinical predictors of early second event in patients with clinically isolated syndrome. J Neurol 2009;256:1061–6.

70. Vukusic S, Confavreux C. Natural history of multiple sclerosis: risk factors and prognostic indicators. Curr Opin Neurol 2007;20:269–74.

Promising Emerging Therapies for Multiple Sclerosis

Gavin Giovannoni, MBBCh, PhD, FCP(SA), FRCP, FRCPath

KEYWORDS

- Alemtuzumab • Daclizumab • BG-12 • Fumarate • Cladribine
- Fingolimod • Laquinimod • Teriflunomide

Multiple sclerosis (MS) is the most common disabling neurologic condition to affect young adults in the developed world. MS is believed to be an autoaggressive disease mediated by autoreactive T and B cells (**Table 1**).[1] Putative autoantigens include myelin basic protein (MBP), proteolipid protein, myelin oligodendrocyte glycoprotein, myelin-associated glycoprotein, and αB-crystallin.[2]

MS is characterized pathologically by inflammation, demyelination, and variable degrees of axonal loss and gliosis.[3] Although it is frequently classified as a white matter disease, gray matter involvement is well described, with both prominent cortical and deep gray matter involvement.[4]

The specific cause of MS remains to be defined.[5] Most investigators accept, however, that MS is complex disease that is triggered in genetically susceptible individuals by a complex interplay of genes, epigenetics, and the environment.[6] Whether or not the triggering event is due to single factor or numerous sequential environmental exposures is unknown.[6] Environmental factors that are well recognized include viral infections, in particular Epstein-Barr virus, sunlight/vitamin D, and smoking.[7] The immunopathogenesis of MS has been largely defined using the animal model, experimental allergic encephalomyelitis (EAE), which is also used for screening putative disease-modifying therapies (DMTs).[8] In EAE, and by inference in acute MS lesions, activated autoreactive T-cells produce proinflammatory cytokines, which stimulate other T cells and B cells, which, in parallel with cells of the innate immune system,

Disclosures: Professor Giovannoni has received consulting fees from Bayer Schering Healthcare, Biogen-Idec, FivePrime Therapeutics, Genzyme, GlaxoSmithKline, GW Pharma, Ironwood Pharmaceuticals, Merck-Serono, Novartis, Protein Discovery Laboratories, Roche, Teva-Aventis, Vertex Pharmaceuticals, and UCB Pharma; lecture fees from Bayer Schering Healthcare, Biogen-Idec, Pfizer, Teva-Aventis, and Vertex Pharmaceuticals; and grant support from Bayer Schering Healthcare, Biogen-Idec, GW Pharma, Merck-Serono, Merz, Novartis, Teva-Aventis, and UCB Pharma.
Neuroscience and Trauma Centre, Blizard Institute of Cell and Molecular Science, Barts and The London School of Medicine and Dentistry, Queen Mary University of London, 4 Newark Street, London E1 2AN, UK
E-mail address: g.giovannoni@qmul.ac.uk

Neurol Clin 29 (2011) 435–448
doi:10.1016/j.ncl.2011.01.003
0733-8619/11/$ – see front matter © 2011 Elsevier Inc. All rights reserved.

Table 1
Promising disease-modifying therapies in late phase development for multiple sclerosis

Agents	Route and Dose	Mechanisms of Action	Side Effects
Monoclonal antibodies			
Anti-CD52 Alemtuzumab (formerly Campath-1H)	12 or 24 mg IV, 3 to 5 per week	Partially humanized mAb that targets CD52 on leukocytes Rapid leukopenia (rapid return of neutrophils and monocytes) B-cell rebound to supranormal levels T-cell depletion, long-lasting Immune reconstitution associated with increased frequencies of T-regulatory cells	Acute cell lysis with cytokine release syndrome (fever, chills, skin rash, etc.) Autoimmune hyperthyroidism (30%) ITP (2%) Infections (herpes and varicella) Goodpasture syndrome Possibly increased incidence of secondary malignancies
Anti-CD20 Rituximab Ocrelizumab Ofatumumab	Rituximab—1g IVI, 2 weeks apart Ocrelizumab—600 mg or 2000 mg IVI, 2 weeks apart Ofatumumab—100 mg, 300 mg, or 700 mg IVI	Chimeric and humanized mAbs against CD20 B-cell depletion Reduced antigen presentation	Impaired antibody responses Infection PML Fever Chills Systemic inflammatory syndrome
Anti-CD25 Daclizumab	2 mg/kg subcutaneously every 2 weeks	Modulates cells expressing CD25 or the high-affinity IL-2 receptor Increase regulatory CD56^{bright} NK cells Reduced activated T-cell populations	Skin rash Injection-site reactions Infections Possible increased incidence of secondary malignancies
Oral therapies			
BG-12 (dimethyl fumarate)	Oral 240 mg twice a day or 3 times a day	Neuroprotective via the upregulation of Nrf2 transcription factor Anti-inflammatory (via nuclear factor κB pathway Antioxidant (reduced reactive oxygen radicals) Immunomodulatory (increased T$_h$2 cytokines)	Flushing Headache Nausea Diarrhea

Drug	Route/Dose	Mechanism	Adverse Effects
Cladribine	Oral 3.5 or 5.25 mg/kg	Lymphotoxic Prolonged reduction in CD4 and CD8 T cells and to a lesser extent B cells Reduction in production of proinflammatory cells	Lymphopenia Infections Herpes zoster (2%) Headache Nasopharyngitis Possibly increased incidence of secondary malignancies
Fingolimod	Oral 0.5 mg daily	Partial agonist at the sphingosine-1-phosphate receptor 1 (internalizes receptor preventing it of being recycled back to the surface) Sequesters lymphocytes in lymphoid tissue Binds SP-1 receptors in the CNS that may promote remyelination	First-dose effect results in bradycardia and the potential for heart block Lymphopenia Hypertension Reduced FeV1 Infections Macular edema Hepatoxicity Possibly increased incidence of secondary malignancies
Laquinimod	Oral 0.6 mg daily	Immunomodulatory (T_h1 to T_h2 shift) Reduced immune cell entry into CNS Alteration of antigen presentation Reduced MHC expression Reduced cell adhesion molecule expression	Increase of liver enzymes Arthralgia Possible venous thrombosis
Teriflunomide	Oral 7 or 14 mg daily	Inhibits dihydroorotate dehydrogenase Reduced nitric oxide production Decreases B- and T-cell proliferation Reduced IL-1 and TNF-α production	Hepatoxicity Infection Headaches Alopecia Diarrhea Arthralgia Rhabdomyolysis

Abbreviations: BID, twice daily; IV, intravenous; TID, three times per day.

such as natural killer (NK) cells, macrophages, and microglia, augment and perpetuate the inflammatory process. Cytokines increase blood-brain barrier (BBB) permeability, upregulate and activate endothelial adhesion molecule expression, increase production of antibodies, activate microglia and astrocytes, and recruit peripheral macrophages, which in turn produce a plethora of bioactive mediators. Activated microglia, macrophages, and T cells (both CD4+ and CD8+) are seen in MS lesions[9] and clonotypic B cells, and CD8+ T cells are seen in lesions and the CSF.[10] The inflammatory microenvironment in MS lesions is complex, with potential roles described for T helper (T_h)1, Th_{17}, T_h2, and T-regulatory CD4+ cells; cytotoxic CD8+ cells; macrophages; NK cells; microglia/macrophages; and astrocytes. Secretion of pro- and anti-inflammatory molecules, proteases, nitric oxide derivatives, reactive oxygen species, and cytokines (IL-6, tumor necrosis factor [TNF]-α, interleukin [IL]-4, IL-10, and IL-17) may occur in the same lesion. In addition, cytokines are involved in central nervous system (CNS) repair.[11] T_h17 CD4+ T cells have recently emerged as being important in the pathogenesis of MS.[12]

Although demyelination is the defining feature of the MS lesion, neuroaxonal loss is well described.[13,14] Damage to axons is probably mediated by cytotoxic T-cells, macrophages, antibodies, oxidative stress, and loss of trophic support by oligodendrocytes.[9,15] Axonal transection in MS lesions is related to inflammation in MS lesions.[13,14] Redistribution of Na^+ channels, increased energy requirements, mitochondrial failure, and Ca^{2+}-mediated toxicity all contribute to axonal degeneration in MS.[16,17] Remyelination, mediated by oligodendrocytes that are derived from local progenitors, depends on many factors: the local microenvironment has to switch from a proinflammatory autodestructive one to one that promotes repair. Immunomodulatory cytokines and growth factors, such as IL-4, IL-10, brain-derived neurotrophic factor, and transforming growth factor β, are believed to play a role in promoting recovery. Defining the mechanisms that promote remyelination and designing appropriate clinical trials are key to developing treatments that will have an effect on the neurodegenerative component of MS and, importantly, repair.[18,19]

POTENTIAL TARGETS FOR TREATING MULTIPLE SCLEROSIS

Targets for treating MS include immune dysfunction (anti–T- and anti–B-cell therapies), immune regulation (enhancing T-regulatory function), reducing permeability of BBB, preventing transmigration of cells across the BBB (antiadhesion molecule therapies), targeting key mediators of the inflammatory cascade (anticytokine therapies), putative autoantigens (immune tolerance), reducing demyelination, preventing neuroaxonal loss (neuroprotection), promoting remyelination, and augmenting regenerative processes (growth factors). Several DMTs in development have an impact on one or more of these targets. The remainder of this article focuses on the DMTs that are in late-phase development (phase III) with the promise of being licensed within the next 5 years. Broadly, these therapies can be classified into biologic therapies or monoclonal antibodies (mAbs) and small molecule or oral therapies.

MONOCLONAL ANTIBODIES
Anti-CD52 (Alemtuzumab [Campath-1H])

Alemtuzumab (Genzyme and Bayer Schering) is currently in late phase III development. Alemtuzumab is a humanized IgG1 mAb that binds to CD52 on leukocytes. It rapidly depletes CD52-bearing leukocytes, which include T cells, B cells, NK cells, monocytes and macrophages, and some granulocytes.[20] Whether or not it functions by depleting autoreactive cells directly involved in the autoaggressive cascade is a moot point. Other actions of alemtuzumab include stabilization the BBB and possible "rebooting" or "resetting" of the immune system. Immune reconstitution postalemtuzumab is characterized by enrichment of the CD4+ CD25+ FoxP3+ T-regulatory cell population,[21] which reduces proliferation of autoreactive T cells. The brisk rebound of B cell counts, which typically overshoots pretreatment B-cell levels by more than 50%, is another indicator that alemtuzumab fundamentally changes the immune system in people with MS.[22]

Alemtuzumab is currently licensed for chronic lymphocytic leukemia. Treatment is given annually as infusions over a 3- to 5-day period. Initial trials evaluated alemtuzumab in relapsing secondary progressive MS subjects. Although alemtuzumab suppressed relapses and MRI activity, it did not prevent or reverse disease progression in secondary progressive MS.[23] When alemtuzumab was used early to treat subjects with active relapsing-remitting MS (RRMS), however, patients were observed to improve. The latter observations prompted a single-blind phase 2 trial to evaluate alemtuzumab in early active RRMS (<3 years postonset) as compared with interferon beta-1a (Rebif) (44 μg, subcutaneously, 3 times per week), one of the main first-line treatment (CAMS223 study).[24]

Compared to interferon beta-1a, alemtuzumab significantly reduced the rate of sustained accumulation of disability (9.0% vs 26.2%; hazard ratio 0.29; 95% CI, 0.16 to 0.54; $P<.001$) and the annualized relapse rate (0.10 versus 0.36; hazard ratio 0.26; 95% CI, 0.16 to 0.41; $P<.001$).[25] Remarkably, the *Expanded Disability Status Scale* (EDSS) score improved by 0.39 points in the alemtuzumab group and worsened by 0.38 point in the interferon beta-1a group ($P<.001$). Alemtuzumab also had a dramatic reduction in MRI activity (gadolinium [Gd]-enhancing lesions and T2 lesion load) and atrophy measures.[25] The majority of subjects who receive alemtuzumab develop infusion reactions secondary to cytokine release, which is typically characterized by pyrexia, malaise, and rash. This reaction is markedly improved by pretreatment with corticosteroids and antihistamines. An unexpected serious adverse event was the development of immune thrombocytopenic purpura (ITP) in 6 study subjects. Unfortunately, one of the patients who developed ITP died as a result of an intracranial hemorrhage. In the other 5 subjects, the ITP responded to standard therapy. Another side effect of alemtuzumab therapy in subjects with MS is the development of autoimmune thyroid disease that occurs in approximately 30% of treated subjects and, more rarely, Goodpasture syndrome, which has recently been reported in 2 patients.[26] The phenomenon of delayed B-cell autoimmunity in the setting of immune reconstitution is not unique to alemtuzumab and occurs in association with bone marrow transplantation, HIV-AIDS, and highly-active antiretroviral therapy.[27] Based on observations in these settings, other antibody-mediated autoimmune diseases (eg, hemolytic anemia, immune neutropenia, thrombotic thrombocytopenic purpura, acquired hemophilia, and other disorders) should be expected to occur post–alemtuzumab therapy. It seems that the B-cell overshoot postalemtuzumab correlates with circulating B-cell activating factor levels, a B-cell growth factor.[22] Subjects who develop delayed B-cell–related autoimmunity postalemtuzumab have greater T-cell apoptosis and cell cycling in response to alemtuzumab-induced lymphocyte depletion, a phenomenon that seems to be driven by higher levels of IL-21; subjects who subsequently develop secondary autoimmunity have more than 2-fold greater levels of baseline serum IL-21 than the nonautoimmune group.[28] Because IL-21 expression seems to be genetically predetermined, it may become an important biomarker to predict which patients are more likely to develop autoimmunity post alemtuzumab therapy.[28]

Patients treated with alemtuzumab also experienced higher rates of infections, in particular, recrudescence of latent herpes infections. Two large phase III trials are under way evaluating alemtuzumab in treatment-naïve MS patients and in those who have failed first-line therapy.

Anti-CD20 mAbs (Rituximab, Ocrelizumab, and Ofatumumab)

A central pathogenic role of B cells in MS diseases is supported by the efficacy of rituximab[29] and more recently of ocrelizumab[30] and ofatumumab,[31] which all target CD20 that is expressed on mature B cells and not on plasma cells. Anti-CD20 therapy causes a transient but prolonged depletion of peripheral circulating B cells (>6 months). The peripheral B-cell depletion has indirect effects on macrophages and T-cell–mediated immune responses and results in repopulation of the peripheral circulating B-cell pool from the bone marrow with naïve B cells. Clinical trials have demonstrated a rapid reduction in disease activity on MRI, which was sustained in a 72-week open-label study[32] and subsequently confirmed in a 48-week, double-blind, phase II trial.[29] In primary progressive MS, rituximab showed a trend in reducing time to sustained progression in treated patients.[33] There was a reduction in accumulation of T2 lesions, however, suggestive of biologic response, and a subgroup analysis showed time to confirmed disease progression was delayed in rituximab-treated subjects less than 51 and in those with Gd-enhancing lesions during the study, when compared with placebo.[33] Two phase II studies of ocrelizumab and ofatumumab have recently reported promising results in RRMS.[30,31] As a result, several phase III trials are planned or are currently under way to assess the efficacy of ocrelizumab and ofatumumab in MS. Progressive multifocal leukoencephalopathy (PML) has been reported in rheumatology patients treated with rituximab and cases have been reported in patients treated for lymphoma.[34] The development of ocrelizumab for the treatment of rheumatoid arthritis and lupus has recently been suspended, reportedly due to serious opportunistic infections, several of which were fatal in more than 2000 patients treated in trials combining methotrexate with the agent.[35]

Anti-CD25 (Daclizumab)

Daclizumab has been widely used in prevention of transplant rejection and blocks CD25, which forms part of the high-affinity IL-2 receptor (Tac epitope). In resting T cells, the level of CD25 is low but is significantly upregulated in activated T cells.[36] The scientific rationale behind the development of daclizumab was to reduce T-cell proliferation by blocking the formation of the high-affinity IL-2 receptor. How daclizumab exerts its therapeutic effect is speculative; rather than a rapid depletion of lymphocytes, its effect may be mediated via the expansion of the pool of regulatory CD56[bright] NK cells, which have a role in killing activated T cells in inflammatory lesions.[37] Daclizumab also inhibits survival of CD4+ CD25+ FoxP3+ T-regulatory cells and this may play a role in some of the associated side effects. Three phase II trials have been completed investigating the role of daclizumab in patients who have failed interferon beta treatment or as an adjunct to interferon beta.[38–40] In these trials, daclizumab was successful in stabilizing disease activity and was effective in reducing the number of Gd-enhancing lesions on MRI. The Daclizumab in Active Relapsing Multiple Sclerosis study compared interferon beta alone with interferon beta and daclizumab and found the addition of daclizumab significantly reduced the number of new or Gd-enhancing lesions on MRI.[40] Extension and additional studies to further explore both efficacy and safety profiles of daclizumab are under way.

ORAL AGENTS

Current first-line DMTs are administered as subcutaneous or intramuscular (IM) injections and are associated with frequent side effects, including injection site reactions, flu-like symptoms, and lipoatrophy, although the more effective natalizumab and the mAbs (discussed previously) require regular parenteral administration and come with potential life-threatening side effects and/or undefined long-term risks. Therefore, the holy grail of MS has been to develop oral agents that are at least as efficacious as the parenteral therapies but with fewer side effects. There are currently 5 promising oral drugs in late-stage clinical development: BG-12 (dimethyl fumarate), cladribine, fingolimod, laquinimod, and teriflunomide. Recently, cladribine has been licensed in Russia and Australia and fingolimod in Russia and the United States for use in relapsing-remitting MS.

BG-12

BG-12 (Biogen-Idec), or dimethyl fumarate, is a new formulation of a commonly used agent for the treatment of psoriasis (Fumaderm). An advantage of dimethyl fumarate over the other agents is the extensive experience of the drug in psoriasis and its known safety profile. The fumarates seem to function via NF-E2–related factor 2 (Nrf2), a transcriptional pathway, which controls phase 2 detoxifying enzyme gene expression, and plays a role in the oxidative stress response and immune homeostasis.[41,42] Activation of the Nrf2 pathway reduces oxidative stress–induced neuronal death,[43,44] protects the BBB,[45] and protects myelin integrity in the CNS.[46] Dimethyl fumarate induces changes astroglial and microglial cells and inhibits expression of proinflammatory cytokines and adhesion molecules; these effects suggest that BG-12 may have both neuroprotective and anti-inflammatory effects.[47,48] In a phase II study, oral BG-12 (240 mg 3 times per day) reduced Gd-enhancing lesions by 69% compared with placebo and reduced new T2 and T1 hypointense lesions over a 24-week period. The annualized relapse rate tended to be reduced; due to the short duration of the study this did not reach significance.[49] Two phase III trials are ongoing, one of which is a head-to-head study against glatiramer acetate.

Cladribine

Cladribine (2-chlorodeoxyadenosine) is a synthetic purine nucleoside analog prodrug, which accumulates and is incorporated into the DNA of lymphocytes as a result of a high ratio of deoxycytidine kinase to 5' nucleotidase activity in lymphocytes.[50] It selectively induces apoptosis in lymphocytes and targets bot proliferating and non-proliferating lymphocytes.[50] Cladribine causes reduction in B and T lymphocytes (CD4+ T cells and CD8+ T cells)[51] but only causes a transient reduction in neutrophils and monocytes.[52] Cladribine crosses the BBB[53] and has been shown to reduce levels of proinflammatory chemokines in the cerebrospinal fluid.[54] A recent pivotal phase III study was completed comparing the efficacy of 2 doses of cladribine (3.5 mg/kg vs 5.25 mg/kg) and placebo in patients with relapsing-remitting MS over 96 weeks.[55] Cladribine tablets are taken orally as short course with a need for only 8 to 20 days per year of treatment. Relapse rate was the primary endpoint and was reduced by 58% and 55%, respectively, in the treatment arms. The proportion remaining relapse-free was higher in the treatment arms and there was reduction in progression as measured by sustained progression of the EDSS score at 3 months (33% and 31%, respectively).[55] Secondary outcomes included MRI parameters: Gd+ lesions and T2 lesions with a combined 73% reduction in MRI activity. The drug was well tolerated with a low withdrawal rate due to adverse events. As expected from its mechanism of action, lymphopenia was a frequent adverse event. The rates of infection were marginally higher in subjects who received cladribine, with the majority graded as mild or moderate. Twenty subjects developed herpes zoster infection; all were uncomplicated and dermatomal. Three subjects who received cladribine in the study developed malignancy; the malignancies were heterogeneous and spread across organs systems. Until more safety data emerge, whether or not cladribine treatment predisposes users to secondary malignancies cannot be assessed. A long-term follow-up (median 5.1 years) study on 5979 subjects treated with cladribine for hairy cell or chronic lymphoid leukemia, however, revealed that the observed-to-expected frequency of secondary malignancies when compared with age-adjusted rates for the general population was 1.50 (95% CI, 1.14 to 1.93),[56] a value consistent with the increase rate of secondary malignancies already associated with these diseases. The investigators of the study concluded that cladribine did not significantly increase risk of secondary malignancies.[56] A blinded extension study and a phase III trial in patients with clinically isolated syndromes are ongoing.

Fingolimod

Fingolimod (FTY720) is a structural analog of sphingosine-1-phosphate, which plays an important role in lymphocyte migration from lymph nodes into the periphery. Fingolimod readily crosses the BBB and interacts with S1P receptors in the CNS.[57] Fingolimod has also been shown to prevent demyelination and promote remyelination in animal models.[58] Fingolimod downregulates expression of inflammatory genes and vascular adhesion molecules, reducing matrix metalloproteinase gene (MMP-9) and increasing tissue inhibitor of metalloproteinase (TIMP-1), resulting in an environment that favors preservation of BBB integrity.[59] Late-stage rescue therapy with fingolimod reverses BBB permeability, reduces demyelination, and results in clinical improvement in neurologic functioning. In a phase III study, 2 doses (0.5 mg and 1.25 mg) of oral FTY720 demonstrated superiority over interferon beta-1a IM at 12 months with regard to relapse rate (52% and 38% reduction with FTY720 versus interferon beta-1a IM ($P<.0001$). Both doses reduced MRI inflammatory activity compared with interferon beta-1a IM.[60] Fingolimod was generally well tolerated and the overall safety profile of the fingolimod 0.5-mg dose seemed better than 1.25-mg dose, including lower rates of serious infections. The FTY720 Research Evaluating Effects of Daily Oral Therapy in Multiple Sclerosis phase III study compared high- and low-dose fingolimod with placebo and showed reduced relapse rate, disability progression, and MRI lesion load.[61] Mild side effects occurred in greater than 90% of subjects and serious events in approximately 10%. Bradycardia and atrioventricular conduction block, complications associated with the first dose, were reported more frequently in the high-dose group. Other adverse events included macular edema, infections, hypertension, and a reduction in forced expiratory volume in the first second of expiration (FEV_1). Whether or not fingolimod increases the incidence of secondary malignancies will require data from postmarketing surveillance studies.

Laquinimod

Laquinimod is an oral immunomodulatory agent derived from linomide and is better tolerated than the latter. Linomide was poorly tolerated in trials of MS with frequent side effects, including fatigue, malaise, flu-like symptoms, and several reports of serositis and neuropathy.[62–64] Laquinimod has been shown effective in animal models.[65] It is thought to be effective in MS by inducing the release of transforming growth factor, a shift of the immune response toward a T_h2 type profile rather than suppressing the immune system, a reduced leukocyte infiltration in the CNS, and the induction of a deviation of MBP-specific cells from a T_h1 to T_h2/T_h3 pattern.[66]

Two phase I trials with laquinimod demonstrated that the drug was well tolerated by healthy volunteers and patients with MS. A phase II study tested 2 different doses of oral laquinimod (0.1 mg/d and 0.3 mg/d) versus placebo in 180 with RRMS.[67] Mean cumulative number of active MRI lesions was the primary outcome measure treating subjects with laquinimod (0.3 mg) or placebo and showed a 44% reduction. Clinical outcome parameters (relapse rate and disability) were not different between the groups. A subsequent phase II study evaluated the effect of 2 doses of laquinimod (0.3 mg and 0.6 mg) compared with placebo and primary outcome was MRI-monitored disease activity over 36 weeks. Compared with placebo, laquinimod (0.6 mg) per day showed a 40.4% reduction of the baseline adjusted mean cumulative number of Gd+ lesions per scan, whereas treatment with 0.3 mg per day showed no significant effects.[68] In the open-label extension study of this latter study, the proportion patients free of Gd-enhancing lesions on MRI increased from a baseline of 31% to 47% by the end of the extension.[69] The most prominent adverse event with laquinimod is a moderate elevation of liver enzymes that seems to be reversible with cessation of therapy. Laquinimod (0.6 mg) is currently being further evaluated in two phase III trials; one is a head-to-head study against interferon beta-1a IM (Avonex) and the other is comparing it to placebo.

Teriflunomide

Teriflunomide is the active metabolite of leflunomide, which is an approved treatment for rheumatoid arthritis, and acts by reversibly inhibiting the mitochondrial enzyme dihydroorotate dehydrogenase, which plays a crucial role in pyrimidine synthesis.[70] Teriflunomide has an anti-inflammatory effect by interfering with T- and B-cell proliferation.[71] In EAE, leflunomide suppresses disease activity by inhibition TNF-α and IL-2.[72,73] In EAE, prophylactic or therapeutic dosing of teriflunomide (at 3 or 10 mg/kg) delays disease onset and reduces maximal and cumulative scores compared with vehicle-treated animals.[74] A phase II study comparing 2 doses of teriflunomide (7 and 14 mg once daily) compared with placebo for a period of 36 weeks has been reported[75]; the primary endpoint of the study was the number of active MS lesions and new lesions on MRI which were significantly reduced in both treatment arms. EDSS progression was delayed in the high-dose arm and a trend toward reduction in relapses was observed.[75] It is reassuring, in the extensions study, that teriflunomide seems well tolerated over 8 years of treatment.[76] The first double-blind, placebo-controlled, phase III trial of oral teriflunomide in relapsing multiple sclerosis was recently reported.[77] Of the 1088 patients randomized to study treatment, 73% completed study treatment (71% on placebo, 75% in the 7-mg arm, and 73% in the 14-mg arm). Both doses of teriflunomide reduced the annualized relapse rate compared with placebo with relative risk reductions of 31% and 32% for the 7-mg and 14-mg groups, respectively. The proportions of patients with 12-week confirmed disability progression were 27%, 22%, and 20% for placebo, 7-mg, and 14-mg groups, respectively. The risk for disability progression was reduced by 24% $(P = .08)$ and 29.8% $(P = .03)$ in the 7-mg and 14-mg groups. Teriflunomide was well tolerated with similar numbers of patients reporting treatment-emergent adverse events (88%, 89%, and 91%), serious treatment-emergent adverse events (13%, 14%, and 16%), and treatment-emergent adverse events leading to treatment discontinuation (8%, 10%, and 11%) for placebo, 7-mg, and 14-mg groups, respectively.[76] No deaths were reported.

There are several on-going phase III trials to evaluate the efficacy of teriflunomide alone or as an add-on agent to interferon beta or glatiramer acetate. Based on reproductive studies in animals, female patients are advised to avoid pregnancy when taking teriflunomide because it is known to be teratogenic.

SUMMARY

Not all patients respond to interferon beta and glatiramer acetate treatment. For suboptimal or nonresponders, current options include switching between classes or escalating therapy to natalizumab or mitoxantrone. The recent licensing of cladribine and fingolimod in some countries expands the options of treatment for patients who are treatment-naïve and those who are failing parenteral therapies because of lack of efficacy, poor tolerance, or unacceptable risks (eg, PML on natalizumab). The use of these new therapies will have to be tempered with the lack of long-term safety data. When comparing agents, it is difficult to compare individual trials because the patient cohorts often differ regarding duration of disease, baseline relapse rates, exposure to prior DMT, protocol definitions of relapses, and what constitutes sustained disease progression; in many instances the primary outcome measures of the various trials differ. Head-to-head studies against established therapies are ongoing or planned with many of the emerging agents. In early active MS, alemtuzumab has been shown to outperform interferon beta-1a (Rebif, 44 µg three times per day). There will always be a trade-off between efficacy and safety, with many of the more-effective agents carrying a higher risk for serious adverse events. Subjects with MS, however, are frequently willing to take more risk than their physicians in the hope of preventing relapses and disease progression in the long-term. What is clear is that there remains a large unmet need for DMTs with improved efficacy, tolerability, and safety and lower cost. Several of the emerging agents discussed previously promise better efficacy. Unfortunately, improved efficacy usually comes with increased toxicity and undefined long-term side effects.

REFERENCES

1. Compston A, Coles A. Multiple sclerosis. Lancet 2008;372(9648):1502–17.
2. Steinman L. Multiple sclerosis. Presenting an odd autoantigen. Nature 1995; 375(6534):739–40.
3. Stadelmann C, Wegner C, Bruck W. Inflammation, demyelination, and degeneration - Recent insights from MS pathology. Biochim Biophys Acta 2011;1812(2): 275–82.
4. Stadelmann C, Albert M, Wegner C, et al. Cortical pathology in multiple sclerosis. Curr Opin Neurol 2008;21(3):229–34.
5. Giovannoni G, Cutter GR, Lunemann J, et al. Infectious causes of multiple sclerosis. Lancet Neurol 2006;5(10):887–94.
6. Ramagopalan SV, Dobson R, Meier UC, et al. Multiple sclerosis: risk factors, prodromes, and potential causal pathways. Lancet Neurol 2010;9(7):727–39.
7. Giovannoni G, Ebers G. Multiple sclerosis: the environment and causation. Curr Opin Neurol 2007;20(3):261–8.
8. Steinman L, Zamvil SS. How to successfully apply animal studies in experimental allergic encephalomyelitis to research on multiple sclerosis. Ann Neurol 2006; 60(1):12–21.
9. Sospedra M, Martin R. Immunology of multiple sclerosis. Annu Rev Immunol 2005;23:683–747.

10. Jacobsen M, Cepok S, Quak E, et al. Oligoclonal expansion of memory CD8+ T cells in cerebrospinal fluid from multiple sclerosis patients. Brain 2002;125(Pt 3): 538–50.

11. Hohlfeld R, Kerschensteiner M, Meinl E. Dual role of inflammation in CNS disease. Neurology 2007;68(22 Suppl 3):S58–63 [discussion: S91–6].

12. Bowman EP, Chackerian AA, Cua DJ. Rationale and safety of anti-interleukin-23 and anti-interleukin-17A therapy. Curr Opin Infect Dis 2006;19(3):245–52.

13. Trapp BD, Peterson J, Ransohoff RM, et al. Axonal transection in the lesions of multiple sclerosis. N Engl J Med 1998;338(5):278–85.

14. Ferguson B, Matyszak MK, Esiri MM, et al. Axonal damage in acute multiple sclerosis lesions. Brain 1997;120(Pt 3):393–9.

15. Sayre LM, Perry G, Smith MA. Oxidative stress and neurotoxicity. Chem Res Toxicol 2008;21(1):172–88.

16. Waxman SG. Axonal conduction and injury in multiple sclerosis: the role of sodium channels. Nat Rev Neurosci 2006;7(12):932–41.

17. Waxman SG. Ions, energy and axonal injury: towards a molecular neurology of multiple sclerosis. Trends Mol Med 2006;12(5):192–5.

18. Hemmer B, Cepok S, Nessler S, et al. Pathogenesis of multiple sclerosis: an update on immunology. Curr Opin Neurol 2002;15(3):227–31.

19. Franklin RJ, Ffrench-Constant C. Remyelination in the CNS: from biology to therapy. Nat Rev Neurosci 2008;9(11):839–55.

20. Coles AJ, Thompson S, Cox AL, et al. Dehydroepiandrosterone replacement in patients with Addison's disease has a bimodal effect on regulatory (CD4+CD25hi and CD4+FoxP3+) T cells. Eur J Immunol 2005;35(12):3694–703.

21. Bloom DD, Chang Z, Fechner JH, et al. CD4+ CD25+ FOXP3+ regulatory T cells increase de novo in kidney transplant patients after immunodepletion with Campath-1H. Am J Transplant 2008;8(4):793–802.

22. Thompson SA, Jones JL, Cox AL, et al. B-cell reconstitution and BAFF after alemtuzumab (Campath-1H) treatment of multiple sclerosis. J Clin Immunol 2010; 30(1):99–105.

23. Coles AJ, Cox A, Le Page E, et al. The window of therapeutic opportunity in multiple sclerosis: evidence from monoclonal antibody therapy. J Neurol 2006; 253(1):98–108.

24. CAMMS223 Trial Investigators, Coles AJ, Compston DA, Selmaj KW, et al. Alemtuzumab vs. interferon beta-1a in early multiple sclerosis. N Engl J Med 2008; 359(17):1786–801.

25. Coles AJ, Compston DA, Selmaj KW, et al. Alemtuzumab vs. interferon beta-1a in early multiple sclerosis. N Engl J Med 2008;359(17):1786–801.

26. Clatworthy MR, Wallin EF, Jayne DR. Anti-glomerular basement membrane disease after alemtuzumab. N Engl J Med 2008;359(7):768–9.

27. Jillella AP, Kallab AM, Kutlar A. Autoimmune thrombocytopenia following autologous hematopoietic cell transplantation: review of literature and treatment options. Bone Marrow Transplant 2000;26(8):925–7.

28. Jones JL, Phuah CL, Cox AL, et al. IL-21 drives secondary autoimmunity in patients with multiple sclerosis, following therapeutic lymphocyte depletion with alemtuzumab (Campath-1H). J Clin Invest 2009;119(7):2052–61.

29. Hauser SL, Waubant E, Arnold DL, et al. B-cell depletion with rituximab in relapsing-remitting multiple sclerosis. N Engl J Med 2008;358(7):676–88.

30. Kappos L, Calabresi P, O'Connor P, et al. Efficacy and safety of ocrelizumab in patients with relapsing–remitting multiple sclerosis: results of a phase II randomised placebo-controlled multicentre trial. Mult Scler 2010;16(Suppl 7):S33.

31. Soelberg-Sorensen P, Drulovic J, Havrdova E, et al. Magnetic resonance imaging (MRI) efficacy of ofatumumab in relapsing-remitting multiple sclerosis (RRMS)—24-week results of a phase II study. Mult Scler 2010;16(Suppl 7):S37–8.

32. Bar-Or A, Calabresi PA, Arnold D, et al. Rituximab in relapsing-remitting multiple sclerosis: a 72-week, open-label, phase I trial. Ann Neurol 2008;63(3):395–400.

33. Hawker K, O'Connor P, Freedman MS, et al. Rituximab in patients with primary progressive multiple sclerosis: results of a randomized double-blind placebo-controlled multicenter trial. Ann Neurol 2009;66(4):460–71.

34. Calabrese LH, Molloy ES. Therapy: rituximab and PML risk-informed decisions needed! Nat Rev Rheumatol 2009;5(10):528–9.

35. Nhs. Investigational rheumatoid arthritis treatment ocrelizumab suspended following safety concerns. 2010. Available at: http://www.library.nhs.uk/musculoskeletal/ViewResource.aspx?resID=345559. Accessed November 26, 2010.

36. Granucci F, Feau S, Angeli V, et al. Early IL-2 production by mouse dendritic cells is the result of microbial-induced priming. J Immunol 2003;170(10):5075–81.

37. Bielekova B, Catalfamo M, Reichert-Scrivner S, et al. Regulatory CD56(bright) natural killer cells mediate immunomodulatory effects of IL-2Ralpha-targeted therapy (daclizumab) in multiple sclerosis. Proc Natl Acad Sci U S A 2006; 103(15):5941–6.

38. Bielekova B, Richert N, Howard T, et al. Humanized anti-CD25 (daclizumab) inhibits disease activity in multiple sclerosis patients failing to respond to interferon beta. Proc Natl Acad Sci U S A 2004;101(23):8705–8.

39. Rose JW, Burns JB, Bjorklund J, et al. Daclizumab phase II trial in relapsing and remitting multiple sclerosis: MRI and clinical results. Neurology 2007; 69(8):785–9.

40. Wynn D, Kaufman M, Montalban X, et al. Daclizumab in active relapsing multiple sclerosis (CHOICE study): a phase 2, randomised, double-blind, placebo-controlled, add-on trial with interferon beta. Lancet Neurol 2010;9(4):381–90.

41. Itoh K, Chiba T, Takahashi S, et al. An Nrf2/small Maf heterodimer mediates the induction of phase II detoxifying enzyme genes through antioxidant response elements. Biochem Biophys Res Commun 1997;236(2):313–22.

42. Chen XL, Dodd G, Thomas S, et al. Activation of Nrf2/ARE pathway protects endothelial cells from oxidant injury and inhibits inflammatory gene expression. Am J Physiol Heart Circ Physiol 2006;290(5):H1862–70.

43. Calabrese V, Ravagna A, Colombrita C, et al. Acetylcarnitine induces heme oxygenase in rat astrocytes and protects against oxidative stress: involvement of the transcription factor Nrf2. J Neurosci Res 2005;79(4):509–21.

44. Li J, Johnson D, Calkins M, et al. Stabilization of Nrf2 by tBHQ confers protection against oxidative stress-induced cell death in human neural stem cells. Toxicol Sci 2005;83(2):313–28.

45. Zhao J, Moore AN, Redell JB, et al. Enhancing expression of Nrf2-driven genes protects the blood brain barrier after brain injury. J Neurosci 2007;27(38): 10240–8.

46. Hubbs AF, Benkovic SA, Miller DB, et al. Vacuolar leukoencephalopathy with widespread astrogliosis in mice lacking transcription factor Nrf2. Am J Pathol 2007;170(6):2068–76.

47. Wierinckx A, Breve J, Mercier D, et al. Detoxication enzyme inducers modify cytokine production in rat mixed glial cells. J Neuroimmunol 2005;166(1–2):132–43.

48. Schilling S, Goelz S, Linker R, et al. Fumaric acid esters are effective in chronic experimental autoimmune encephalomyelitis and suppress macrophage infiltration. Clin Exp Immunol 2006;145(1):101–7.

49. Kappos L, Gold R, Miller DH, et al. Efficacy and safety of oral fumarate in patients with relapsing-remitting multiple sclerosis: a multicentre, randomised, double-blind, placebo-controlled phase IIb study. Lancet 2008;372(9648):1463–72.

50. Carson DA, Wasson DB, Taetle R, et al. Specific toxicity of 2-chlorodeoxyadenosine toward resting and proliferating human lymphocytes. Blood 1983;62(4):737–43.

51. Beutler E, Sipe J, Romine J, et al. Treatment of multiple sclerosis and other auto-immune diseases with cladribine. Semin Hematol 1996;33(1 Suppl 1):45–52.

52. Rice GP, Filippi M, Comi G. Cladribine and progressive MS: clinical and MRI outcomes of a multicenter controlled trial. Cladribine MRI Study Group. Neurology 2000;54(5):1145–55.

53. Liliemark J. The clinical pharmacokinetics of cladribine. Clin Pharmacokinet 1997;32(2):120–31.

54. Bartosik-Psujek H, Belniak E, Mitosek-Szewczyk K, et al. Interleukin-8 and RANTES levels in patients with relapsing-remitting multiple sclerosis (RR-MS) treated with cladribine. Acta Neurol Scand 2004;109(6):390–2.

55. Giovannoni G, Comi G, Cook S, et al. A placebo-controlled trial of oral cladribine for relapsing multiple sclerosis. N Engl J Med 2010;362(5):416–26.

56. Cheson BD, Vena DA, Barrett J, et al. Second malignancies as a consequence of nucleoside analog therapy for chronic lymphoid leukemias. J Clin Oncol 1999; 17(8):2454–60.

57. Brinkmann V. FTY720 (fingolimod) in multiple sclerosis: therapeutic effects in the immune and the central nervous system. Br J Pharmacol 2009;158(5): 1173–82.

58. Jung CG, Kim HJ, Miron VE, et al. Functional consequences of S1P receptor modulation in rat oligodendroglial lineage cells. Glia 2007;55(16):1656–67.

59. Foster CA, Mechtcheriakova D, Storch MK, et al. FTY720 rescue therapy in the dark agouti rat model of experimental autoimmune encephalomyelitis: expression of central nervous system genes and reversal of blood-brain-barrier damage. Brain Pathol 2009;19(2):254–66.

60. Cohen JA, Barkhof F, Comi G, et al. Oral fingolimod or intramuscular interferon for relapsing multiple sclerosis. N Engl J Med 2010;362(5):402–15.

61. Kappos L, Radue EW, O'Connor P, et al. A placebo-controlled trial of oral fingo-limod in relapsing multiple sclerosis. N Engl J Med 2010;362(5):387–401.

62. Karussis DM, Meiner Z, Lehmann D, et al. Treatment of secondary progressive multiple sclerosis with the immunomodulator linomide: a double-blind, placebo-controlled pilot study with monthly magnetic resonance imaging evaluation. Neurology 1996;47(2):341–6.

63. Andersen O, Lycke J, Tollesson PO, et al. Linomide reduces the rate of active lesions in relapsing-remitting multiple sclerosis. Neurology 1996;47(4):895–900.

64. Wolinsky JS, Narayana PA, Noseworthy JH, et al. Linomide in relapsing and secondary progressive MS: part II: MRI results. MRI Analysis Center of the University of Texas-Houston, Health Science Center, and the North American Linomide Investigators. Neurology 2000;54(9):1734–41.

65. Brunmark C, Runstrom A, Ohlsson L, et al. The new orally active immunoregulator laquinimod (ABR-215062) effectively inhibits development and relapses of experimental autoimmune encephalomyelitis. J Neuroimmunol 2002;130(1/2): 163–72.

66. Yang JS, Xu LY, Xiao BG, et al. Laquinimod (ABR-215062) suppresses the development of experimental autoimmune encephalomyelitis, modulates the Th1/Th2 balance and induces the Th3 cytokine TGF-beta in Lewis rats. J Neuroimmunol 2004;156(1/2):3–9.

67. Polman C, Barkhof F, Sandberg-Wollheim M, et al. Treatment with laquinimod reduces development of active MRI lesions in relapsing MS. Neurology 2005; 64(6):987–91.
68. Comi G, Pulizzi A, Rovaris M, et al. Effect of laquinimod on MRI-monitored disease activity in patients with relapsing-remitting multiple sclerosis: a multicentre, randomised, double-blind, placebo-controlled phase IIb study. Lancet 2008;371(9630): 2085–92.
69. Comi G, Abramsky O, Arbizu T, et al. Oral laquinimod in patients with relapsing-remitting multiple sclerosis: 36-week double-blind active extension of the multi-centre, randomized, double-blind, parallel-group placebo-controlled study. Mult Scler 2010;16(11):1360–6.
70. Xu X, Blinder L, Shen J, et al. In vivo mechanism by which leflunomide controls lymphoproliferative and autoimmune disease in MRL/MpJ-lpr/lpr mice. J Immunol 1997;159(1):167–74.
71. Korn T, Magnus T, Toyka K, et al. Modulation of effector cell functions in experimental autoimmune encephalomyelitis by leflunomide—mechanisms independent of pyrimidine depletion. J Leukoc Biol 2004;76(5):950–60.
72. Korn T, Toyka K, Hartung HP, et al. Suppression of experimental autoimmune neuritis by leflunomide. Brain 2001;124(Pt 9):1791–802.
73. Smolen JS, Emery P, Kalden JR, et al. The efficacy of leflunomide monotherapy in rheumatoid arthritis: towards the goals of disease modifying antirheumatic drug therapy. J Rheumatol Suppl 2004;71:13–20.
74. Merrill JE, Hanak S, Pu SF, et al. Teriflunomide reduces behavioral, electrophysiological, and histopathological deficits in the Dark Agouti rat model of experimental autoimmune encephalomyelitis. J Neurol 2009;256(1):89–103.
75. O'Connor PW, Li D, Freedman MS, et al. A Phase II study of the safety and efficacy of teriflunomide in multiple sclerosis with relapses. Neurology 2006;66(6): 894–900.
76. Confavreux C, O'Connor PW, Freedman MS, et al. Safety of teriflunomide in the treatment of relapsing multiple sclerosis: results over an 8-year extension. Mult Scler 2010;16:S291.
77. O'Connor P, Wolinsky JS, Confavreux C, et al. A placebo-controlled phase III trial (TEMSO) of oral teriflunomide in relapsing multiple sclerosis: clinical efficacy and safety outcomes. Mult Scler 2010;16:S23.

Symptomatic Management in Multiple Sclerosis

Lawrence M. Samkoff, MD, Andrew D. Goodman, MD*

KEYWORDS

• Multiple sclerosis • Immunomodulatory therapies
• Symptom management • Urinary tract dysfunction

The development of immunomodulatory therapies for multiple sclerosis (MS) has had significant impact in altering the natural history of the disease. Although these agents reduce relapse rate and MRI-associated disease activity, they are only partially effective and do not ameliorate irreversible axonal injury, which produces much of the symptomatic burden of MS. Treatment of MS-associated symptoms remains an essential cornerstone of comprehensive care of patients with MS and, arguably, more favorably enhances quality of life than do the disease-modifying medications.[1] This article reviews strategies of symptom management in patients with MS.

NEUROGENIC BLADDER

Urinary tract dysfunction is present in more than 70% of patients with MS and is a cause of substantial morbidity.[1–3] Symptoms of bladder dysfunction occur on average 6 years after diagnosis but may be present in up to 10% of patients at initial presentation.[2]

Physiologic micturition is dependent on adequate bladder storage of urine and coordinated contraction of detrusor muscle and relaxation of the external sphincter at socially appropriate times. This requires integration of neuronal centers in the cerebral hemispheres, pons, and sacral spinal cord and their interconnections that are frequently affected by demyelinating lesions of MS.[2,3] Briefly, the lower motor neurons of the sacral spinal cord innervate the smooth detrusor muscle of the bladder wall and striated external sphincter; afferent signals from stretch receptors in the detrusor wall are also processed in the sacral cord, resulting in reflexive detrusor contraction. Concomitantly, sensory input ascends in the spinal cord to synapse in the pontine tegmentum. The pontine micturition center efferent pathway traverses adjacent to the corticospinal tract and synapses in the sacral cord, producing relaxation of the external sphincter. Pontine output is inhibited by cortical neurons in the frontal lobes, thereby allowing for micturition to occur in the appropriate setting.

Department of Neurology, University of Rochester School of Medicine and Dentistry, Rochester, NY, USA
* Corresponding author.
E-mail address: Andrew_Goodman@URMC.Rochester.edu

Neurol Clin 29 (2011) 449–463
doi:10.1016/j.ncl.2011.01.008
0733-8619/11/$ – see front matter © 2011 Elsevier Inc. All rights reserved.

neurologic.theclinics.com

In MS, bladder dysfunction can be categorized as either failure to store or failure to empty abnormalities.[1] Three types of neurogenic bladder dysfunction occur in patients with MS.[3] Detrusor hyperreflexia is associated with either suprasacral cord lesions or suprapontine cerebral lesions, which produce disinhibition of the detrusor reflex. This results in a small, poorly compliant bladder, with a failure-to-store abnormality, which presents symptomatically with urinary urgency, frequency, and with or without urge incontinence. Detrusor-sphincter dyssynergia (DSD) also occurs with suprasacral lesions, resulting in inadequate relaxation of the external urinary sphincter during detrusor contraction. In DSD, the bladder fails to empty due to co-contraction of the detrusor and external sphincter muscles, leading to overall urinary retention. Patients with DSD may also complain of urinary urgency, frequency, and incontinence as well as urinary hesitancy and a sensation of bladder fullness after voiding.[4] Less commonly, sacral cord demyelinating lesions produce a hypotonic, overly compliant bladder that fails to empty. Patients may present with urinary frequency, overflow incontinence, and signs of incomplete emptying.[3,4]

The type of neurogenic bladder present in any individual patient cannot be accurately determined by presenting symptoms, which are similar among the subtypes.[1,3] Initially, it is desirable to obtain a urinalysis and urine culture to determine whether or not there is a urinary tract infection. Treatment with antibiotics may produce long-lasting resolution of urinary symptoms in some patients. If there is no improvement, it is then necessary to obtain a postvoid residual (PVR) urine volume by ultrasound to determine therapeutic options, which differ between failure-to-empty and failure-to-store dysfunction.[2–4] In general, a PVR urine volume of less than or equal to 100 mL is categorized as failure to store, whereas a PVR urine volume of greater than 100 mL is indicative of failure to empty.[3]

The mainstay treatment of failure-to-store bladder disorder is anticholinergic agents, including the nonselective muscarinics, oxybutynin (Ditropan), tolterodine (Detrol), trospium (Sanctura), and fesoterodine (Toviaz). Alternatively, the selective M2-antimuscarinics and M3-antimuscarinics, darifenacin (Enablex) and solifenacin (Vesicare), may be used. Common side effects of these agents include dry mouth and constipation. They are contraindicated in patients with angle-closure glaucoma and mechanical bladder outlet obstruction. In general, the nonselective agents should be avoided in patients with cognitive dysfunction, because these drugs may cross the blood-brain barrier and potentially exacerbate these abnormalities.[3] More recently, detrusor muscle botulinum toxin A injection has demonstrated sustained efficacy in reducing urinary urgency, frequency, and incontinence in patients with detrusor hyperreflexia.[5] Intranasal desmopressin (DDAVP) has also been shown to reduce nocturia but requires monitoring for hyponatremia and serum osmolality.[6]

Patients with failure-to-empty bladder dysfunction are best treated with clean intermittent straight catheterization (CISC), which should be performed on at least a once-daily basis.[3] An α-adrenergic medication, such as tamsulosin, may reduce PVR urine volume in some patients and may be effective in some patients with failure-to-empty bladder dysfunction.[3] Patients with DSD, who have symptoms of both failure-to-store and failure-to-empty bladder dysfunction, may benefit from a combination of CISC and anticholinergic agents in controlling their urinary symptoms (**Fig. 1**).

NEUROGENIC BOWEL

Bowel dysfunction, either constipation, fecal incontinence, or a combination of both, occurs in 39% to 73% of individuals with MS.[7,8] In one survey of 155 people with MS, 34% spent more than 30 minutes daily managing their bowel symptoms, and bowel

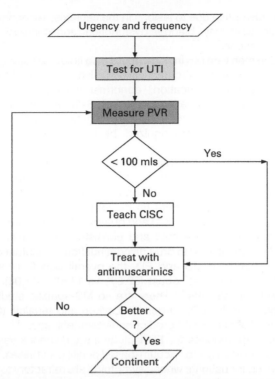

Fig. 1. An algorithm of the approach to neurogenic bladder in patients with MS. (*Reproduced from* Fowler CJ, Panicker JN, Drake M, et al. A UK consensus on the management of the bladder in multiple sclerosis. Postgrad Med J 2009;85(1008):552–9; with permission.)

dysfunction was rated as equally impacting as mobility difficulty on quality-of-life measures.[9]

The pathophysiology of bowel dysfunction in MS is uncertain but is dependent on the integrity of bowel transit, pelvic floor musculature, anorectal sensation, and executive control.[7] MS lesions in the frontal lobes, brainstem, and spinal cord may all disrupt afferent and efferent pathways relevant to autonomic and voluntary regulation of bowel function. Coexisting spasticity, gait mobility, and fatigue may also contribute to bowel dysfunction.[7] Anticholinergic medications that are commonly used to manage MS-associated neurogenic bladder may exacerbate constipation, as can antispasticity and antidepressant agents that are often prescribed.[7]

Treatment of constipation in MS includes conservative measures, such as timed bowel evacuation, dietary fiber, bulk-forming agents, biofeedback, and maintenance of physical activity and adequate hydration.[1,7,10,11] Medical therapies include stool softeners, rectal stimulants (glycerol or bisacodyl suppositories), laxatives, and enemas.[7] Fecal incontinence related to impaction can be addressed by manual disimpaction and strategies to reduce constipation.[7] Isolated fecal incontinence with urgency may be addressed with antidiarrheal agents (eg, loperamide) or anticholinergic medications.[7]

SEXUAL DYSFUNCTION

Sexual dysfunction (SD) in patients with MS is common, affecting up to 50% to 90% of men and 40% to 85% of women.[12,13] The causes of SD in MS are multifactorial and include physiologic disruption due to lesions in the neuraxis; secondary effects due to concomitant fatigue, spasticity, bladder dysfunction, and depression; and adverse reactions from medications.[1,12,14]

Symptoms of SD in men with MS include decreased libido, erectile dysfunction (ED), and ejaculatory disturbance.[12,15] Women with MS also complain of reduced libido as well as decreased vaginal lubrication, abnormal vaginal sensation, and anorgasmia.[12,15,16] In a study of 109 patients with MS, 84% of men and 85% of women had at least one symptom of SD, with resultant negative impact on quality of life.[15] Unfortunately, SD is frequently unrecognized, because patients and physicians are reluctant to discuss these problems.[12]

The treatment of SD in men with MS is primarily pharmacologic, directed at ED. Sildenafil citrate (Viagra) is a peripherally acting phosphodiesterase-5 (PDE5) inhibitor that enhances neurogenic ED.[17] In a randomized, placebo-controlled study of 217 men with MS and ED, sildenafil citrate (in doses from 25 to 100 mg) significantly improved both ED (89% vs 24%, P<.001) and quality of life compared with placebo.[17] Adverse effects of sildenafil were mild and consisted of headache, flushing, and dyspepsia, none of which resulted in drug discontinuation. In another controlled study of sildenafil in 203 men with MS and ED, the overall benefit of sildenafil on ED compared with placebo was less robust (32.8% vs 17.6%, P<.04). Cardiovascular events occurred in three patients.[18] There are no MS-specific studies of the other approved PDE5 inhibitors for ED, vardenafil (Levitra) and tadalafil (Cialis), but their similar mechanisms of action would predict equivalent efficacy.[1,12]

Nonpharmacologic approaches for ED include intracavernous vasodilator agents (eg, papaverine and alpostadil) and vacuum-based penile prostheses.[12] These modalities can be considered for patients whose symptoms are refractory to PDE5 inhibitors or for whom adverse drug effects are intolerable.

There is no established medical therapy for SD in women with MS. In one double-blind, placebo-controlled, crossover study of 19 women with MS-associated SD, sildenafil failed to demonstrate significant benefit, although there was some improvement in vaginal lubrication in the sildenafil group.[19] Treatment of SD in women with MS relies mostly on nonpharmacologic modalities. Vaginal lubricants may be useful to enhance perineal sensation and vaginal dryness.[12] External vibratory stimulation of the vagina and clitoris may augment physiologic vasocongestion and orgasm.[12]

COGNITIVE DYSFUNCTION

Cognitive impairment is common in MS, with prevalence rates ranging from 43% to 70% in both early and late disease.[20,21] Cognitive domains that are commonly affected in MS include sustained attention, recent memory, verbal fluency, information processing, executive function, and visuospatial perception.[20,22] These deficits can vary over the clinical course among patients and within individuals.[1,20]

The severity of cognitive impairment in MS correlates weakly with disease duration and physical disability.[1] Poor performance on neuropsychological testing, however, has been demonstrated on cranial MRI to be associated with increasing burden of disease, using measures of whole brain atrophy, cortical atrophy, and white matter lesion volume.[20,23] A minority of patients with MS present with a predominant cognitive syndrome, without associated visual, motor, sensory, or cerebellar involvement.[24] Furthermore, cognitive dysfunction in MS can be exacerbated by concomitant depression and fatigue.[20]

Cognitive impairment in MS is often unrecognized but has significant adverse impact on driving, cooking, and using public transportation.[20,25] Rao and coworkers[26] reported that MS patients with cognitive disorders were more likely to be unemployed, socially withdrawn, and prone to psychiatric morbidity and have difficulty performing routine household tasks. Cognitive dysfunction should thus be suspected in individuals whose work or social performance declines disproportionately to their physical disability.[1]

Patients with MS whose symptoms raise concern for cognitive dysfunction should be referred for neuropsychological testing, which is an effective tool for identifying abnormalities in the domains affected by the disease.[20] The minimal assessment of cognitive function in MS is a testing battery that measures verbal fluency, visuospatial skills, verbal memory, working memory, processing speed, and executive function and has been found to reliably detect MS-associated cognitive impairment.[27]

Treatment of MS cognitive dysfunction has been addressed in two studies with acetylcholinesterase inhibitors used in Alzheimer disease. In a single-center, double-blind, placebo-controlled study of 69 MS patients with cognitive dysfunction, subjects treated with donepezil (10 mg twice a day) for 24 weeks had significant improvement ($P<.043$) in quantitative memory performance compared with the placebo cohort.[28] Subjective improvement in memory was reported by both clinicians (54.3% vs 29.4%) and patients (65.7% vs 32.4%) for the donepezil group.[28,29] A 12-week treatment with rivastigmine (3 mg twice a day), however, failed to demonstrate significant benefit on memory in another placebo-controlled study.[30]

Memantine, an N-methyl-D-aspartate (NMDA) glutamate antagonist also approved for symptomatic treatment of Alzheimer disease, has been investigated as a potential agent for MS-associated cognitive impairment. A placebo-controlled study of memantine (15 mg twice a day) was halted when 7 of 9 subjects in the treatment group reported worsening neurologic symptoms, including blurred vision, fatigue, muscle weakness, and gait instability; patients returned to their baseline neurologic status several days after stopping memantine.[31] Lovera and colleagues[32] conducted a double-blind, placebo-controlled study of memantine (10 mg twice a day, titrated over 4 weeks). Patients in the treatment group performed worse on the primary outcome measures, the Paced Auditory Serial Addition Test and the California Verbal Learning Test–Second Edition, compared with the placebo cohort. In addition, patients in the memantine group had more fatigue and worsening of baseline neurologic symptoms as well as subjectively poorer cognitive and neuropsychiatric outcomes compared with the placebo subjects.

Nonpharmacologic therapy of MS-associated cognitive dysfunction with rehabilitative strategies has produced conflicting results.[20] O'Brien and colleagues[33] performed a meta-analysis of cognitive rehabilitation studies in patients with MS-associated cognitive impairment and found some benefit with therapies targeting the domains of verbal learning and memory, although further research was deemed warranted.

PAIN

Pain and pain syndromes are prevalent in MS, affecting up to 86% of patients during their course of illness.[34–39] In one community-based study that surveyed 180 patients with MS, those afflicted with pain were more likely to report greater MS disease severity, poorer psychological functioning, and poorer health than persons with MS without pain.[38] A cross-sectional analysis of 94 patients in an Australian community with MS found that individuals with chronic pain had lower scores on several quality-of-life measures, including psychological well-being and independent living.[40]

Pain in MS can be classified into four categories: neuropathic (central) pain due to lesions of MS, pain indirectly related to MS, pain related to MS treatment, and pain unrelated to MS.[35] It is important to discriminate among these entities to ensure appropriate therapeutic intervention.

Central pain from MS includes dysesthetic limb pain, trigeminal neuralgia (TN), and Lhermitte phenomenon, which are the most common forms of neuropathic pain in MS.[33] Dysesthetic limb pain affects 14% to 29% of MS patients,[35] usually manifests as chronic burning discomfort involving the arms, legs, or trunk, and is typically bilateral and more prominent in the lower extremities.[34] It is postulated to result from lesions in the spinal cord nociceptive pathways.[34] TN in MS occurs at approximately 20 times the prevalence of that in the general population[34] and is usually due to lesions in the intrapontine trigeminal tract or root entry zone.[41] In MS, up to 31% of TN is bilateral, a rate much higher than TN in the non-MS population.[34] Lhermitte phenomenon is characterized by a paroxysmal sensory disturbance related to neck flexion felt centrally down the neck and back, usually also involving the limbs, and is due to lesions in the cervical posterior column.[34] Pain from Lhermitte phenomenon is typically brief, lasting seconds, and "electrical" in nature.

Treatment of central pain in MS has not been well studied and generally consists of strategies used in other forms of neuropathic pain.[1,34,35] First-line drugs for dysesthetic limb pain include tricyclic antidepressants (amitriptyline and nortriptyline), anticonvulsants (gabapentin, pregabalin, and lamotrigine), and the serotonin-norepinephrine reuptake inhibitors, duloxetine and venlafaxine.[1,34,35] First-line medical therapy for TN includes carbamazepine, and oxcarbazepine; baclofen, gabapentin, and lamotrigine can be used as second-line agents.[42] In patients with medically refractory TN, surgical options include percutaneous gasserian rhizotomy and, possibly, stereotactic gamma knife radiosurgery.[42,43] Both gabapentin and carbamazepine may be used in patients with disruptive Lhermitte phenomenon.[35]

Pain indirectly due to MS is primarily related to spasticity and musculoskeletal disturbances associated with limb weakness and immobility.[1,35] (Treatment of spasticity is discussed later.) Musculoskeletal pain in MS generally responds to modalities used for the specific condition in the non-MS population. Pain related to MS treatment includes local reactions from the injectable immunomodulatory agents and headaches and flu-like symptoms from interferon-β (IFN-β). Injection site pain can be relieved with cooling of the underlying skin; headaches and flu-like symptoms from IFN-β usually respond to acetaminophen or nonsteroidal anti-inflammatory agents.[44] Both low-back pain and headache are frequent in patients with MS, although their treatment is no different from the general population.[34,45]

MOOD DISORDERS

Psychiatric disorders are common in patients with MS, the most frequent of which are depression and anxiety.[46–48] Other behavioral disturbances seen in MS include pseudobulbar affect, agitation, and irritability.[46]

Major depression is the most common mood disorder in MS, with prevalence of up to 50% during the disease course.[47,49,50] Lifetime risk of anxiety syndromes in MS has been reported as high as 35.7%.[48] The rate of depression in MS seems higher than that seen in other chronic systemic and neurologic illnesses, implying in part a neuroanatomic basis to its pathophysiology.[1,47,49]

There has been concern that treatment with IFN-β may increase the risk of depression in MS patients.[51] In the pivotal trial of IFNβ-1b for relapsing-remitting MS,[52] risk of suicide and suicide attempt was higher in the treatment cohort compared with the placebo group. Similarly, depression was significantly greater in subjects treated with IFN-β1a compared with placebo (2% vs 13%, P<.05) in the Controlled High-Risk

Subjects Avonex Multiple Sclerosis Prevention Study (CHAMPS).[53] A Canadian national study, however, found no difference in the use of antidepressants in patients treated with IFN-β or glatiramer acetate.[54] A review of the literature by Goeb and colleagues[51] concluded that the association of IFN-β and depression was at best uncertain, although patients with a history of depression may be at higher risk of developing depression on IFN-β therapy.

Depression in MS is both underreported and underdetected.[55] Recognition of depression in MS is important, because its presence has a negative impact on quality of life, cognitive function, and adherence to medical treatment.[49] In a 7-year longitudinal investigation of 607 persons with MS, depressive symptoms were more common in younger subjects and in those with longer duration of illness, with progressive disease, and with greater level of functional disability.[56] Moreover, suicide risk is increased in individuals with MS, with rates reported from 2 to 7.5 times that of the age-matched general population.[57–59] A Danish study found the risk of suicide in MS highest in men, individuals with disease onset before age 30, and those diagnosed under age 40.[59] In a report of 445 veterans with MS,[60] 29.4% of subjects admitted suicidal ideation. Suicidal ideation was associated with younger age, earlier disease onset, progressive disease course, low income, single marital status, higher levels of disability, and depression. In another study of 140 patients with MS, 28.6% had suicidal intent, which was strongly associated with major depression, alcohol abuse, and social isolation.[61] One-third of suicidal patients had not received psychotherapy and two-thirds of patients with major depression had not been prescribed an antidepressant.

The Beck Depression Inventory,[62] a self-report scale of 21 items, is the most commonly used tool to screen for depression in MS. A recent consensus statement by a panel of MS experts advocates routine screening of patients with the BDI, with a cutoff score of 13 as diagnostic of significant depression.[49] Mohr and colleagues[63] reported that a simple, two-question screening assessment of mood and anhedonia reliably identified MS patients with major depressive disorder.

Once a diagnosis of depression is made, treatment should be initiated. Both pharmacologic and psychotherapeutic modalities are effective in the treatment of depression in the MS population.[49] There have been few rigorous studies of the medical treatment of MS-associated depression. Both desipramine, a tricyclic antidepressant, and sertraline, a selective serotonin reuptake inhibitor, have demonstrated benefit in controlled analyses.[64,65] Individualized cognitive-behavioral psychotherapy was more beneficial than supportive group therapy for MS-associated depression in one study.[65] Combination antidepressant medication and behavioral psychotherapy may be more efficacious than either alone.[49]

In general, selective serotonin reuptake inhibitors are the first-line agents used for MS-associated depression based on their favorable side-effect profile.[1] Tricyclic antidepressants and duloxetine may be useful in patients with comorbid neuropathic pain.[1] Unfortunately, despite the availability of established therapy, more than 50% of MS patients with depression are not prescribed antidepressants.[49,66]

FATIGUE

Fatigue in MS is defined as an overwhelming sense of tiredness, lack of energy, or exhaustion exceeding the expected; it is difficult to measure objectively. Although the underlying pathophysiologic mechanisms are poorly understood, there may be a relation to overproduction of inflammatory cytokines systemically or within the central nervous system.[67] Prevalence of fatigue among the MS population has been estimated up to 92%, with 33% considering it the most troubling of all symptoms, distinct but often in conjunction with depression. The impact of fatigue in the MS population is profound and pervasive. It includes effects on employment (it may be the leading cause of disability claims) and disruption of family life and social roles.[68,69] A variety of both physical and pharmacologic treatment strategies are used, often simultaneously and synergistically. Energy conservation measures include ensuring adequate sleep, daytime naps, and assistive devices for mobility and household chores. Tactics should be used to avoid or manipulate detrimental environmental influences, such as heat and humidity, with cooling devices, fans, dehumidifiers, and air conditioning.[70] Carefully implemented exercise programs have been demonstrated to benefit some aspects of fatigue.[71] Amantadine demonstrated efficacy in various controlled clinical trials. The relevant mechanism of action is undefined but possibly relates to dopaminergic properties having an impact on the reticular activating system.[72–74] In practice it is given once or twice a day (usually in a 100-mg dose) but timing needs to be individually adjusted to avoid insomnia as a side effect. Other potential side effects are reversible: mental confusion, hallucinations, and livedo reticularis. Studies of modafinil have yielded conflicting results.[75–77] It seems that modafinil may be helpful in some individuals who do not get satisfactory relief of fatigue with amantadine alone. Other drugs that may be helpful include methylphenidate and dextroamphetamine, although there are few if any rigorous data that establish efficacy. These drugs are not specifically approved for use in MS.

SPASTICITY

Spasticity can be defined as a state of increased muscle tone with velocity-dependent increased resistance to passive movement, often associated with spasms. Prevalence estimates of spasticity range up to 70% to 80% of MS patients. The pathophysiologic mechanism is interruption of descending pathways' inhibitory control of group II spinal interneurons resulting in overactivity of alpha motor neurons.[78] In general, the therapeutic approach to spasticity should be multidimensional: physical and occupational therapy, stretching, and exercise in addition to pharmacotherapy.

The first medication usually prescribed is baclofen. Its mechanism of action is as an agonist of γ-aminobutyric acid (GABA) receptors on spinal interneurons resulting in decreased alpha motor neuron activity. It is approved for spasticity in MS with demonstrated efficacy in various trials.[79,80] Side effects that limit the effectiveness are daytime sedation and increased muscle weakness that may have a negative impact on limb function, especially gait. The short half-life also limits its effectiveness to 3 to 4 hours.

Tizanidine is an α_2-adrenergic agonist that reduces release of excitatory transmitters, effectively reducing muscle tone. It is approved for reducing spasticity and spasms. Clinical trials showed efficacy without the limiting significant weakness.[81–84] Its effectiveness is limited by sedation and dizziness that in some cases is associated with hypotension because tizanidine is similar to the antihypertensive, clonidine, in its pharmacology.

Diazepam binds to the benzodiazepine–GABA A receptor, increasing presynaptic inhibition in the spinal cord. Efficacy was assessed in several trials and is similar to the baclofen effect. Effectiveness in practice is limited by sedation and the addictive potential, in the authors' experience.

Gabapentin is also a GABAergic. Efficacy in spasticity has been suggested in small trials but this drug has not been approved for spasticity.[85,86] It may be most useful in practice as adjunctive therapy with other spasticity medications, such as baclofen. It is not protein bound or metabolized, making it relatively safe to take along with other drugs. Effectiveness again can be limited by sedation.

Botulinum toxin blocks presynaptic acetylcholine release at the neuromuscular junction in skeletal muscle. Although not specifically approved for spasticity, efficacy was assessed in several trials.[87–89] Its main use in practice may be in smaller muscles in the hands and feet. Effectiveness is limited by size of involved muscle and thus the dose required.

The baclofen pump works by directly delivering liquid baclofen to the lower cord through the cerebrospinal fluid. It has been approved by the Food and Drug Administration for spasticity and several trials demonstrated efficacy in otherwise intractable cases.[90] Its effectiveness is sustained over time but can be limited by muscle weakness and technical difficulties such as kinking of the catheter. It is not limited by sedation.[91,92]

TREMOR

The pathophysiology of tremor is presumably related to dysfunction in cerebellar efferent pathways (eg, dentatorubrothalamic). It may affect up to 80% of all MS patients. The impact of tremor not only is often a social embarrassment but also in more severe cases can be severely disabling with respect to performance of activities of daily living. Approaches to treatment include physical means to dampen the tremor, such as joint stabilization maneuvers and limb weights. In addition, compensation strategies, such as large-handled utensils, may be used. Unfortunately, tremor is often resistant to pharmacotherapy intervention. Clinical trial data are extremely limited. Among the drugs that are commonly attempted are clonazepam and β-blockers; the effectiveness of both may be limited by sedation. Other agents sometimes used are primidone and gabapentin (both may also be limited by sedation). Isoniazid was demonstrated in a small trial to be of benefit but its utility may be limited by liver toxicity.[93–96] Surgical approaches have been used at selected centers. Stereotactic thalamotomy of ventral intermediate nucleus has shown of benefit as reported in several case series. Adverse effects have included hemiparesis, dysphasia, and dysphagia. Deep brain stimulation has been achieved through stereotactic implantation of microelectrodes in ventral intermediate nucleus and has shown some efficacy. Potential advantages include reversibility and adjustability. Disadvantages have been adverse effects, such as paresthesias, reported by many patients, and sometimes short-lived effectiveness.[97–99]

IMPAIRED GAIT

Gait difficulties are among the commonest and troubling impairments resulting from MS, which historically have not adequately been treated by drugs, such as those for spasticity. Among 1011 people with MS surveyed in a study commissioned by the National Multiple Sclerosis Society, 64% experienced trouble walking at least twice weekly and, of these, 70% reported it the most challenging aspect of their MS. Dalfampridine (4-aminopyridine) is a potassium channel blocker previously known in the literature as fampridine.[100,101] Extended-release dalfampridine was shown to result in an average 25% increase in walking speed in approximately 37% of patients overall in phase 3 trials of patients receiving the drug who met prescribed criteria as consistent responders.[102,103] In addition, among those patients who were responders, there was significant subjective improvement in gait-related MS symptoms.[104] The most concerning adverse events that have emerged from various dalfampridine trials include seizures, acute encephalopathy, and confusional episodes. The Food and Drug Administration approved the extended-release formulation of dalfampridine (daily oral dose of 10 mg given approximately 12 hours apart) for use in MS to enhance walking in patients with existing gait impairment in 2010. Patients with a history of seizures or more than mildly impaired renal function should be excluded because of safety concerns. In practice, a trial period of 2 to 4 weeks is usually sufficient to assess individual effectiveness and tolerability in the authors' experience.

REFERENCES

1. Boissy AR, Cohen JA. Multiple sclerosis symptom management. Expert Rev Neurother 2007;7(9):1213–22.
2. de Seze M, Ruffion A, Denys P, et al. The neurogenic bladder in multiple sclerosis: review of the literature and proposal of management guidelines. Mult Scler 2007;13(7):915–28.
3. Fowler CJ, Panicker JN, Drake M, et al. A UK consensus on the management of the bladder in multiple sclerosis. Postgrad Med J 2009;85(1008):552–9.
4. Del Popolo G, Panariello G, Del Corso F, et al. Diagnosis and therapy for neurogenic bladder dysfunctions in multiple sclerosis patients. Neurol Sci 2008; 29(Suppl 4):S352–5.
5. Kalsi V, Gonzales G, Popat R, et al. Botulinum injections for the treatment of bladder symptoms of multiple sclerosis. Ann Neurol 2007;62(5):452–7.
6. Bosma R, Wynia K, Havlikova E, et al. Efficacy of desmopressin in patients with multiple sclerosis suffering from bladder dysfunction: a meta-analysis. Acta Neurol Scand 2005;112(1):1–5.
7. Wiesel PH, Norton C, Glickman S, et al. Pathophysiology and management of bowel dysfunction in multiple sclerosis. Eur J Gastroenterol Hepatol 2001; 13(4):441–8.
8. Hinds JP, Eidelman BH, Wald A. Prevalence of bowel dysfunction in multiple sclerosis. A population survey. Gastroenterology 1990;98(6):1538–42.
9. Norton C, Chelvanayagam S. Bowel problems and coping strategies in people with multiple sclerosis. Br J Nurs 2010;19(4):220 221–6.
10. Bywater A, While A. Management of bowel dysfunction in people with multiple sclerosis. Br J Community Nurs 2006;11(8):333–4, 336–7, 340–1.
11. Wiesel PH, Norton C, Roy AJ, et al. Gut focused behavioural treatment (biofeedback) for constipation and faecal incontinence in multiple sclerosis. J Neurol Neurosurg Psychiatry 2000;69(2):240–3.
12. Fletcher SG, Castro-Borrero W, Remington G, et al. Sexual dysfunction in patients with multiple sclerosis: a multidisciplinary approach to evaluation and management. Nat Clin Pract Urol 2009;6(2):96–107.
13. Demirkiran M, Sarica Y, Uguz S, et al. Multiple sclerosis patients with and without sexual dysfunction: are there any differences? Mult Scler 2006;12(2): 209–14.
14. Kessler TM, Fowler CJ, Panicker JN. Sexual dysfunction in multiple sclerosis. Expert Rev Neurother 2009;9(3):341–50.
15. Tepavcevic DK, Kostic J, Basuroski ID, et al. The impact of sexual dysfunction on the quality of life measured by MSQoL-54 in patients with multiple sclerosis. Mult Scler 2008;14(8):1131–6.
16. Gruenwald I, Vardi Y, Gartman I, et al. Sexual dysfunction in females with multiple sclerosis: quantitative sensory testing. Mult Scler 2007;13(1):95–105.
17. Fowler CJ, Miller JR, Sharief MK, et al. A double blind, randomised study of sildenafil citrate for erectile dysfunction in men with multiple sclerosis. J Neurol Neurosurg Psychiatry 2005;76(5):700–5.

18. Safarinejad MR. Evaluation of the safety and efficacy of sildenafil citrate for erectile dysfunction in men with multiple sclerosis: a double-blind, placebo controlled, randomized study. J Urol 2009;181(1):252–8.

19. Dasgupta R, Wiseman OJ, Kanabar G, et al. Efficacy of sildenafil in the treatment of female sexual dysfunction due to multiple sclerosis. J Urol 2004; 171(3):1189–93 [discussion: 1193].

20. Chiaravalloti ND, DeLuca J. Cognitive impairment in multiple sclerosis. Lancet Neurol 2008;7(12):1139–51.

21. Amato MP, Portaccio E, Goretti B, et al. Cognitive impairment in early stages of multiple sclerosis. Neurol Sci 2010;31(Suppl 2):S211–4.

22. Rao SM, Leo GJ, Bernardin L, et al. Cognitive dysfunction in multiple sclerosis. I. Frequency, patterns, and prediction. Neurology 1991;41(5):685–91.

23. Filippi M, Rocca MA. MRI and cognition in multiple sclerosis. Neurol Sci 2010; 31(Suppl 2):S231–4.

24. Staff NP, Lucchinetti CF, Keegan BM. Multiple sclerosis with predominant, severe cognitive impairment. Arch Neurol 2009;66(9):1139–43.

25. Staples D, Lincoln NB. Intellectual impairment in multiple sclerosis and its relation to functional abilities. Rheumatol Rehabil 1979;18(3):153–60.

26. Rao SM, Leo GJ, Ellington L, et al. Cognitive dysfunction in multiple sclerosis. II. Impact on employment and social functioning. Neurology 1991;41(5):692–6.

27. Benedict RH, Cookfair D, Gavett R, et al. Validity of the minimal assessment of cognitive function in multiple sclerosis (MACFIMS). J Int Neuropsychol Soc 2006;12(4):549–58.

28. Krupp LB, Christodoulou C, Melville P, et al. Donepezil improved memory in multiple sclerosis in a randomized clinical trial. Neurology 2004;63(9):1579–85.

29. Christodoulou C, Melville P, Scherl WF, et al. Effects of donepezil on memory and cognition in multiple sclerosis. J Neurol Sci 2006;245(1/2):127–36.

30. Shaygannejad V, Janghorbani M, Ashtari F, et al. Effects of rivastigmine on memory and cognition in multiple sclerosis. Can J Neurol Sci 2008;35(4): 476–81.

31. Villoslada P, Arrondo G, Sepulcre J, et al. Memantine induces reversible neurologic impairment in patients with MS. Neurology 2009;72(19):1630–3.

32. Lovera JF, Frohman E, Brown TR, et al. Memantine for cognitive impairment in multiple sclerosis: a randomized placebo-controlled trial. Mult Scler 2010; 16(6):715–23.

33. O'Brien AR, Chiaravalloti N, Goverover Y, et al. Evidenced-based cognitive rehabilitation for persons with multiple sclerosis: a review of the literature. Arch Phys Med Rehabil 2008;89(4):761–9.

34. O'Connor AB, Schwid SR, Herrmann DN, et al. Pain associated with multiple sclerosis: Systematic review and proposed classification. Pain 2008;137(1): 96–111.

35. Pollmann W, Feneberg W. Current management of pain associated with multiple sclerosis. CNS Drugs 2008;22(4):291–324.

36. Bermejo PE, Oreja-Guevara C, Diez-Tejedor E. Pain in multiple sclerosis: Prevalence, mechanisms, types and treatment. Rev Neurol 2010;50(2):101–8.

37. Svendsen KB, Jensen TS, Overvad K, et al. Pain in patients with multiple sclerosis: a population-based study. Arch Neurol 2003;60(8):1089–94.

38. Ehde DM, Osborne TL, Hanley MA, et al. The scope and nature of pain in persons with multiple sclerosis. Mult Scler 2006;12(5):629–38.

39. Ehde DM, Gibbons LE, Chwastiak L, et al. Chronic pain in a large community sample of persons with multiple sclerosis. Mult Scler 2003;9(6):605–11.

40. Khan F, Pallant J. Chronic pain in multiple sclerosis: prevalence, characteristics, and impact on quality of life in an australian community cohort. J Pain 2007;8(8): 614–23.
41. Cruccu G, Biasiotta A, Di Rezze S, et al. Trigeminal neuralgia and pain related to multiple sclerosis. Pain 2009;143(3):186–91.
42. Cruccu G, Gronseth G, Alksne J, et al. AAN-EFNS guidelines on trigeminal neuralgia management. Eur J Neurol 2008;15(10):1013–28.
43. Zorro O, Lobato-Polo J, Kano H, et al. Gamma knife radiosurgery for multiple sclerosis-related trigeminal neuralgia. Neurology 2009;73(14):1149–54.
44. Langer-Gould A, Moses HH, Murray TJ. Strategies for managing the side effects of treatments for multiple sclerosis. Neurology 2004;63(11 Suppl 5): S35–41.
45. Polman CH, O'Connor PW, Havrdova E, et al. A randomized, placebo-controlled trial of natalizumab for relapsing multiple sclerosis. N Engl J Med 2006;354(9): 899–910.
46. Paparrigopoulos T, Ferentinos P, Kouzoupis A, et al. The neuropsychiatry of multiple sclerosis: Focus on disorders of mood, affect and behaviour. Int Rev Psychiatry 2010;22(1):14–21.
47. Siegert RJ, Abernethy DA. Depression in multiple sclerosis: a review. J Neurol Neurosurg Psychiatry 2005;76(4):469–75.
48. Korostil M, Feinstein A. Anxiety disorders and their clinical correlates in multiple sclerosis patients. Mult Scler 2007;13(1):67–72.
49. Goldman Consensus Group. The Goldman consensus statement on depression in multiple sclerosis. Mult Scler 2005;11(3):328–37.
50. Sollom AC, Kneebone II. Treatment of depression in people who have multiple sclerosis. Mult Scler 2007;13(5):632–5.
51. Goeb JL, Even C, Nicolas G, et al. Psychiatric side effects of interferon-beta in multiple sclerosis. Eur Psychiatry 2006;21(3):186–93.
52. Interferon beta-1b is effective in relapsing-remitting multiple sclerosis. I. Clinical results of a multicenter, randomized, double-blind, placebo-controlled trial. The IFNB multiple sclerosis study group. Neurology 1993;43(4):655–61.
53. Jacobs LD, Beck RW, Simon JH, et al. Intramuscular interferon beta-1a therapy initiated during a first demyelinating event in multiple sclerosis. CHAMPS study group. N Engl J Med 2000;343(13):898–904.
54. Patten SB, Williams JV, Metz LM. Anti-depressant use in association with interferon and glatiramer acetate treatment in multiple sclerosis. Mult Scler 2008; 14(3):406–11.
55. Chwastiak LA, Ehde DM. Psychiatric issues in multiple sclerosis. Psychiatr Clin North Am 2007;30(4):803–17.
56. Beal CC, Stuifbergen AK, Brown A. Depression in multiple sclerosis: a longitudinal analysis. Arch Psychiatr Nurs 2007;21(4):181–91.
57. Bronnum-Hansen H, Stenager E, Nylev Stenager E, et al. Suicide among danes with multiple sclerosis. J Neurol Neurosurg Psychiatry 2005;76(10): 1457–9.
58. Sadovnick AD, Eisen K, Ebers GC, et al. Cause of death in patients attending multiple sclerosis clinics. Neurology 1991;41(8):1193–6.
59. Stenager EN, Stenager E, Koch-Henriksen N, et al. Suicide and multiple sclerosis: An epidemiological investigation. J Neurol Neurosurg Psychiatry 1992; 55(7):542–5.
60. Turner AP, Williams RM, Bowen JD, et al. Suicidal ideation in multiple sclerosis. Arch Phys Med Rehabil 2006;87(8):1073–8.

61. Feinstein A. An examination of suicidal intent in patients with multiple sclerosis. Neurology 2002;59(5):674–8.
62. Beck AT, Ward CH, Mendelson M, et al. An inventory for measuring depression. Arch Gen Psychiatry 1961;4:561–71.
63. Mohr DC, Hart SL, Julian L, et al. Screening for depression among patients with multiple sclerosis: two questions may be enough. Mult Scler 2007;13(2): 215–9.
64. Schiffer RB, Wineman NM. Antidepressant pharmacotherapy of depression associated with multiple sclerosis. Am J Psychiatry 1990;147(11):1493–7.
65. Mohr DC, Boudewyn AC, Goodkin DE, et al. Comparative outcomes for individual cognitive-behavior therapy, supportive-expressive group psychotherapy, and sertraline for the treatment of depression in multiple sclerosis. J Consult Clin Psychol 2001;69(6):942–9.
66. Cetin K, Johnson KL, Ehde DM, et al. Antidepressant use in multiple sclerosis: epidemiologic study of a large community sample. Mult Scler 2007;13(8): 1046–53.
67. Schwid SR, Thornton CA, Pandya S, et al. Quantitative assessment of motor fatigue and strength in MS. Neurology 1999;53(4):743–50.
68. Stroud NM, Minahan CL. The impact of regular physical activity on fatigue, depression and quality of life in persons with multiple sclerosis. Health Qual Life Outcomes 2009;7:68.
69. Krupp LB, Alvarez LA, LaRocca NG, et al. Fatigue in multiple sclerosis. Arch Neurol 1988;45:435–7.
70. Schwid SR, Petrie MD, Murray R, et al. A randomized controlled study of the acute and chronic effects of cooling therapy for MS. Neurology 2003;60: 1955–60.
71. Petajan JH, Gappmaier E, White AT. Impact of aerobic training on fitness and quality of life in multiple sclerosis. Ann Neurol 1996;39:432–41.
72. The Canadian MS Research Group. A randomized controlled trial of amantadine in fatigue associated with multiple sclerosis. Can J Neurol Sci 1987;14: 273–8.
73. Cohen RA, Fisher M. Amantadine treatment of fatigue associated with multiple sclerosis. Arch Neurol 1989;46:676–80.
74. Krupp LB, Coyle PK, Doscher C, et al. Fatigue therapy in multiple sclerosis: results of a double-blind, randomized, parallel trial of amantadine, pemoline, and placebo. Neurology 1995;45:1956–61.
75. Zifko UA, Rupp M, Schwarz S, et al. Modafinil in treatment of fatigue in multiple sclerosis. Results of an open-label study. J Neurol 2002;249:983–7.
76. Rammohan KW, Rosenberg JH, Lynn DJ, et al. Efficacy and safety of modafinil (Provigil) for the treatment of fatigue in multiple sclerosis: a two centre phase 2 study. J Neurol Neurosurg Psychiatry 2002;72:179–83.
77. Stankoff B, Waubant E, Confavreux C, et al. Modafinil for fatigue in MS: a randomized placebo-controlled double-blind study. Neurology 2005;64: 1139–43.
78. Shakespeare DT, Boggild M, Young C. Anti-spasticity agents for multiple sclerosis. Cochrane Database Syst Rev 2003;4:CD001332.
79. Feldman RG, Kelly-Hayes M, Conomy JP, et al. Baclofen for spasticity in multiple sclerosis. Double-blind crossover and three-year study. Neurology 1978;28: 1094.
80. Smith CR, LaRocca NG, Giesser BS, et al. High-dose oral baclofen: experience in patients with multiple sclerosis. Neurology 1991;41:1829–31.

81. United Kingdom Tizanidine Trial Group. A double-blind, placebo-controlled trial of tizanidine in the treatment of spasticity caused by multiple sclerosis. Neurology 1994;44(11 Suppl 9):70–8.

82. Nance PW, Sheremata WA, Lynch SG, et al. Relationship of the antispasticity effect of tizanidine to plasma concentration in patients with multiple sclerosis. Arch Neurol 1997;54:731–6.

83. Smith C, Birnbaum G, Carter JL, et al. US Tizanidine Study Group. Tizanidine treatment of spasticity caused by multiple sclerosis: results of a double-blind, placebo-controlled trial. Neurology 1994;44(11 Suppl 9):34–42.

84. From A, Heltberg A. A double-blind trial with baclofen (Lioresal) and diazepam in spasticity due to multiple sclerosis. Acta Neurol Scand 1975;51(2): 158–66.

85. Mueller ME, Gruenthal M, Olson WL, et al. Gabapentin for relief of upper motor neuron symptoms in multiple sclerosis. Arch Phys Med Rehabil 1997;78:521–4.

86. Cutter NC, Scott DD, Johnson JC, et al. Gabapentin effect on spasticity in multiple sclerosis: a placebo-controlled, randomized trial. Arch Phys Med Rehabil 2000;81:164–9.

87. Dolly JO, Aoki KR. The structure and mode of action of different botulinum toxins. Eur J Neurol 2006;13(Suppl 4):1–9.

88. Giovannelli M, Borriello G, Castri P, et al. Early physiotherapy after injection of botulinum toxin increases the beneficial effects on spasticity in patients with multiple sclerosis. Clin Rehabil 2007;21:331–7.

89. Hyman N, Barnes M, Bhakta B, et al. Botulinum toxin (Dysport) treatment of hip adductor spasticity in multiple sclerosis: a prospective, randomised, double blind, placebo controlled, dose ranging study. J Neurol Neurosurg Psychiatry 2000;68:707–12.

90. Penn RD, Savoy SM, Corcos D, et al. Intrathecal baclofen for severe spinal spasticity. N Engl J Med 1989;320:1517–21.

91. Zahavi A, Geertzen JH, Middel B, et al. Long term effect (more than five years) of intrathecal baclofen on impairment, disability, and quality of life in patients with severe spasticity of spinal origin. J Neurol Neurosurg Psychiatry 2004;75: 1553–7.

92. Boviatsis EJ, Kouyialis AT, Korfias S, et al. Functional outcome of intrathecal baclofen administration for severe spasticity. Clin Neurol Neurosurg 2005;107: 289–95.

93. Mills RJ, Yap L, Young CA. Treatment for ataxia in multiple sclerosis. Cochrane Database Syst Rev 2007;1:CD005029.

94. Hallett M, Lindsey JW, Adelstein BD, et al. Controlled trial of isoniazid therapy for severe postural cerebellar tremor in multiple sclerosis. Neurology 1985;35:1374–7.

95. Duquette P, Pleines J, du Souich P. Isoniazid for tremor in multiple sclerosis: a controlled trial. Neurology 1985;35:1772–5.

96. Koller WC. Pharmacologic trials in the treatment of cerebellar tremor. Arch Neurol 1984;41:280–1.

97. Bittar RG, Hyam J, Nandi D, et al. Thalamotomy versus thalamic stimulation for multiple sclerosis tremor. J Clin Neurosci 2005;12:638–42.

98. Schuurman PR, Bosch DA, Bossuyt PM, et al. A comparison of continuous thalamic stimulation and thalamotomy for suppression of severe tremor. N Engl J Med 2000;342:461–8.

99. Schuurman PR, Bosch DA, Merkus MP, et al. Long-term follow-up of thalamic stimulation versus thalamotomy for tremor suppression. Mov Disord 2008;23: 1146–53.

100. Goodman AD, Cohen JA, Cross A, et al. Fampridine-SR in multiple sclerosis: a randomized, double-blind, placebo-controlled, dose-ranging study. Mult Scler 2007;13:357–68.

101. Goodman AD, Brown TR, Cohen JA, et al. Dose comparison trial of sustained-release fampridine in multiple sclerosis. Neurology 2008;71:1134–41.

102. Goodman AD, Brown TR, Krupp LB, et al. Sustained-release oral fampridine in multiple sclerosis: a randomised, double-blind, controlled trial. Lancet 2009; 373:732–8.

103. Goodman AD, Brown TR, Edwards KR, et al. A phase 3 trial of extended release oral dalfampridine in multiple sclerosis. Ann Neurol 2010;68:494–502.

104. Hobart JC, Riazi A, Lamping DL, et al. Measuring the impact of MS on walking ability: the 12-Item MS Walking Scale (MSWS-12). Neurology 2003;60(1):31–6.

Complementary and Alternative Medicine and Multiple Sclerosis

Allen C. Bowling, MD, PhD[a,b,c,*]

KEYWORDS

- Complementary and alternative medicine
- Unconventional medicine • Multiple sclerosis
- Demyelinating disease

There is widespread use of complementary and alternative medicine (CAM) among multiple sclerosis (MS) patients. However, conventional health providers may have limited awareness and understanding of CAM therapies. Some of these therapies may be harmful or may interact with conventional MS medications, whereas others are low risk and may provide therapeutic effects. The quality of MS care may be improved if clinicians are able to provide objective CAM information to patients and, when appropriate, direct patients away from therapies that are ineffective or harmful and toward those that are low risk and possibly effective.

This article provides clinically relevant information about CAM therapies that are likely to be encountered in day-to-day practice. Reviews with broader scopes, more detailed information, and critical analyses may be found in other publications.[1–5]

TERMINOLOGY AND DEFINITIONS

There are many different terms and definitions in the area of unconventional medicine.[6] In fact, one of the most common terms, *alternative medicine*, is frequently used incorrectly.

Unconventional medicine is a broad term that usually refers to forms of medicine that are not widely taught in medical schools or generally available in hospitals.

The author has nothing to disclose.
[a] MS Service, Colorado Neurological Institute (CNI), 701 East Hampden Avenue, #320, Englewood, CO 80113, USA
[b] Complementary and Alternative Medicine Service, Colorado Neurological Institute (CNI), 701 East Hampden Avenue, #320, Englewood, CO 80113, USA
[c] Department of Neurology, University of Colorado, Denver, CO, USA
* MS Service, Colorado Neurological Institute (CNI), 701 East Hampden Avenue, #320, Englewood, CO 80113.
E-mail address: abneurocare@qwestoffice.net

Neurol Clin 29 (2011) 465–480
doi:10.1016/j.ncl.2010.12.006
0733-8619/11/$ – see front matter © 2011 Elsevier Inc. All rights reserved.

Complementary and alternative refer to the ways in which these unconventional therapies are used. Complementary indicates that they are used in conjunction with conventional medicine, while alternative signifies that they are used instead of conventional medicine. In lay and professional publications, the term alternative medicine is sometimes used incorrectly to refer to unconventional medicine generally. Complementary and alternative medicine, or CAM, refers to both approaches. The use of conventional medicine in combination with unconventional medicine is known as integrative medicine.[6]

CONVENTIONAL AND UNCONVENTIONAL MEDICINE

In the past two decades, there have been remarkable breakthroughs in understanding, diagnosing, and treating MS. There are now many effective disease-modifying as well as symptomatic therapies. Despite these advances, conventional MS therapies have limitations. For example, both symptomatic and disease-modifying therapies may produce side effects or may be ineffective or only partially effective. In addition, proven therapies may be limited or nonexistent, especially for progressive forms of MS and for specific symptoms, such as tremors, weakness, and incoordination.

The limitations of conventional medicine, as well as other factors, drive many MS patients to pursue CAM. In studies in the United States and other Western countries, one-half to three-fourths of those with MS use CAM.[5–7] Among MS patients, as well as the general population, the majority of those who use CAM do so in a complementary manner. In other words, unconventional medicine is used in conjunction with conventional medicine.[5,6]

MS-RELEVANT CAM THERAPIES
Acupuncture, Chinese Herbal Medicine, and Traditional Chinese Medicine

Acupuncture is one of several components of an ancient healing method, traditional Chinese medicine (TCM) (**Box 1**). Other TCM components include herbs, nutrition, exercise, tai chi, stress reduction, and massage.[1]

Efficacy
Although acupuncture is a popular CAM therapy, studies of TCM in MS are scant. Clinical trials of acupuncture for symptomatic treatment in MS are too limited to provide definitive information.[1–5,8,9] In other conditions, acupuncture may alleviate pain, nausea, and vomiting.[1,10] There are no high-quality trials that have evaluated the safety or efficacy of Chinese herbal medicine in MS.[1]

Safety
Acupuncture is generally well tolerated when it is provided by a well-trained practitioner.[1] By contrast, the safety of Chinese herbal medicine is unknown for MS and many other medical conditions. Of concern, activation of T cells or macrophages, a theoretical risk for worsening MS or decreasing the efficacy of immune-modulating and immune-suppressing medications, may be caused by multiple Chinese herbs, including Asian ginseng, astragalus, and maitake and reishi mushrooms.[1,3]

Summary
Acupuncture is a low-risk component of TCM. Although it has not been rigorously studied in MS, clinical trials in other conditions indicate that it may relieve pain. By contrast, Chinese herbal medicine, which is also a component of TCM, poses theoretical risks and is of unknown efficacy in MS. TCM is an excellent example of the diverse, and sometimes confusing, risk-benefit profiles of CAM therapies—for MS

Box 1
MS-relevant CAM therapies
Acupuncture, Chinese Herbal Medicine, and Traditional Chinese Medicine
Bee Venom Therapy
Cooling
Dental Amalgam Therapy
Dietary Supplements:
Antioxidants
Cranberry
Echinacea and other immune-stimulating supplements
Ginkgo biloba
St John's wort
Vitamin B12
Vitamin D
Diets: The Swank Diet and Other Polyunsaturated Fatty Acid–Enriched Diets
Guided Imagery
Hyperbaric Oxygen
Low-Dose Naltrexone (LDN)
Marijuana
Massage
Reflexology
Tai Chi
Yoga

patients, the single healing system of TCM includes one therapy (acupuncture) that may be reasonable and another therapy (Chinese herbal medicine) that should probably be avoided.

Bee Venom Therapy

With bee venom therapy (BVT), bee stings are administered to specific body parts by placing bees on the skin with tweezers.[1]

Efficacy

In the highest quality clinical trial of BVT in MS, a randomized crossover design was used to evaluate the effects of this therapy on multiple outcome measures (attack frequency, neurologic disability, magnetic resonance imaging [MRI] activity, fatigue, and overall quality of life) in 26 patients with relapsing-remitting or secondary-progressive MS.[11] In this trial, BVT did not produce any symptomatic or disease-modifying effects.

Safety

BVT is usually well tolerated.[11,12] Rarely, bee stings may cause anaphylaxis. In addition, periorbital bee stings, which are sometimes claimed to improve MS-related visual dysfunction, may actually cause optic neuritis, and thus should be avoided.[13]

Summary

BVT is a generally well-tolerated therapy but has not been shown to produce any therapeutic effects in MS. Unlike many forms of CAM for which no MS clinical trials have been conducted and consequently there is not any MS-specific safety and efficacy information, BVT has been formally investigated in a small MS study and has been shown to be ineffective.

Cooling Therapy

Cooling, an unconventional therapy that is unique to MS, makes therapeutic use of the temperature sensitivity that occurs in MS. For years, it has been recognized that small increases in body temperature (0.5°C) may worsen MS symptoms and that small decreases in body temperature may alleviate symptoms.[1] This fact has led to the development of various cooling methods, which range from simple approaches, such as staying in air-conditioned areas and drinking cold beverages, to complex methods, such as wearing specially designed cooling garments.[1]

Efficacy

Several small studies of variable quality have found that cooling garments alleviate multiple MS symptoms.[1] There is one rigorous clinical trial of cooling in MS.[14] In this randomized, controlled, blinded study, cooling was associated with objective improvement in visual function and walking after 1 hour of cooling. There was also subjective improvement in fatigue, cognitive function, and strength reported over a 1-month period. Cooling may be especially effective in those who are known to be heat sensitive.

Safety

Cooling is usually well tolerated. For some patients, the garments are cumbersome. There may be mild discomfort at the onset of cooling. For the rare MS patients who are cold sensitive, cooling may worsen symptoms.[1]

Summary

Cooling is a low-risk therapy that may transiently relieve multiple MS symptoms.

Dental Amalgam Removal

There are claims that dental amalgam removal is an effective treatment for MS. It has been proposed that amalgam causes MS or worsens MS through a variety of mechanisms, including mercury-generated electrical currents, allergic reactions to mercury, or the slow release of solid mercury or mercury vapors.[1]

Efficacy

There are anecdotal accounts of amalgam removal producing beneficial effects in MS patients. However, there are no studies that convincingly demonstrate that mercury causes MS or that amalgam removal has symptomatic or disease-modifying effects in MS.[1,15,16]

Safety

Amalgam removal is usually well tolerated. Rarely, the procedure damages tooth structure or injures nerves. Also, the levels of mercury in the blood may actually increase shortly after amalgam removal.[17,18]

Summary

Amalgam removal is generally safe, but has not been shown to produce symptomatic or disease-modifying effects in MS.

Dietary Supplements: Antioxidants

The pathophysiologic processes that cause myelin and axonal injury in MS may include free radical–induced oxidative damage. Hence, there are claims that antioxidants may have disease-modifying effects in MS.[19]

Efficacy

Several different antioxidant compounds have produced therapeutic effects in experimental autoimmune encephalitis (EAE).[20,21] Small, short-term MS clinical trials with various antioxidants, including α-lipoic acid[22] and a combination of selenium and vitamins C and E,[23] suggest that these approaches are well tolerated; however, these studies have not been powered adequately to assess efficacy. A small study of inosine produced suggestive immunologic, MRI, and clinical effects,[24] while a large, well-designed trial found that interferon-inosine combination therapy did not have any greater effect on disability progression than interferon therapy alone.[25]

Safety

Through mechanisms that have not been fully characterized, many antioxidants activate immune cells, including T cells and macrophages.[2] As a result, these compounds carry theoretical risks in MS. However, as noted, antioxidants have generally been well tolerated in the limited clinical studies to date. Inosine use has been associated with kidney stones.[24]

Summary

Based on theoretical and animal model evidence, antioxidant compounds could have therapeutic effects in MS. Some antioxidant products are specifically marketed to MS patients. However, at this time there are no well-designed clinical trials that demonstrate definitive efficacy in MS. Additional studies in this area, especially clinical trials, should provide information about the safety and efficacy of antioxidants in MS.

Dietary Supplements: Cranberry

Patients with MS may be prone to urinary tract infections (UTIs) caused by MS-associated bladder dysfunction. Cranberry may prevent UTIs through a unique mechanism of action: compounds in cranberry appear to inhibit the adhesion of specific bacteria to the uroepithelium.[1]

Efficacy

Cranberry may prevent UTIs, especially in young to middle-aged women with normal urinary function.[26] However, there is no evidence that cranberry is effective for treating UTIs. Because UTIs may cause pseudoexacerbations in MS, clinicians should be vigilant for UTIs. When UTIs are diagnosed, they should be treated promptly with antibiotics, not cranberry.

Safety

Cranberry is generally safe. Long-term use has been associated with kidney stones. Cranberry may increase the anticoagulant effect of warfarin.[27]

Summary

Cranberry is a low-risk therapy that may be effective for preventing, but not for treating, UTIs.

Dietary Supplements: Echinacea and Other "Immune-Stimulating" Supplements

Lay publications on alternative medicine sometimes claim that because MS is an immune disease, those with MS should take echinacea and other dietary supplements that are known to activate immune cells, including T cells and macrophages.[28] This information is incorrect and potentially dangerous.

Efficacy

Studies of "immune stimulation" by dietary supplements are generally restricted to in vitro or animal model studies. As a result, the concerns with these supplements in MS are generally theoretical. Popular herbs that stimulate T cells or macrophages include echinacea, alfalfa, ashwagandha (*Withania somnifera*), Asian ginseng, astragalus, cat's claw, garlic, maitake mushroom, mistletoe, shiitake mushroom, Siberian ginseng, and stinging nettle.[2] Other supplements that activate T cells or macrophages include zinc, melatonin, and antioxidant vitamins and minerals (see Dietary Supplements: Antioxidants).[2]

Safety

In MS, immune-stimulating supplements carry theoretical risks. In addition, echinacea may increase the hepatotoxic effects of medications, which include some MS medications such as methotrexate and interferons.[2,27]

Summary

There is no evidence that echinacea or other immune-stimulating supplements produce any therapeutic effects in MS. On the contrary, these supplements, which may be quite expensive, actually pose theoretical risks in MS.

Dietary Supplements: Ginkgo Biloba

Ginkgo biloba, an extract of the leaf of the *Ginkgo biloba* tree, has been suggested to exert symptomatic and disease-modifying effects in MS. Constituents of the herb are known to have both anti-inflammatory and antioxidant effects.[2,27]

Efficacy

In animal model experiments, ginkgo has decreased disease severity in some, but not all, studies.[2] Ginkgo does not appear to be an effective treatment for MS attacks.[29] It has not been studied for attack prevention. Ginkgo improved cognitive function[30] and fatigue[31] in small clinical trials.

Safety

Ginkgo is generally safe. Because it exerts anticoagulant effects and may rarely increase the risk of seizures, it should be avoided or used cautiously by patients with seizures and those who take antiplatelet or anticoagulant medications, have coagulopathies, or are undergoing surgery. Ginkgo may also produce dizziness, headaches, rashes, nausea, vomiting, diarrhea, and flatulence.[2,27]

Summary

Ginkgo is a generally well tolerated herbal therapy that, in limited clinical studies, alleviated MS-associated fatigue and cognitive dysfunction. Additional studies are needed to more definitively assess the safety and efficacy of ginkgo in MS.

Dietary Supplements: St John's Wort

St John's wort has been used to treat depression, a common MS symptom, for thousands of years.[1,27]

Efficacy

Clinical trials and meta-analyses indicate that St John's wort is an effective treatment for mild to moderate, but not severe, depression.[27,32]

Safety
St John's wort is usually safe. Rarely, it causes fatigue and photosensitivity. Its potential interactions with medications generally raise more concern than its side effects. Because St John's wort induces multiple cytochrome P-450 enzymes, it may alter blood levels of many medications, including anticonvulsants, warfarin (Coumadin), antidepressants, and oral contraceptives.[27]

Summary
St John's wort may be effective for mild to moderate depression. It is generally well tolerated, but may potentially interact with many different medications.

Dietary Supplements: Vitamin B12

Lay publications on alternative medicine sometimes recommend vitamin B12 supplements for MS.

Efficacy
There is no evidence that vitamin B12 supplements produce clinically meaningful therapeutic effects in MS patients generally.[33–35] There is a small subset of MS patients who have vitamin B12 deficiency.[36] These patients should be treated with vitamin B12 supplementation.

Safety
Vitamin B12 supplements are generally safe. Rarely they may produce diarrhea, rashes, and itching.[36]

Summary
Vitamin B12 supplements are usually well tolerated. However, contrary to what is sometimes stated in lay publications, there is no evidence that vitamin B12 supplementation produces meaningful therapeutic effects in MS patients generally. MS patients with documented vitamin B12 deficiency should be treated with intramuscular or oral vitamin B12.

Dietary Supplements: Vitamin D

There are several ways in which vitamin D is relevant to MS. First, MS patients are prone to osteopenia and osteoporosis, and vitamin D is essential for maintaining bone density.[37] Also, because vitamin D exerts immune-regulating effects, it could have preventive and disease-modifying effects.[38,39]

Efficacy
Low levels and low intake of vitamin D have been associated with increased risk for developing MS.[39] In addition, low vitamin D levels have been associated with increased relapse rate[40,41] and more severe levels of disability.[39] Limited intervention studies in MS suggest that vitamin D supplements are generally well tolerated in MS. These studies have produced suggestive immunologic and therapeutic effects, but do not provide rigorous evidence for disease-modifying effects.[42,43]

Safety
Vitamin D is generally safe. High doses may cause fatigue, abdominal cramps, nausea, vomiting, renal damage, hypertension, and several other side effects. The appropriate daily intake for vitamin D and calcium were revised in November 2010 through a report by the Institute of Medicine (IOM).[44] In adults, the recommended daily amount (RDA) for vitamin D is now 600–800 international units (IU) and that for calcium is 1,000–1,

300 milligrams (mg). The tolerable upper intake level (UL), which is the safe upper limit for regular daily use, is 4,000 IU for vitamin D and 2,000–3,000 mg for calcium.

Summary

Reasonable doses of vitamin D supplements are generally well tolerated. Vitamin D3 supplements should be considered in MS patients who have low vitamin D levels, have risk factors for low bone density, or are known to have decreased bone density. Vitamin D could have preventive and disease-modifying effects in MS, but additional research, especially high-quality intervention trials, are needed.

Diets: The Swank Diet and Other Polyunsaturated Fatty Acid–Enriched Diets

In MS patients, diets are among the most popular CAM therapies. Epidemiologic, in vitro, animal model, and clinical trial studies over the past several decades suggest that diets that are relatively low in saturated fats and relatively high in polyunsaturated fatty acids (PUFAs), such as omega-3 and omega-6 fatty acids, may produce disease-modifying effects in MS.[45,46]

Efficacy

The "Swank diet," developed by Swank and Dugan, is low in saturated fat and high in PUFAs. Although this diet was reported to have dramatic disease-modifying effects in an MS clinical trial, this trial was not controlled, randomized, or blinded.[45,47]

Subsequently, more rigorous trials were undertaken with PUFA supplementation.[45] There are 3 randomized controlled trials of omega-6 supplements, 2 of which reported statistically significant reductions in attack severity and duration. The available data from all 3 trials was later pooled and found to slow disability progression in those with mild MS at the onset of the trial.[45]

There are more limited published studies of omega-3 supplementation. The most rigorous study to date was a large, randomized, double-blind, controlled trial that did not report a statistically significant treatment effect.[48] However, for disability progression, there was a trend in favor of the treatment group ($P<.07$). Another small randomized trial of omega-3 fatty acid supplements in combination with glatiramer acetate or interferons reported a trend for improved physical and emotional functioning in those taking omega-3 fatty acids.[49] A well-designed Norwegian study of interferon treatment in combination with omega-3 supplements or placebo has been reported recently in preliminary form.[50] This study, which monitored MRI activity, relapse rate, disability progression, and multiple symptoms, did not find any evidence for a therapeutic effect of omega-3 supplements.

Safety

Omega-3 and omega-6 supplements are usually well tolerated. The Food and Drug Administration (FDA) has classified fish oil, a rich source of omega-3 fatty acids, as "generally regarded as safe."[27] The safety of long-term supplementation with other omega-3 fatty acids and omega-6 fatty acids generally is not known. Omega-6 fatty acids may raise triglyceride levels and may rarely cause seizures. Omega-3 and omega-6 fatty acids may exert mild anticoagulant effects. Because PUFA supplementation (omega-3 or omega-6) may cause vitamin E deficiency, supplementation with modest doses of vitamin E may be indicated.[27,45]

Summary

PUFA-enriched diets are generally safe. These approaches have produced suggestive results in several MS clinical trials over the past few decades. However, the negative results in a recent preliminary report of a well-conducted Norwegian study raise concerns about the efficacy of these strategies—this study has not yet been published in a peer-reviewed journal. PUFA-enriched diets should not be used instead of conventional disease-modifying medications. The safety and effectiveness of these diets in combination with disease-modifying medications (interferons, glatiramer acetate, mitoxantrone, and natalizumab) has not been rigorously studied.

Guided Imagery

In guided imagery, a form of mind-body medicine, an individual creates relaxing mental images. Guided imagery may be used in combination with other relaxation methods, such as progressive muscle relaxation.[1]

Efficacy
One small MS study found that guided imagery alleviated anxiety but not depression or multiple other MS symptoms.[51] In other medical conditions, limited clinical trials of guided imagery have reported possible therapeutic effects on anxiety, depression, pain, and insomnia.[1]

Safety
Guided imagery is generally safe. Relaxation may increase spasticity. Guided imagery may produce anxiety, disturbing thoughts, and fear of losing control, especially in those with psychiatric conditions.[1]

Summary
Guided imagery is generally well tolerated, and may decrease anxiety and possibly other MS-associated symptoms.

Hyperbaric Oxygen

Lay books on alternative medicine and commercial centers that specialize in hyperbaric oxygen (HBO) sometimes claim that HBO is an effective therapy for MS and many other diseases. While HBO is indeed a recognized medical therapy, it has proven effectiveness for only a limited number of conditions, including burns, severe infections, decompression sickness, and carbon monoxide poisoning.[1]

Efficacy
A study published in the *New England Journal of Medicine* in 1983 reported that HBO produced therapeutic effects in MS.[52] This study is sometimes used as evidence that HBO is an effective MS therapy. However, multiple subsequent trials did not generally find clinically significant therapeutic effects. In addition, independent reviews of the published clinical trials conclude that HBO does not produce consistent therapeutic effects in MS and that HBO should not be used to treat MS.[53–55]

Safety
HBO is generally well tolerated. It may produce mild visual symptoms, and rarely causes cataracts, seizures, tympanic membrane rupture, and pneumothorax.[1]

Summary
Unlike many forms of CAM, HBO has actually been extensively studied in MS. These studies indicate that HBO does not produce any consistent therapeutic effects in MS. Nevertheless, HBO is sometimes heavily marketed to MS patients. HBO is generally safe, but may rarely cause serious side effects.

Low-Dose Naltrexone

For MS, low doses of oral naltrexone, an opiate antagonist, have been claimed to relieve symptoms, prevent attacks, and slow disability progression. It has been proposed that LDN could be therapeutic for MS through several possible mechanisms, including partial opiate agonist, excitotoxic, and antioxidant effects.[1,56]

Efficacy

Although there are many anecdotal reports about LDN efficacy in MS, published studies of this therapy are limited and inconsistent. In the animal model of MS, LDN decreases the severity of disease on the basis of pathologic and clinical measures.[57] In 2 similar short-term crossover trials in MS, one study found no beneficial effects[58] whereas the other, reported preliminarily, found that LDN had no effect on physical functioning but did improve pain and mental health.[59] A 6-month, open-label study of 40 people with primary progressive MS found that LDN improved spasticity, worsened pain, and had no effect on depression, fatigue, or overall quality of life.[56]

Safety

In the limited MS studies to date, LDN has generally been well tolerated. Neurologic worsening occurred in one patient in the study of primary progressive MS.[56] LDN may produce opiate withdrawal if used in patients who are being treated chronically with opiates.

Summary

LDN appears to be generally safe. In the MS clinical trials to date, LDN has produced variable and inconsistent efficacy results. Additional studies are needed to determine the safety and efficacy of LDN in MS.

Marijuana (Cannabis)

Marijuana, also known as cannabis, contains a class of compounds known as cannabinoids (CBs). Tetrahydrocannabinol (THC), a constituent of marijuana, is a cannabinoid. CBs have multiple pharmacologic effects. CBs suppress excessive neuronal activity and could thereby relieve some MS symptoms, including pain and spasticity. Also, through neuroprotection and immune modulation, CBs could theoretically be disease modifying in MS.[60]

Efficacy

CBs produce symptomatic and disease-modifying effects in EAE.[60] Suggestive, but not definitive, results have been obtained in clinical trials. In the most rigorous clinical trial to date, THC, but not cannabis oil, produced a small therapeutic effect on spasticity and a possible effect on disability.[61] Sativex, an orally administered form of cannabis, has been shown to relieve multiple MS symptoms, including pain, spasticity, and sleeping difficulties in some,[62] but not all,[63] studies.

Safety

Marijuana has many potential side effects, including sedation, seizures, nausea, vomiting, impaired driving, incoordination, poor pregnancy outcomes, impaired lung function, dependence, and increased risk of cancer of the head, neck, and lung.[1,3]

Summary

There is suggestive evidence that marijuana may relieve symptoms and modify the disease course in MS. However, these findings are not definitive. Marijuana use is associated with significant side effects and is illegal in many countries. In the United States, "medical marijuana" laws in some states allow patients with MS (and certain other medical conditions) to use marijuana legally. It is important for MS patients to be aware that, even though it may be legal for use in MS in some states, the safety and efficacy of marijuana in MS has not been definitively established. Additional, high-quality clinical trials of marijuana in MS are needed and are currently being conducted in the United Kingdom.

Massage

Massage, an ancient form of bodywork, involves the use of traction and pressure to manipulate soft tissue.[1]

Efficacy

There are only a few formal studies of massage in MS. In the largest study to date, 24 MS patients were treated for 5 weeks with either "standard medical care" or standard medical care in combination with twice-weekly massage therapy.[64] The treatment group showed improvement in anxiety, depression, self-esteem, body image, social functioning, and "image of disease progression."

Safety

Massage is generally safe. Mild side effects include myalgias, headaches, and lethargy. Massage may rarely produce more serious side effects, such as bone fractures and hepatic bleeding. Massage should be avoided or used cautiously by pregnant women and by those with thrombosis, burns, skin infections, open wounds, bone fractures, osteoporosis, cancer, and heart disease.[1]

Summary

Massage is a generally safe therapy that has produced promising results in limited studies. Further studies are needed to more definitively determine the safety and effectiveness of massage in MS.

Reflexology

In reflexology, a type of bodywork, manual pressure is applied to specific sites, which are usually on the feet and are believed to correspond to specific organs or organ systems. There are multiple mechanisms by which reflexology has been claimed to produce therapeutic effects.[65]

Efficacy

In one controlled study, 71 people with MS were treated with either reflexology or nonspecific calf massage. The treated group exhibited significant improvement in paresthesias, urinary symptoms, and spasticity. There was a relatively high dropout rate.[66] In another controlled study, 73 MS patients with pain were treated with reflexology or nonspecific foot massage. Both interventions were associated with improvement in pain, the primary outcome measure, and other symptoms, including fatigue and overall quality of life.[67]

Safety

Reflexology is generally well tolerated. Mild side effects include fatigue, foot pain, and changes in bowel and bladder function. Reflexology should be avoided or used cautiously by patients with significant foot conditions, including bone or joint disorders, gout, ulcers, and vascular disease.[1]

Summary

Reflexology is a low-risk therapy that has produced promising results in one controlled MS study. However, another controlled trial found that similar beneficial effects occurred with reflexology and sham foot massage. It has been proposed that some of the benefits noted with reflexology may be a result of nonspecific effects, including the relaxing effects of foot massages and the advice and support provided by therapists.[65,67,68] More rigorous trials are needed to determine whether reflexology has therapeutic effects in MS.

Tai Chi

Tai chi is one of several components of the ancient multimodal healing method known as TCM. Tai chi, which has been practiced for centuries in China, has undergone limited investigation in MS.[1]

Efficacy

In small, nonblinded trials in MS, tai chi has improved spasticity, walking stability, and social and emotional functioning.[69,70]

Safety

Tai chi is generally safe. There is a risk of falling, and it may strain joints and muscles. For those with disabilities, tai chi may be modified. Tai chi should be avoided or used cautiously by patients with fractures, severe osteoporosis, acute low back pain, and significant joint injuries.[1]

Summary

Tai chi is a generally safe therapy that has improved multiple MS symptoms in limited studies. Larger and more rigorous trials of tai chi in MS are needed.

Yoga

Yoga was developed in India thousands of years ago and is a component of the ancient Indian healing tradition known as Ayurveda. Although yoga is now widely practiced around the world, it has actually undergone only limited clinical investigation.[1]

Efficacy

One well-designed, controlled trial in MS reported that, relative to controls, those who practiced yoga or did conventional exercise had less fatigue.[71] Another smaller study found that yoga improved attention in MS patients.[72]

Safety

Yoga is generally safe. As with tai chi, it may be modified for those with disabilities. Vigorous exercise and difficult postures should be avoided or done cautiously by pregnant women and by patients with gait instability, fatigue, heat sensitivity, or significant bone, lung, or heart conditions.[1]

Summary

Yoga is a generally well tolerated therapy that may decrease fatigue and increase attention in MS. Additional studies of yoga and MS are needed.

SUMMARY

MS is a complex, potentially disabling disease for which we have only partial pathologic understanding and partially effective therapies. These features of the disease may lead patients with MS to use CAM. These very same features of MS make it essential for patients as well as clinicians to thoughtfully and critically consider CAM therapies. In MS, some CAM therapies may be generally safe, produce therapeutic effects, and be underused and underrecognized. On the other hand, other CAM therapies are not effective, produce harmful side effects, or have never been studied. Clinicians may improve the quality of MS care by helping patients differentiate CAM therapies with reasonable risk-benefit profiles from those that are ineffective, dangerous, or unstudied.

REFERENCES

1. Bowling AC. Complementary and alternative medicine and multiple sclerosis. New York: Demos Medical Publishing; 2007.
2. Bowling AC, Stewart TM. Current complementary and alternative therapies of multiple sclerosis. Curr Treat Options Neurol 2003;5:55–68.
3. Bowling AC, Stewart TM. Dietary supplements and multiple sclerosis: a health professional's guide. New York: Demos Medical Publishing; 2004.
4. Polman CH, Thompson AJ, Murray TJ, et al. Multiple sclerosis: the guide to treatment and management. New York: Demos Medical Publishing; 2006. p. 117–79.
5. Bowling AC. Unconventional medicine and multiple sclerosis: the role of conventional health providers. In: Lucchinetti CF, Hohlfeld R, editors. Multiple sclerosis 3 (blue books of neurology series). Philadelphia: Saunders; 2010. p. 355–70.
6. Eisenberg D, Davis R, Ettner S, et al. Trends in alternative medicine use in the United States, 1990–1997. JAMA 1998;280:1569–75.
7. Shinto L, Yadav V, Morris C, et al. Demographic and health-related factors associated with complementary and alternative medicine (CAM) use in multiple sclerosis. Mult Scler 2006;12:94–100.
8. Soe STE, Kopsky DJ, Jongen PJ, et al. Multiple sclerosis patients with bladder dysfunction have decreased symptoms after electro-acupuncture. Mult Scler 2009;15:1376–7.
9. Donnelan CP, Shanley J. Comparison of the effect of two types of acupuncture on quality of life in secondary progressive multiple sclerosis: a preliminary, single-blind randomized controlled trial. Clin Rehabil 2008;22:195–205.
10. NIH consensus development panel on acupuncture. JAMA 1998;280:1518–24.
11. Wesselius T, Heersema DJ, Mostert JP, et al. A randomized crossover study of bee sting therapy for multiple sclerosis. Neurology 2005;65:1764–8.
12. Castro HJ, Mendez-Inocencio JI, Omidvar B, et al. A phase I study of the safety of honeybee venom extract as a possible treatment for patients with progressive forms of multiple sclerosis. Allergy Asthma Proc 2005;26:470–6.
13. Song H-S, Wray SH. Bee sting optic neuritis. J Clin Neuroophthalmol 1991;11: 1145–9.
14. NASA/MS Cooling Study Group. A randomized controlled study of the acute and chronic effects of cooling therapy for MS. Neurology 2003;60:1955–60.
15. Casetta I, Invernizzi M, Granieri E. Multiple sclerosis and dental amalgam: case control study in Ferrara, Italy. Neuroepidemiology 2001;20:134–7.
16. NIH Conference Assessment. Effects and side-effects of dental restorative materials. Adv Dent Res 1992;6:1–144.
17. Ekstrand J, Bjorkman L, Edlund C, et al. Toxicological aspects on the release and systemic uptake of mercury from dental amalgam. Eur J Oral Sci 1998;106: 678–86.
18. Eley BM, Cox SW. The release, absorption, and possible health effects of mercury from dental amalgam: a review of recent findings. Br Dent J 1993; 175:355–62.
19. Van Meeteren ME, Teunissen CE, Dijkstra A, et al. Antioxidants and polyunsaturated fatty acids in multiple sclerosis. Eur J Clin Nutr 2005;59:1347–61.

20. Marracci GH, Jones RE, McKeon GP, et al. Alpha lipoic acid inhibits T cell migration into the spinal cord and suppresses and treats experimental autoimmune encephalomyelitis. J Neuroimmunol 2002;131:104–14.

21. Scott GS, Spitsin SV, Kean RB, et al. Therapeutic intervention in experimental allergic encephalomyelitis by administration of uric acid precursors. Proc Natl Acad Sci U S A 2002;99:16303–8.

22. Yadav V, Marracci G, Lovera J, et al. Lipoic acid in multiple sclerosis: a pilot study. Mult Scler 2005;11:159–65.

23. Mai J, Sorenson P, Hansen J. High dose antioxidant supplementation to MS patients: effects on glutathione peroxidase, clinical safety, and absorption of selenium. Biol Trace Elem Res 1990;24:109–17.

24. Markowitz CE, Spitsin S, Zimmerman V, et al. The treatment of multiple sclerosis with inosine. J Altern Complement Med 2009;15:619–25.

25. Gonsette RE, Sindic C, D'hooge MB, et al. Boosting endogenous neuroprotection in multiple sclerosis: the association of inosine and interferon-beta in relapsing-remitting multiple sclerosis (ASIIMS) trial. Mult Scler 2010;16:455–62.

26. Guay DR. Cranberry and urinary tract infections. Drugs 2009;69:775–807.

27. Jellin JM, Gregory PJ, Batz F, et al. Pharmacist's letter/prescriber's letter natural medicines comprehensive database. 8th edition. Stockton (CA): Therapeutic Research Faculty; 2010.

28. Bowling AC, Ibrahim R, Stewart TM. Alternative medicine and multiple sclerosis: an objective review from an American perspective. Int J MS Care 2000;2:14–21.

29. Brochet B, Guinot P, Orgogozo J, et al. Double-blind, placebo controlled, multi-centre study of ginkgolide B in treatment of acute exacerbations for multiple sclerosis. The Ginkgolide Study Group in multiple sclerosis. J Neurol Neurosurg Psychiatry 1995;58:360–2.

30. Lovera J, Bagert B, Smoot K, et al. Ginkgo biloba for the improvement of cognitive performance in multiple sclerosis: a randomized, placebo-controlled trial. Mult Scler 2007;13:376–85.

31. Johnson SK, Diamond BJ, Rausch S, et al. The effect of Ginkgo biloba on functional measure in multiple sclerosis: a pilot randomized controlled trial. Explore (NY) 2006;2:19–24.

32. Werneke U, Horn O, Taylor DM. How effective is St. John's wort? The evidence revisited. J Clin Psychiatry 2004;65:611–7.

33. Kira J, Tobimatus S, Goto I. Vitamin B12 metabolism and massive-dose methyl vitamin B12 therapy in Japanese patients with multiple sclerosis. Intern Med 1994;33:82–6.

34. Loder C, Allawi J, Horrobin DF. Treatment of multiple sclerosis with lofepramine, L-phenylalanine, and vitamin B-12: mechanism of action and clinical importance: roles of the locus coeruleus and central noradrenergic systems. Med Hypotheses 2002;59:594–602.

35. Wade DT, Young CA, Chaudhuri KR, et al. A randomized placebo controlled exploratory study of vitamin B-12, lofepramine, and L-phenylalanine (the "Cari Loder regime") in the treatment of multiple sclerosis. J Neurol Neurosurg Psychiatry 2002;73:246–9.

36. Goodkin D, Jacobsen D, Galvez N, et al. Serum cobalamin deficiency is uncommon in multiple sclerosis. Arch Neurol 1994;51:1110–4.

37. Weinstock-Guttman B, Gallagher E, et al. Risk of bone loss in men with multiple sclerosis. Mult Scler 2004;10:170–5.

38. Smolders J, Damoiseaux J, Menheere P. Vitamin D as an immune modulator in multiple sclerosis, a review. J Neuroimmunol 2008;194:7–17.

39. Ascherio A, Munger KL, Simon KC. Vitamin D and multiple sclerosis. Lancet Neurol 2010;9:599–612.
40. Mowry EM, Krupp LB, Milazzo M, et al. Vitamin D status is associated with relapse rate in pediatric-onset multiple sclerosis. Ann Neurol 2010;67:618–24.
41. Simpson S, Taylor B, Blizzard L, et al. Higher 25-hydroxyvitamin D is associated with lower relapse risk in multiple sclerosis. Ann Neurol 2010;68:193–203.
42. Burton JM, Kimball S, Vieth R, et al. A Phase I/II dose-escalation trial of vitamin D3 and calcium in multiple sclerosis. Neurology 2010;74:1852–9.
43. Wingerchuk DM, Lesaux J, Rice GP, et al. A pilot study of oral calcitriol (1,25-dihydroxyvitamin D3) for relapsing-remitting multiple sclerosis. J Neurol Neurosurg Psychiatry 2005;76:1294–6.
44. Ross AC, Taylor CL, Yaktine AL, et al, editors. Dietary reference intakes for calcium and vitamin D. Washington, DC: The National Academies Press; 2010.
45. Stewart TM, Bowling AC. Polyunsaturated fatty acid supplementation in MS. Int MS J 2005;12:88–93.
46. Mehta LR, Dworkin RH, Schwid SR. Polyunsaturated fatty acids and their potential therapeutic role in multiple sclerosis. Nat Clin Pract Neurol 2009;5:82–92.
47. Swank R, Dugan B. Effect of low saturated fat diet in early and late cases of multiple sclerosis. Lancet 1990;336:37–9.
48. Bates D, Cartlidge N, French J, et al. A double-blind controlled trial of long chain n-3 polyunsaturated fatty acids in the treatment of multiple sclerosis. J Neurol Neurosurg Psychiatry 1989;52:18–22.
49. Weinstock-Guttman B, Baier M, Park Y, et al. Low fat dietary intervention with omega-3 fatty acid supplementation in multiple sclerosis patients. Prostaglandins Leukot Essent Fatty Acids 2005;73:392–404.
50. Myhr K-M, Reinertsen S, Beiske AG, et al. Omega-3 fatty acids treatment in relapsing-remitting multiple sclerosis. Neurology 2010;74(Suppl2):A370.
51. Maguire BL. The effects of imagery on attitudes and moods in multiple sclerosis patients. Altern Ther Health Med 1996;2:75–9.
52. Fischer BH, Marks M, Reich T. Hyperbaric oxygen treatment of multiple sclerosis. A randomized, placebo-controlled, double-blind study. N Engl J Med 1983;308:181–6.
53. Bennett M, Heard R. Hyperbaric oxygen therapy for multiple sclerosis. Cochrane Database Syst Rev 2004;1:CD003057.
54. Kleijnen J, Knipschild P. Hyberbaric oxygen for multiple sclerosis: review of controlled trials. Acta Neurol Scand 1995;91:330–4.
55. Bennett M, Heard R. Hyperbaric oxygen therapy for multiple sclerosis. CNS Neurosci Ther 2010;16:115–24.
56. Gironi M, Martinelli-Boneschi F, Sacerdote P, et al. A pilot trial of low-dose naltrexone in primary progressive multiple sclerosis. Mult Scler 2008;14:1076–83.
57. Zagon IS, Rahn KA, Turel AP, et al. Endogenous opioids regulate expression of experimental autoimmune encephalomyelitis: a new paradigm for the treatment of multiple sclerosis. Exp Biol Med (Maywood) 2009;234:1383–92.
58. Sharafaddinzadeh N, Moghtaderi A, Kashipazha D, et al. The effect of low-dose naltrexone on quality of life of patients with multiple sclerosis: a randomized placebo-controlled trial. Mult Scler 2010;16(8):964–9.
59. Cree BA, Kornyeyeva E, Goodin DS. Pilot trial of low-dose naltrexone and quality of life in multiple sclerosis. Ann Neurol 2010;68:145–50.
60. Bowling AC. Cannabinoids in MS—are we any closer to knowing how best to use them? Mult Scler 2006;12:523–5.

61. Zajicek J, Sanders HP, Wright DE, et al. Cannabinoids in multiple sclerosis (CAMS) study: safety and efficacy data for 12 months follow-up. J Neurol Neurosurg Psychiatry 2005;76:1664–9.

62. Barnes MP. Sativex: clinical efficacy and tolerability in the treatment of symptoms of multiple sclerosis and neuropathic pain. Expert Opin Pharmacother 2006;7: 607–15.

63. Centonze D, Mori F, Koch G, et al. Lack of effect of cannabis-based treatment on clinical and laboratory measures in multiple sclerosis. Neurol Sci 2009;30:531–4.

64. Hernandez-Reif M, Field T, Field T, et al. Multiple sclerosis patients benefit from massage therapy. J Bodyw Mov Ther 1998;2:168–74.

65. Ernst E. Is reflexology an effective intervention? A systematic review of randomized controlled trials. Med J Aust 2009;191:263–6.

66. Siev-Nur I, Gamus D, Lerner-Geva L, et al. Reflexology treatment relieves symptoms of multiple sclerosis: a randomized controlled study. Mult Scler 2003;9: 356–61.

67. Hughes CM, Smyth S, Lowe-Strong AS. Reflexology for the treatment of pain in people with multiple sclerosis: a double-blind randomized sham-controlled clinical trial. Mult Scler 2009;15:1329–38.

68. Mackereth PA, Booth K, Hillier VF, et al. What do people talk about during reflexology? Analysis of worries and concerns expressed during sessions for patients with multiple sclerosis. Complement Ther Clin Pract 2009;15:85–90.

69. Husted C, Pham L, Hekking A. Improving quality of life for people with chronic conditions: the example of t'ai chi and multiple sclerosis. Altern Ther Health Med 1999;5:70–4.

70. Mills M, Allen J. Mindfulness of movement as a coping strategy in multiple sclerosis. A pilot study. Gen Hosp Psychiatry 2000;22:425–31.

71. Oken BS, Kishiyama S, Zajdel D, et al. Randomized controlled trial of yoga and exercise in multiple sclerosis. Neurology 2004;62:2058–64.

72. Velikonja O, Curic K, Ozura A, et al. Influence of sports climbing and yoga on spasticity, cognitive function, mood and fatigue in patients with multiple sclerosis. Clin Neurol Neurosurg 2010;112(7):597–601.

Pediatric Multiple Sclerosis

Tanuja Chitnis, MD[a], Lauren Krupp, MD[b], Ann Yeh, MD[c],
Jennifer Rubin, MD[d], Nancy Kuntz, MD[d], Jonathan B. Strober, MD[e],
Dorothee Chabas, MD, PhD[f], Bianca Weinstock-Guttmann, MD[g],
Jayne Ness, MD, PhD[h],*, Moses Rodriguez, MD[i],
Emmanuelle Waubant, MD, PhD[f]

KEYWORDS

• Multiple sclerosis • Children • Pediatric • Treatment

In the past 5 years, there has been an exponential growth in the knowledge about multiple sclerosis (MS) in children and adolescents. Recent publications have shed light on its diagnosis, pathogenesis, clinical course, and treatment. However, there remain several key areas that require further exploration. This article summarizes the current state of knowledge on pediatric MS and discusses future avenues of investigation.

DEFINITIONS

The awareness that MS can affect children (ie, before the age of 18 years) and the interest in pediatric MS have increased during the past 20 years. When the first cohort

[a] Harvard Medical School, Partners Pediatric Multiple Sclerosis Center, Massachusetts General Hospital for Children, 55 Fruit Street, Boston, MA 02114, USA
[b] Department of Neurology, National Pediatric Multiple Sclerosis Center, SUNY Stony Brook, Stony Brook, NY, USA
[c] Pediatric Multiple Sclerosis Center of Excellence, Jacobs Neurological Institute, SUNY-Buffalo, 219 Bryan Street, Buffalo, NY 14222, USA
[d] Department of Pediatric Neurology, Children's Memorial Hospital, Northwestern Feinberg School of Medicine, 2300 Children's Plaza, Chicago, IL 60614, USA
[e] Pediatric Muscular Dystrophy Association Clinic, Neurology and Pediatrics UCSF, Division of Child Neurology, Department of Neurology, University of California, San Francisco, Suite 609, 350 Parnassus Avenue, San Francisco, CA 94117, USA
[f] Department of Neurology, UCSF Regional Pediatric Multiple Sclerosis Center, University of California, San Francisco, San Francisco, CA, USA
[g] SUNY University of Buffalo, Baird Multiple Sclerosis Center and Pediatric Multiple Sclerosis Center of Excellence, Jacobs Neurological Institute, SUNY-Buffalo, 219 Bryan Street, Buffalo, NY, USA
[h] University of Alabama at Birmingham, Center for Pediatric Onset Demyelinating Disease, Children's Hospital of Alabama, 1600 7th Avenue South, CHB 314, Birmingham, AL 35233-1711, USA
[i] Mayo Clinc Pediatric Multiple Sclerosis Center, Mayo Clinic, 200 1st Street SW, Rochester, MN 55905, USA
* Corresponding author.
E-mail address: jness@uab.edu

Neurol Clin 29 (2011) 481–505
doi:10.1016/j.ncl.2011.01.004
0733-8619/11/$ – see front matter © 2011 Elsevier Inc. All rights reserved.

neurologic.theclinics.com

of pediatric MS[1] was published in 1987, there was no consensus definition. Until 2001, the criteria used to diagnose MS in adults were mostly based on the clinical dissemination of symptoms in time and space.[2] Consensus MS criteria including magnetic resonance imaging (MRI) findings were published[3] in 2001 and refined in 2005.[4] However, these criteria may have a limited applicability in the pediatric population. In fact, MS is a challenging diagnosis in children, especially those who have not yet reached puberty, because of the atypical clinical, biologic, and MRI presentations and the broader spectrum of potential differential diagnoses specific to that age range.[5] In particular, differentiating a first episode of MS from acute disseminated encephalomyelitis (ADEM) in children who present with an initial demyelinating event can be an issue for any clinician, given the clinical overlap between the 2 entities and the absence of a reliable biomarker or MRI criteria.

Because pediatric MS affects a limited number of children, multicentered, international collaborations became necessary to move forward in the field. In 2002, an International Pediatric MS Study Group was created (www.ipmssg.org), and in 2007, it framed operational definitions for acquired demyelinating diseases of the central nervous system (CNS) in children, to facilitate the diagnosis and improve communication between researchers in the field.[6]

Diagnosis of an Initial Demyelinating Event

According to these definitions, ADEM (monophasic) requires the presence of both encephalopathy and polysymptomatic presentation. ADEM may last up to 3 months, with fluctuating symptoms or MRI findings. In contrast, a clinically isolated syndrome (CIS) can be either monofocal or polyfocal but usually does not include encephalopathy.

INCIDENCE AND PREVALENCE/DEMOGRAPHIC FEATURES

Although the worldwide prevalence of pediatric MS is unknown, data are available from individual countries or MS centers. Several large series[7–10] report prevalence rates of MS onset in childhood or adolescence ranging from 2.2% to 4.4% of all MS cases, whereas some MS referral centers report that up to 10% of the patients with MS experienced symptom onset before age 18 years.[11] Population-based studies suggest even lower rates, with pediatric MS comprising 1.7% of MS cases.[12,13] MS incidence in the California pediatric cohort was about 2 per 100,000 person-years (vs 14.2 per 100,000 person-years overall). A multicenter Asian study found that overall 12.5% of the patients were younger than 18 years at disease onset. About 42% of these patients had an opticospinal form of MS.[14] In general, pediatric MS onset before age 10 years is rare and constitutes approximately 20% of the reported pediatric cases in large series.[15] It is unclear whether the incidence of pediatric MS has increased in the past decades or is merely being increasingly recognized because of improved diagnostic criteria and medical awareness.

Demographic Features

The male to female ratio of pediatric MS varies by age. Before age 6 years, the ratio of girls to boys is 0.8:1. It increases from age 6 to 10 years to 1.6:1, to 2.1:1 in children older than 10 years and 1:3 in adolescents.[16] Although MS in adults is more common in non-Hispanic whites, several studies have pointed out significant racial and ethnic variability in the pediatric population in North America. Two pediatric MS centers in the United States have reported higher proportions of blacks/African Americans (7.4% vs 4.3%)[8] and Hispanic and first-generation Americans (Krupp and colleagues, unpublished data 2009) than in the adult MS population and, in 1 study, the general population. Studies from a Canadian and US center showed that the pediatric patients were more likely to report Caribbean, Asian, or Middle-Eastern ancestry and less likely to report European ancestry[17] (Krupp and colleagues, unpublished data, 2009). The reasons behind this greater diversity in ethnicity, race, and ancestry in pediatric MS remain unclear, but it likely represents a combination of genetic and environmental influences, in addition to changing regional demographic factors affecting that age range in North America (ie, increased influx of immigrants of non-European ancestry across North America in recent years).

PATHOPHYSIOLOGY/IMMUNOLOGY

There are few reports of pathologic changes in cases of pediatric MS and ADEM. Most are cases of tumefactive demyelination, which may represent a bias in the tendency to biopsy these particular cases.[18–22] Those cases with a detailed pathologic evaluation report a dense accumulation of lymphocytes and macrophages in a prominently perivascular distribution, with rare B cells. Demyelination is present in a predominantly perivascular pattern, whereas axonal damage is typically absent.[19] It is unclear whether pathologic changes are similar to or different from those of the subtypes described in adult MS.[23]

T cells play a key role in the pathophysiology of MS. Current immunologic models of the disease indicate that activated T cells cross the blood-brain barrier and incite an inflammatory reaction within the CNS.[24] Several groups have studied T-cell responses to various antigenic stimuli in pediatric MS. A recent study of a large cohort of children with CNS inflammatory demyelination, type I diabetes, and CNS injury demonstrated that these children exhibited heightened peripheral T-cell responses to a wide array of self-antigens compared with healthy controls. Children with autoimmune diseases and CNS injury also exhibited abnormal T-cell responses against multiple cow-milk proteins.[25]

The role of circulating antimyelin antibodies has been debated extensively in adult MS studies. Myelin oligodendrocyte glycoprotein (MOG) is an attractive target because it is expressed on the outer myelin membrane and may be easily targeted by the immune response. Using a tetramer approach, the levels of anti-MOG antibodies were higher in the serum of the younger children with MS and in children with an initial attack that was clinically indistinguishable from ADEM, whether or not they were subsequently found to have MS.[26] Using myelin-transfected cells as a detection system, 38.7% of patients younger than 10 years at disease onset were found to have MOG antibodies, compared with 14.7% of patients in the 10- to 18-year age group.[27] A study examining antimyelin basic protein antibodies in the serum and cerebrospinal fluid (CSF) found that approximately 20% of pediatric patients with MS as well as healthy controls had high-affinity, high-titer antibodies. In the pediatric patients with MS, these antibodies were also found in the CSF, and the presence of antibodies was associated with an encephalopathic type of onset.[28] These studies reiterate an emerging theme, which suggests that antimyelin antibodies may not be exclusive to pediatric MS; however, their presence is associated with an encephalopathic onset of disease, which in turn may be a product of a "younger" immune system.

Studies examining markers of axonal damage in the CSF found minimal changes in most children with MS; however, a subgroup with prominent clinical symptoms at the time of CSF examination exhibited elevated levels of tau protein,[29] which may reflect increased CNS damage.

Additional investigations are needed to further understand the immunobiology of pediatric MS to identify appropriate therapeutic targets in this population. In addition, validated biomarkers will greatly help in the diagnosis and prognosis of MS in children.

ENVIRONMENTAL AND GENETIC RISK FACTORS FOR PEDIATRIC MS SUSCEPTIBILITY

Several environmental factors have been shown to play a pivotal role in MS suscepti- bility in adults. In children, very few studies have addressed these issues. Determining the role of viral exposures in the development of adult MS has been difficult because of the lag time between the exposures and disease onset. Studying the role of common viruses in the pediatric MS population provides a unique opportunity, given the close temporal relationship between the infection and MS onset and the fact that exposure to those viruses is lesser in children than in adults. Several studies examining viral exposures in pediatric MS have consistently identified significantly increased frequen- cies of Epstein-Barr virus (EBV) seropositivity in children with MS compared with matched controls.[16,30–32] Although there was no difference between the pediatric MS and control groups in regard to seropositivity to cytomegalovirus (CMV), herpes simplex virus type 1 (HSV-1), varicella-zoster virus, and parvovirus B19, EBV seropos- itivity has been reported to be associated with an almost 3 times increased likelihood of MS.[16] Data from the US Pediatric MS Network confirms the substantial association between EBV and increased pediatric MS susceptibility (odds ratios between 3.14 and 7.60 according to the model). This association is independent of the age at blood draw, sex, race and ethnicity, and HLA-DRB1 status.[33] The novel observations in this study are that a remote infection with CMV decreases the risk to develop MS by more than 70%, and in HLA-DRB1 positive individuals, a remote infection with HSV-1 decreased MS risk by 70%.[33] In contrast, in HLA-DRB1 negative individuals, HSV-1 seropositivity had a 4 times higher risk of MS. The protective role of these remote infections questions the timing of viral encounters and their effect on the immune response, more specifically the response to EBV.

Concern over the use of vaccinations, most recently hepatitis B vaccine, and the subsequent development of MS has been raised. Mikaeloff[34] found that there was no increased risk of developing a first episode of childhood MS up to 3 years postvac- cination in the French population.[34] However, these investigators showed a trend for the Engerix B vaccine to increase the risk in the longer term. This finding needs to be confirmed in the future.

The same group evaluated the risk of childhood-onset MS as related to exposure to passive smoking.[34] The relative risk for a first episode of MS was found to be more than twice that of the control population and was even higher for those with a pro- longed exposure of 10 years or more.

Unlike in adult MS, the effect of vitamin D status on MS susceptibility is unknown, although levels of 25-hydroxyvitamin D_3 have been found to be independently associ- ated with the subsequent relapse rate in pediatric patients with MS (for each 10 ng/mL increment of 25-hydroxyvitamin D_3, risk of subsequent MS relapse was decreased by 34%).[35]

There are few studies evaluating genetic risk factors in pediatric MS. The US Pedi- atric MS Network has also reported that HLA-DRB1, like in adult MS, may be a risk factor for pediatric MS. In multivariate models adjusted for age, race, ethnicity, and remote viral exposures, the risk of having MS if carrying at least 1 HLA-DRB1 allele was increased by 2 to 4, depending on the model used.[33] This is in line with another study of adolescents with MS.[36]

Further studies exploring genetic and environmental risk factors are required to explore the precise mechanisms leading to disease onset. The discovery of gene-environment interactions may also shed new light on the understanding of molecular mechanisms involved in the disease processes and might lead to the development of new therapeutic strategies.

DIFFERENTIAL DIAGNOSIS

In general, atypical features include the presence of fever, encephalopathy, progressive symptoms or disease course, other organ system involvement (including the peripheral nervous system), absence of CSF oligoclonal IgG, and markedly elevated CSF leukocyte counts.[37] The more the number of atypical features present and the younger the child, the more the consideration necessary before making the diagnosis of MS. A summary of the differential diagnosis of pediatric MS is listed in **Table 1**.

A thorough history and physical examination, serum and cerebrospinal fluid testing, and neuroimaging likely provide the diagnostic specificity desired to differentiate between acquired demyelinating disorders of the CNS in children and the other disorders outlined in this section. Approaches to specific presentations are summarized in **Box 1**.

CLINICAL PRESENTATION AND CLINICAL COURSE OF PEDIATRIC MS
Clinical Presentation

Retrospective versus prospective studies demonstrate considerable variability in the frequency of initial MS symptoms, although most differences may be because of symptoms that could not be well recorded (ie, sensory deficits), whereas the reported frequencies of symptoms associated with clear objective changes on examination (ie, motor findings, ataxia) are fairly consistent among studies. A young age of onset may also interfere with data accuracy (ie, anterior visual pathway dysfunction) and, often, additional abnormalities are identified only when sensitive paraclinical measures such as visual evoked potentials (VEPs) and/or optical coherence tomography (OCT) are used.[38,39]

Several studies have shown that encephalopathy may also occur with a first episode of MS or neuromyelitis optica (8%–16%), usually reported in younger patients.[40–43] Thus, rather than being disease specific (ie, MS vs ADEM), the presence of encephalopathy may be related to immaturity of the brain or immune system in young patients. Seizures as a first event, as part of the encephalopathy or isolated, were also reported (29%) in the pediatric population, usually in ADEM cases and less frequently in MS.[41–44]

Polysymptomatic presentation was also reported in children diagnosed with MS at the time of their first event with large variances (10%–67%).[9,10] However, the polysymptomatic presentation is seen more often in the self-limited ADEM entity (72%) than in MS (27%).[44]

Clinical Course

The initial clinical course in the vast majority of patients with pediatric MS is relapsing-remitting, in 85.7% to 100% of cases, rates that are somewhat higher than in adults.[1,7,10] Although 62% of patients with relapsing-remitting (RRMS) have been reported to recover completely after relapses,[45] disability can occur as the result of an incomplete recovery from relapses. In some cases, patients later develop a more insidious progression of disability with or without superimposed exacerbations. This phase of the disease is called secondary progressive.

Table 1
Differential diagnosis of pediatric MS by disease subtype

Disease		Presentation	Diagnostic Clues/Evaluation
Systemic Immunologic/ Inflammatory	SLE	Multisystemic autoimmune disorder most commonly affecting the skin, joints, and kidneys Neuropsychiatric symptoms include cerebrovascular events, psychosis, chorea, and encephalopathy[115]	Elevated CSF lymphocyte counts and laboratory studies indicating renal involvement or autoimmune antibodies
	Sarcoidosis	Extremely variable presentation, including seizures in prepubertal children and cranial neuropathies in older children Hypothalamic symptoms such as diabetes insipidus, headaches, motor complaints, and papilledema may be observed[116]	Positive CSF-ACE (when present) and periventricular white matter lesions, cranial nerve involvement or meningeal enhancement noted on brain MRI scans should lead to consideration of tissue biopsy confirmation
	Behçet syndrome	Form of vasculitis that classically produces oral and genital ulcers and uveitis	Pathergy: nodular reaction at needle site
	Sjögren syndrome	Should be suspected when sicca symptoms (including dry eyes, dry mouth) are prominent Sjögren syndrome can affect both the brain and spinal cord	Schirmer test/slit-lamp test for xerophthalmia Nuclear scan of salivary gland or salivary gland biopsy for xerostomia
	Hashimoto encephalitis	May been seen in association with Hashimoto thyroiditis and should be considered when children present with encephalopathy associated with a history of thyroid disorder and elevated levels of intrathecal antithyroid antibodies	Elevated levels of intrathecal antithyroid antibodies
	Langerhans cell histiocytosis	Disorder due to excessive macrophages, which attack multiple organs including the nervous system[117] Onset is usually in childhood, and organ involvement can include skin, bone, muscles, liver, lung, spleen, and bone marrow	CNS lesions most commonly occur in the hypothalamic pituitary region Cerebellar syndrome associated with bilateral symmetric lesions in the dentate nucleus and/or basal ganglia may also be seen[118]

Infections and Neoplasms		
Tuberculosis	Systemic signs of illness, including fever and weight loss, are usually present Basilar meningeal enhancement would suggest TB infection	CSF demonstrates a mild to moderately increased cell count and protein level TB skin testing may not be reliable if the patient lives in an endemic region for TB or has been immunized against BCG or if the child is immunocompromised, which may lead to a false-negative result[119]
HIV	The incidence of CNS involvement with HIV is highest in the first 2 years of life, and can occur before any other signs of immunosuppression and is frequently the first AIDS-defining illness in children[120]	In more advanced disease, CNS imaging shows cortical atrophy and basal ganglia calcifications on CT scans and white matter lesions and central atrophy on MRI of the brain
HTLV	The virus causes a chronic retroviral infection with increased incidence in endemic areas. Infection begins as a chronic relapsing infective dermatitis involving the scalp and usually progresses to an inflammatory myelopathy	CSF demonstrates elevated HTLV antibody titers; the MRI of the spine is usually normal[121]
PML	PML is a progressive neurologic disorder with multifocal lesions caused by primary infection or reactivation of the JC virus, usually in immunocompromised patients	MRI lesions tend to be subcortical and patchy and then spread deeper and become confluent[122]
Herpes virus	Viral encephalitis and cerebral thrombosis can both be initiated by infections with viruses from the herpes family	MRI scan demonstrates involvement of medial temporal, inferior frontal, insular, and cingulate gyrus regions Presence of diffusion abnormalities or hemorrhage suggests herpes
Neuroborreliosis, Lyme disease	Cranial and peripheral nerve involvement is more frequent than CNS involvement[123]	CSF findings include elevated CSF white cell count and protein level, as well as CSF oligoclonal bands[124] MRI abnormalities consist of variable numbers of small, nonenhancing T1-hypointense and T2-hyperintense lesions without mass effect[125]

(continued on next page)

Table 1
(continued)

Disease		Presentation	Diagnostic Clues/Evaluation
	Mycoplasma	Common cause of encephalopathy and transverse myelitis in children. Mycoplasma-associated ADEM rarely includes optic neuritis	MRI demonstrates patchy, asymmetric FLAIR and T2 hyperintensities involving gray and white matter[126]
	Whipple disease	Consider in the setting of a GI illness with unexplained neurologic symptoms, such as supranuclear vertical gaze palsy, rhythmic palatal myoclonus and eye movements, dementia with psychiatric symptoms, and/or hypothalamic manifestations[127]	Diagnostic small bowel biopsy
	Primary CNS lymphoma	Rare in children, but multifocal lesions can be confused for MS lesions. CSF cytology has high specificity but low sensitivity[128]	Fine aspirate cytology or open biopsy is required for definitive diagnosis Diagnostic evaluation should be performed before steroid therapy, as lymphomas are steroid-responsive and diagnostic tests performed after steroid administration may be falsely negative[129]
Vascular disorders	CADASIL	Usually presents in middle age with migraine-like vascular episodes and MRI brain abnormalities Asymptomatic children, whose parents have been diagnosed with CADASIL, have been noted to have MRI abnormalities, including small T2-hyperintense lesions in periventricular and subcortical white matter[130]	Genetic testing for mutations in the NOTCH-3 gene
	Moyamoya syndrome	Cerebrovascular condition characterized by decreased blood flow in the major vessels of the anterior brain circulation leading to collateral vasculature development Presenting symptoms are related to either brain ischemia (strokes, TIAs) or consequences of the compensatory mechanisms for ischemia, including hemorrhages or headaches	MRI findings most suggestive of moyamoya include reduced-flow voids in the anterior circulation in association with prominent collateral-flow voids through the basal ganglia and thalamus

	Migraine headaches	Classical migraines are easy to recognize; however, aura sine migraine and/or atypical presentations are less easily diagnosed	MRI can demonstrate one or more small T2 hyperintensities and, as compared with pediatric MS, these occur in far fewer numbers, particularly infrequent in deep or periventricular white matter or in infratentorial, cerebellar, or brainstem locations[131]
	CNS vasculitis	Presents with multifocal neurologic impairments in association with headaches, seizures, behavior changes, and TIA/stroke[37] Difficult to diagnose because of the absence of cutaneous or systemic signs or symptoms	Abnormal results in cerebral arteriography and brain biopsy are frequently required to make this diagnosis
Leukodystrophies	ALD	Half the cases present in childhood with cerebral dysfunction,[132] whereas the other half present as either a cerebellar form or as an adrenomyeloneuropathy, with the latter more common in female carriers who typically present in the 20s to 40s	ALD tends to affect the parieto-occipital white matter symmetrically Diagnosed by finding elevated very long chain fatty acids in plasma
	Krabbe disease	Most children present before 6 mo of age with extreme irritability followed by rigidity and tonic spasms, with PNS involvement, and MRI scan demonstrating symmetric plaquelike areas in the centrum semiovale[133] The juvenile form usually begins between the ages of 4 and 2C y, presenting with a sensorimotor demyelinating polyneuropathy and normal cognition	MRI: parieto-occipital white matter is often symmetrically involved Diagnosis is made by measuring the deficient galactocerebrosidase enzyme
	MLD	The peripheral nervous system can be involved, more commonly in the younger children, whereas those presenting later often present with behavioral or psychiatric changes[134]	Sulfatides can be measured in the urine as a screening test
	PMD	Most patients present early in life with nystagmus, developmental delay, and progressive spastic paraparesis; the PNS may also be involved	MRI shows diffuse T2 signal in the white matter and rarely shows more discrete lesions

(continued on next page)

Table 1
(continued)

Disease		Presentation	Diagnostic Clues/Evaluation
	Childhood ataxia with diffuse CNS hypomyelination (vanishing white matter disease)	Chronic progressive disease with episodic deterioration brought on by injury or intercurrent illness[135] Older patients tend to present with spasticity and ataxia with fairly well-preserved cognitive function	MRI most often shows symmetric involvement of the cerebral hemispheric white matter. In addition, all or part of the white matter has signal intensity close to, or the same as, CSF on proton density scans
	Alexander disease	Symptoms typically begin between 6 and 15 y of age with bulbar dysfunction and a slowly progressive ataxia and spastic diplegia[132]	MRI bilateral frontal regions are usually affected and show cystic changes[136]
Mitochondrial	LHON	Typically affects men and is most often due to a mtDNA mutation affecting complex I of the ETC[137] Patients present with bilateral acute or subacute visual loss and optic atrophy	Genetic testing identifies most affected individuals
	MELAS	Characterized by episodic vomiting, lactic acidosis, myopathy, seizures, strokelike events, and short stature	Genetic testing available
	Kearns-Sayre syndrome	Triad of progressive external ophthalmoplegia, pigmentary retinal degeneration, and cerebellar dysfunction Associated with elevated CSF protein levels or heart block	MRI findings include progressive leukoencephalopathy and basal ganglia or deep white matter calcifications[37]

Abbreviations: ACE, angiotensin converting enzyme; ALD, adrenoleukodystrophy; BCG, bacille Calmette-Guérin; CADASIL, cerebral autosomal dominant arteriopathy with subcortical infarcts and leukoencephalopathy; CT, computed tomographic; ETC, electron transport chain; FLAIR, fluid attenuation inversion recovery; GI, gastrointestinal; HIV, human immunodeficiency virus; HTLV, human T-lymphotropic virus; LHON, Leber hereditary optic neuropathy; MELAS, mitochondrial encephalopathy with lactic acidosis and strokelike episodes; MLD, metachromatic leukodystrophy; mtDNA, mitochondrial DNA; PML, progressive multifocal leukoencephalopathy; PMD, Pelizaeus-Merzbacher disease; PNS, peripheral nervous system; SLE, sytemic lupus erythematosus; TB, tuberculosis; TIA, transient ischemic attack.

Box 1
Approach to the differential diagnosis of pediatric MS

If other organ system involvement is present, including joints, kidney, lung, and skin, consider systemic inflammatory disorder.

If fever, constitutional symptoms, and enhancing lesions (including leptomeningeal enhancement) are present, consider CNS infections or lymphoma.

If focal neurologic symptoms with headache are present, consider vasculitis.

If progressive course with symmetric changes on MRI and possible peripheral nervous system involvement is present, consider leukodystrophies.

If course is progressive and fluctuating, with myopathy, optic neuropathy, and strokes, consider mitochondrial diseases.

Relapses
The annualized relapse rate in pediatric MS with a mean disease duration of 10 years or more has been estimated to be between 0.38 and 0.87 for the whole relapsing-remitting period in the few studies.[10,46,47] A prospective study of patients with MS seen at a large MS center showed that patients with an onset before 18 years had a higher relapse rate during the first few years of their disease than adults seen at the same institution.[48] The quality of recovery after subsequent relapses during the relapsing-remitting phase has been reported to be good, at least in the very early stages (Fay et, submitted for publication). Recovery from relapses seems to be more rapid in children than in adult patients with MS (mean time of relapse-related symptoms: 4.3 weeks in pediatric MS vs 6–8 weeks in adult MS).[49]

Time to irreversible disability
Although the rate of disability progression varies from individual to individual regardless of the age at onset, a consistent finding in most pediatric MS retrospective studies is lower disability scores compared with adult patients with MS while controlling for disease duration. The median time to reach an Expanded Disability Status Scale (EDSS) of 4 (defined as visible, often irreversible neurologic deficit in a patient who is still able to ambulate at least 500 meters without assistance) was approximately 20 years for pediatric MS versus 10 years for adult MS.[50] Similar data were obtained from the large European database for Multiple Sclerosis (EDMUS) that identified 394 patients with pediatric MS (onset at age <16 years) compared with a cohort of 1775 patients with adult MS.[7] The median times from onset to disability scores of 4, 6 (need to use a cane for a 100-m distance), and 7 (ability to walk no more than 10 m) were 20, 29.9, and 37 years, respectively. The time to reach an EDSS of 4 was 10 years longer than for the adult population with MS and even longer for children younger than 12 years (28 years). However, the pediatric patients with MS reached these disability scores at approximately 10 years earlier (ie, ages 34.6, 42.2, and 50.5 years to reach the respective EDSS of 4, 6, and 7).

Despite a slower development of irreversible disability in pediatric patients with MS, the age when these patients are confronted with disease progression and neurologic deficits is 10 years younger than for the population with adult-onset MS, a time when one is expected to have a family and enter the workforce. The effect of the use of disease-modifying therapies (DMTs) for MS on delaying the disease progression in pediatric MS has yet to be studied.

COGNITIVE AND PSYCHOSOCIAL OUTCOMES

The psychosocial complications of pediatric MS encompass a variety of problems, including feelings of self-consciousness, worries related to the future, problems with family and friends, mood disorders, and cognitive impairment. Children experience a variety of academic difficulties secondary to school absences, severe fatigue, and cognitive complications. Qualitative research, which relies on a combination of open-ended questions and guided discussion, has been performed in pediatric MS and has produced important insights into the concerns and feelings of children with MS.[51–54] Interventions to address these problems are very much needed. Herein the available literature covering psychosocial and cognitive issues in pediatric MS is summarized.

Frequency of Psychiatric Problems

As shown in **Table 2**, there is a wide range in the reported frequency of psychological distress and psychiatric disorders among children with MS. The Schedule for Affective Disorders and Schizophrenia for School-Age Children—Present and Lifetime Version, (KSADS)[55] revealed that approximately 30% to 48% of children with MS or related conditions have affective disorders.[52,56] The most common psychiatric conditions are major depression, anxiety disorder, a combination of anxiety and depressive disorders, panic disorder, bipolar disorder, and adjustment disorder.

Fatigue and quality of life

When the scores from the pediatric MS group were compared with those from age-matched healthy controls and the fifth percentile of the healthy controls was used as the cutoff for fatigue, 73% of the pediatric MS group met this criterion for severe fatigue.[52] In another study, 56% of the youngsters evaluated with the PedsQL Multi-dimensional Fatigue Scale[57] had either mild or severe fatigue.[58]

Cognition

Cognitive impairment occurs in an estimated 30% to 75% of children with MS depending on what definition of impairment is applied and at what point in their course the children undergo evaluations.[52,59,60]

More mild impairment, defined as failing only 1 test, was noted in 59% of subjects.[60] Specific deficits included attention (30%), naming (19%), and receptive language (13%) deficits. Other deficits included delayed recall in tests of verbal memory

Table 2
Psychosocial findings in pediatric MS

Psychosocial Findings	Pediatric MS
Frequency of fatigue	14%–73%[52,58,138,139]
Psychiatric complications	0%–48%[63,138,139]
Frequency of cognitive impairment	0%–77%[52,62,138]
Cognitive domains most affected	Working memory Complex attention Processing speed Executive functioning Language and verbal comprehension[52,59,63,140]
Consequences of cognitive impairment	Failed courses, failed grades, change in college plans, need for in-class assistance

(19%) and visual memory (11%).[60] Many of the findings have been subsequently confirmed.[52]

Compared with controls (recruited from the patients' friends and schoolmates)[52] multiple impairments were noted in pediatric patients with MS. About 31% of patients with MS met the criteria for cognitive impairment (failing at least 3 tests of the battery), and 53% failed at least 2 tests. Similar to prior reports, the domains more frequently affected were memory, complex attention, verbal comprehension, and executive functioning. Of the 19 cognitively impaired patients, 28% had an IQ score of less than 90 and 8% had an IQ score of less than 70. Younger age at symptom onset correlated with lower IQ scores,[52] an association previously described in children with MS.[59] Language problems were detected in 20% to 40% of the cases, with verbal comprehension being among the most frequently failed tests. This result differs from the cognitive profile of individuals with adult MS in whom linguistic problems are rarely reported.[61]

Among children with MS, declines in functioning have been demonstrated in as little as 2 years.[52,60] Up to 40% of the patients worsened on cognitive performance,[62,63] with up to 77% meeting the criteria for cognitive impairment at follow-up. Overall, individuals in the pediatric population with MS seem to be more vulnerable to cognitive decline over short periods compared with adults with MS. Although the basis of cognitive impairment in children affected by MS is not fully understood, it can be expected that future studies will find associations with neuroimaging findings. For example, a preliminary study found an association between cognitive impairment and thalamic and corpus callosal volume.[64] This finding is consistent with that in adults with MS, in which thalamic atrophy and changes in the corpus callosum were closely associated with cognitive impairment.[65-67]

Academic consequences

Cognitive deficits are often associated with a variety of academic difficulties. These include failed courses, failed grades, and, on occasion, the need for in-class assistance. Although it is likely that poor cognitive performance underlies many of these difficulties, other contributing factors include multiple missed school days associated with relapses or treatment, severe fatigue, mood disorders, or other disabling symptoms. Up to 35.1% of the pediatric patients with MS require some type of help or altered school curriculum because of cognitive impairments, and up to 14% are homeschooled because of their illness. Interventions to assist in academic functioning include recognition of the problem and communication of the effects of MS to the teachers and school personnel. Additional time for testing, arranging seating in the front of the class, additional time to get from one class to another can improve day-to-day functioning in school. Some children may also need tutoring and in-class assistance, with implementation of 504 or individualized education plans.

Interventions to improve psychosocial functioning

Based on our experience with a Teen Adventure Program for adolescents with MS, it is clear that programs that can bring teens together to share common experiences and create a support network can be extremely helpful. Programs can take the form of camps, workshops, and webinars and can help children feel less "different," realize they are not alone, and provide tools for better communication with health care professionals. Such steps lead to a greater sense of empowerment. A goal of these programs is to provide a forum for education and means for children to learn from one another. More opportunities need to be developed using the Internet and other forms of social media to link those affected by pediatric MS. Educational materials on pediatric MS for affected individuals and families, created by the National Multiple Sclerosis Society or individual Pediatric MS Centers, are another extremely important tool that facilitate a positive adaptation to the diagnosis.

DIAGNOSTIC TESTING
CSF Analysis

The CSF profile in childhood-onset MS may vary by age. Typically, white blood cell counts range from 0 to 50 cells/μL, with a lymphocytic predominance.[68] However, it has been shown that, children younger than 11 years have more neutrophils in the CSF than older children.[69]

Although 1 study reports oligoclonal bands (OCB) to be present in the CSF of up to 92% of children with MS,[58] another study found OCB to be less frequent in younger children (43% vs 63% in adolescents).[69] By contrast, in ADEM, 0% to 29% of cases were found to have OCB.[40,41,68,70] Within the French KIDMUS cohort, 94% of children with positive OCB (69 of 72) went on to develop MS.[71]

The IgG index has been found to be elevated in 68% of adolescents with MS (>11 years) but in 35% of younger children (<11 years).[69] These features tend to be dependent on age rather than on disease duration. These distinct CSF IgG and cellular profiles in younger children tend to vanish on repeat CSF analysis (mean 19 months after initial analysis), suggesting a transient immunologic phenomenon associated with disease onset.

Visual Testing

The limited ability of standard Snellen charts to distinguish subtle visual dysfunction is well documented in the adult population with MS.[72] Low-contrast letter acuity (LCLA) charts (Sloan charts) have been shown to provide a sensitive and reliable assessment of visual acuity in the pediatric population with MS.

Other tests such as pattern reversal VEPs have been shown to be of diagnostic utility in childhood MS, with almost half of such patients showing increased visual latency, which revealed a second focus of demyelination before a second clinical attack.[68]

OCT, originally used for patients with glaucoma, has been applied to pediatric patients with MS. This procedure uses near infrared light to quantify the thickness of the retinal nerve fiber layer (RNFL) (which contains only nonmyelinated axons). It has been shown to provide a sensitive evaluation of the RNFL thickness in this population, a correlate of optic atrophy.[39] Taken together, VEP, OCT, and LCLA testing can provide objective evidence of previous inflammatory insult to the optic nerve in the pediatric population with MS. These procedures may help to establish a diagnosis of MS and may also be used for disease monitoring on follow-up.

MRI

In a small study, patients with pediatric MS were reported to have fewer brain MRI T2-bright foci and more frequent large MS lesions than reported in adults with MS.[43] However, more recent data collected at disease onset have shown that children with MS may have a higher lesion burden on their initial brain MRI scan than adults, especially in the brainstem and cerebellum. This finding is of concern, as both higher lesion burden and brainstem and cerebellar involvement have been reported to be associated with poorer outcomes in adults. Furthermore, recent evidence points to more inflammatory disease in pediatric patients with MS than in adults with MS. T2 lesion load is higher early in childhood-onset patients.[39]

Brain lesions in younger children (age <11 years) are large, with poorly defined borders and are frequently confluent at disease onset. Such T2-bright foci in younger children may vanish on repeat scans, unlike that seen in teenagers or adults, suggesting that disease processes in the developing brain, including immune response, may be different from those in older patients.[43]

Several studies have evaluated the utility of MRI in the diagnosis of pediatric MS.[73–75] Each of these has been found to have high specificity but relatively low sensitivity.[76] MRI criteria for pediatric MS need to be developed but will need to take into account age-related differences for younger children compared with adolescents.

DMTs IN PEDIATRIC MS

Seven DMTs have been approved for the treatment of RRMS in the adult population, including 4 first-line (glatiramer acetate [GA], intramuscular [IM] and subcutaneous [SC] interferon beta-1a, and SC interferon beta-1b), and 2 second-line (mitoxantrone and natalizumab) therapies. In addition, therapies such as rituximab, daclizumab, and cyclophosphamide (CTX) have been evaluated in phase 2 trials in adults with breakthrough disease, as have add-on therapies such as monthly steroids and intravenous immunoglobulin. Oral therapies, including cladribine[77] and fingolimod,[78] have also been evaluated in the adult population.[77,79–82] The following sections review the currently available evidence for the use of these agents in children with MS.

Interferon Beta

Several retrospective case series have described the use of interferon beta-1a in the pediatric population. Follow-up in these series has ranged from 12 to 48 months. Interferon beta-1a and 1b appear to be safe and well tolerated in this population, although discontinuation rates are in the range of 30% to 50%.[51,83–86] Many children administered interferon (35%–65%) report flulike symptoms. Other relatively frequently observed side effects include leukopenia (8%–27%), thrombocytopenia (16%), anemia (12%) and a transient elevation in the levels of transaminases (10%–62%).

Abnormal results in liver function tests (LFTs) may be more pronounced in younger children taking interferon.[87] Children with elevated results in LFTs were predominantly younger than 10 years.[84,87] Temporary interruption of interferon treatment seems to lead to normalization of LFTs in children and is most often accompanied by safe reintroduction of therapy after a temporary withdrawal of medication.[84,87]

More than two-thirds of the children taking the SC formulation of interferon beta-1a have reported injection-site reactions. About 6% of children on interferon beta-1a SC experienced abscess and 6% injection-site necrosis over an average follow-up of 1.8 years.[87] Of those administered interferon beta-1b, only 20% older than 10 years and 25% younger than 10 years experienced mild injection-site reactions (average follow-up of 33.8 months) that did not lead to discontinuation of therapy.[84]

Dosing of interferon-beta is not established in the pediatric population. However, most patients tolerate doses titrated following adult protocols or a gradual titration to 30 µg once weekly for interferon beta-1a IM and 22 µg or 44 µg thrice weekly for interferon beta-1a SC. Children older than 10 years tolerate full doses of interferon beta-1b, although decreased tolerance may exist in the younger population.[85]

With respect to efficacy, there have been no randomized controlled trials evaluating the efficacy of interferon beta in the pediatric population. However, in a prospective, open-label study, Ghezzi and colleagues[88] followed up 52 patients with pediatric MS who were treated with interferon beta-1a IM and found a reduction in the annualized relapse rate.[89,90] No controlled data are available on whether interferon beta slows down progression of disability in children. Furthermore, no data on the MRI effect of these medications in children are available.

Glatiramer Acetate

Only 3 retrospective studies have been published evaluating the use of GA in pediatrics.[89,91,92] The medication seems to be well tolerated, except for the typical injection-site reactions and rare and transient chest pain.[89,92] The mean annualized relapse rate decreased during treatment.[92] However, conclusions from these studies regarding the efficacy of this medication cannot be drawn, given the small numbers.

Immunomodulatory and Cytotoxic Therapies

A small number of children continue to have MS relapses despite treatment with the first-line DMT described earlier. Consensus criteria for the definition of breakthrough disease in pediatric MS do not exist. In general, practitioners allow at least 6 months of observation on a given treatment before deeming the treatment suboptimal. Although widely debated, some define suboptimal response to therapy as the presence of greater than 1 relapse in 1 year (clinical or MRI) or evidence of progressive disability.

Immunomodulatory and cytotoxic agents that are used in adult MS in the event of suboptimal response to interferon beta and/or GA have been used in a small number of pediatric patients, as discussed later. There are no reports on the use of oral agents in pediatric MS, including cladribine and fingolimod.

Natalizumab

The medication seems to be well tolerated by pediatric patients with MS who have failed first-line therapies. Patients experience fewer clinical relapses, and MRI scans show no enhancing lesions (Yeh E and colleagues, unpublished data, 2009).[93,94] There have been no reports to date of progressive multifocal leukoencephalopathy in association with this young population treated with natalizumab.

Mitoxantrone

There have been no published reports of mitoxantrone use in the pediatric population except for a few cases followed at the US Pediatric MS Centers of Excellence.[95] Caution should be exercised with its use, given the reported significant side effects of leukemia and cardiomyopathy.

Rituximab

In the pediatric population with MS, only 1 case report of rituximab has been published.[96]

Cyclophosphamide

One case series describing a cohort of children with highly inflammatory and aggressive RRMS despite first-line therapy in whom CTX was initiated has been published.[97] Treatment resulted in a reduction or stabilization of the relapse rate and EDSS in most patients. Half of the children who received CTX in this study later required a combination therapy or treatment with another second-line agent. Only one-third of the children were able to go back to a first-line therapy. With regard to tolerability, almost all the children who received CTX experienced side effects, some of which were serious, including infertility, osteoporosis, and transitional cell carcinoma of the bladder. This therapy should therefore be used with caution in this population.

In summary, interferon beta and GA seem to be well tolerated in children. However, appropriate monitoring for potential side effects is required. There are emerging, but still limited, data on the use of second-line agents in pediatric MS. These therapies may need to be considered in the case of refractory disease, taking into account the risk of the adverse effects versus benefit profile for individual agents.

SYMPTOMATIC TREATMENTS IN PEDIATRIC MS

Optimizing quality of life and function can be aided by the treatment of persistent symptoms. Rehabilitative techniques, adaptive equipment, and medications can all contribute. Spasticity, fatigue, tremor, paroxysmal symptoms, cognitive impairment, and bowel and bladder dysfunction can be improved with symptomatic treatment. Very few clinical studies have been performed in children with MS; therefore, the treatments discussed here are empirically derived and, in general, not approved by the US Food and Drug Administration.

Spasticity can be moderated with stretching and range of motion exercises. Greater degrees of spasticity benefit from oral agents, including baclofen, tizanidine, or benzodiazepines; however, dosing may need to be balanced with side effects, including sedation.[98] Botulinum toxin injections have been useful for decreasing spasticity; however, the short duration of benefit (usually 3–6 months), relatively high cost, and possible development of neutralizing antibodies with repeated administration have limited use.[99] Medically intractable spasticity occurs infrequently in children with MS; however, use of intrathecal baclofen has been tried, as it has been effective in adults with MS and children with cerebral palsy.[100]

Fatigue is a frequent symptom in children with MS and is noted more frequently than can be easily explained by depression, exhaustion from physical disability or heat exposure, sleep disturbance, or poor bowel/bladder control. Ameliorating these potential underlying causes of fatigue is a critical first step. Medications that have been anecdotally used to address fatigue in children with MS include amantadine,[101] modafinil,[102,103] and methylphenidate. Acetylsalicylic acid is under study in adults with MS-related fatigue[104] but has not been formally tried in children with MS likely because of the concern about Reye syndrome–type complications. Potassium channel blockers (4 aminopyridine and 3,4 diaminopyridine) have led to improvements in strength and ambulation in adults with MS[105–108] but have not been trialed in children.

Tremor or ataxia caused by cerebellar involvement in MS is difficult to treat. Rehabilitative therapies, adaptive equipment, and even deep brain stimulation have been used to control functional impairment from tremors in adult patients with MS.[109,110]

Bladder dysfunction can be treated with medications to treat or suppress infection and decrease detrusor hyperreflexia. A recent study demonstrated that tolterodine was somewhat better tolerated than oxybutynin by children for treatment of detrusor instability.[111] Intermittent bladder catheterization for urinary retention and desmopressin acetate nasal spray at bedtime for sleep-depriving nocturia unresponsive to fluid management are beneficial to some children. Constipation occurs frequently, particularly in children with MS-related decreases in mobility. Management includes manipulating the diet, increasing fluid intake, maximizing activity levels, and adding stool softeners and additional fiber/bulk to diet.

Symptomatic therapies are likely underutilized in children with MS. Consideration should be given toward their use empirically and toward controlled clinical trials to clarify risks and benefits.

SUMMARY AND FUTURE DIRECTIONS

There are many remaining challenges to improve the care of children with MS. These include an enhanced understanding of the pathophysiology of the disease through immunologic, genetic, and neuroimaging studies, which will identify relevant therapeutic targets. Moreover, because childhood-onset MS may be closer to the inciting events of MS than adult-onset MS, studies in children may provide otherwise untenable insights into the immunopathogenesis of the disease. Biomarkers that facilitate diagnosis and indicate prognosis in cases of a first demyelinating event or that delineate a more aggressive disease course will allow clinicians to tailor and optimize management and potentially reduce long-term disability.

Studies of the clinical disease course and MRI studies have consistently suggested that pediatric MS is a more inflammatory disease than adult MS, with increased relapses and inflammatory lesions on MRI. However, locomotor disability seems to progress slower in children than in adults. Despite this, cognitive disability is apparent in the early stages of disease, and neuropsychological evaluation should be a part of the clinical care plan of all patients. Further strategies to address cognitive disability and depression in children with MS are of utmost importance.

The most challenging area in pediatric MS is the identification and evaluation of safe and therapeutic strategies that target relevant disease processes. At present, there are no regulatory agency–approved therapeutics for pediatric MS in North America or Europe. Strategies to systematically evaluate the place of individual therapies in the armamentarium of the treating physician are needed. Antiinflammatory agents target an important disease process; however, additional strategies are required to prevent progressive disability and enhance repair of the damaged nervous system in pediatric MS. Targeting the cells of the nervous system that are paramount in the demyelinating process, including oligodendrocytes that make myelin and neurons and axons that conduct physiologic responses, may be a unique strategy to reversing acquired disability in MS.[112] Animal studies have shown that there is a greater capacity for repair in younger animals than in older ones.[113,114] Therefore, the young brain should have a greater potential to respond to approaches to salvage oligodendrocytes or neurons. In addition, the young brain may show a greater response to neuronal plasticity that may in the long run turn out to be an essential component of repair.

Future studies in pediatric demyelinating disorders include those investigating the cause of early-onset disease, including studies in genetics and environmental risk factors, particularly in those at high risk, such as children with CIS or ADEM. In addition, there is a need for studies that evaluate the long-term safety and efficacy of existing and new therapeutic agents to modify disease.

REFERENCES

1. Duquette P, Murray TJ, Pleines J, et al. Multiple sclerosis in childhood: clinical profile in 125 patients. J Pediatr 1987;111(3):359–63.
2. Poser CM, Paty DW, Scheinberg L, et al. New diagnostic criteria for multiple sclerosis: guidelines for research protocols. Ann Neurol 1983;13(3):227–31.
3. McDonald WI, Compston A, Edan G, et al. Recommended diagnostic criteria for multiple sclerosis: guidelines from the International Panel on the Diagnosis of Multiple Sclerosis. Ann Neurol 2001;50(1):121–7.
4. Polman CH, Reingold SC, Edan G, et al. Diagnostic criteria for multiple sclerosis: 2005 revisions to the "McDonald Criteria". Ann Neurol 2005;58(6): 840–6.

5. Waubant E, Chabas D. Pediatric multiple sclerosis. Curr Treat Options Neurol 2009;11(3):203–10.
6. Krupp LB, Banwell B, Tenembaum S. International Pediatric MS Study Group. Consensus definitions proposed for pediatric multiple sclerosis and related disorders. Neurology 2007;68(16 Suppl 2):S7–12.
7. Renoux C, Vukusic S, Mikaeloff Y, et al. Natural history of multiple sclerosis with childhood onset. N Engl J Med 2007;356(25):2603–13.
8. Chitnis T, Glanz B, Jaffin S, et al. Demographics of pediatric-onset multiple sclerosis in an MS center population from the Northeastern United States. Mult Scler 2009;15(5):627–31.
9. Ghezzi A, Deplano V, Faroni J, et al. Multiple sclerosis in childhood: clinical features of 149 cases. Mult Scler 1997;3(1):43–6.
10. Boiko A, Vorobeychik G, Paty D, et al. Early onset multiple sclerosis: a longitudinal study. Neurology 2002;59(7):1006–10.
11. Ferreira ML, Machado MI, Dantas MJ, et al. Pediatric multiple sclerosis: analysis of clinical and epidemiological aspects according to National MS Society Consensus 2007. Arq Neuropsiquiatr 2008;66(3B):665–70.
12. Fromont A, Binquet C, Sauleau EA, et al. Geographic variations of multiple sclerosis in France. Brain 2010;133(Pt 7):1889–99.
13. Klein NP, Ray P, Carpenter D, et al. Rates of autoimmune diseases in Kaiser Permanente for use in vaccine adverse event safety studies. Vaccine 2010;28(4):1062–8.
14. Chong HT, Li P, Benjamin ONG, et al. Pediatric multiple sclerosis is similar to adult-onset form in Asia. Neurology Asia 2007;12:37–40.
15. Chitnis T. Pediatric multiple sclerosis. Neurologist 2006;12(6):299–310.
16. Banwell B, Krupp L, Kennedy J, et al. Clinical features and viral serologies in children with multiple sclerosis: a multinational observational study. Lancet Neurol 2007;6(9):773–81.
17. Kennedy J, O'Connor P, Sadovnick AD, et al. Age at onset of multiple sclerosis may be influenced by place of residence during childhood rather than ancestry. Neuroepidemiology 2006;26(3):162–7.
18. McAdam LC, Blaser SI, Banwell BL. Pediatric tumefactive demyelination: case series and review of the literature. Pediatr Neurol 2002;26(1):18–25.
19. Anderson RC, Connolly ES Jr, Komotar RJ, et al. Clinicopathological review: tumefactive demyelination in a 12-year-old girl. Neurosurgery 2005;56(5):1051–7 [discussion: 1051–7].
20. Riva D, Chiapparini L, Pollo B, et al. A case of pediatric tumefactive demyelinating lesion misdiagnosed and treated as glioblastoma. J Child Neurol 2008;23(8):944–7.
21. Dastgir J, DiMario FJ Jr. Acute tumefactive demyelinating lesions in a pediatric patient with known diagnosis of multiple sclerosis: review of the literature and treatment proposal. J Child Neurol 2009;24(4):431–7.
22. Vanlandingham M, Hanigan W, Vedanarayanan V, et al. An uncommon illness with a rare presentation: neurosurgical management of ADEM with tumefactive demyelination in children. Childs Nerv Syst 2010;26:655–61.
23. Lucchinetti C, Bruck W, Parisi J, et al. Heterogeneity of multiple sclerosis lesions: implications for the pathogenesis of demyelination. Ann Neurol 2000;47(6):707–17.
24. Chitnis T. The role of CD4 T cells in the pathogenesis of multiple sclerosis. Int Rev Neurobiol 2007;79:43–72.

25. Banwell B, Bar-Or A, Cheung R, et al. Abnormal T-cell reactivities in childhood inflammatory demyelinating disease and type 1 diabetes. Ann Neurol 2008; 63(1):98–111.

26. O'Connor KC, McLaughlin KA, De Jager PL, et al. Self-antigen tetramers discriminate between myelin autoantibodies to native or denatured protein. Nat Med 2007;13(2):211–7.

27. McLaughlin KA, Chitnis T, Newcombe J, et al. Age-dependent B cell autoimmunity to a myelin surface antigen in pediatric multiple sclerosis. J Immunol 2009; 183(6):4067–76.

28. O'Connor KC, Lopez-Amaya C, Gagne D, et al. Anti-myelin antibodies modulate clinical expression of childhood multiple sclerosis. J Neuroimmunol 2010; 223(1/2):92–9.

29. Rostasy K, Withut E, Pohl D, et al. Tau, phospho-tau, and S-100B in the cerebrospinal fluid of children with multiple sclerosis. J Child Neurol 2005;20(10):822–5.

30. Alotaibi S, Kennedy J, Tellier R, et al. Epstein-Barr virus in pediatric multiple sclerosis. JAMA 2004;291(15):1875–9.

31. Pohl D, Krone B, Rostasy K, et al. High seroprevalence of Epstein-Barr virus in children with multiple sclerosis. Neurology 2006;67(11):2063–5.

32. Lunemann JD, Huppke P, Roberts S, et al. Broadened and elevated humoral immune response to EBNA1 in pediatric multiple sclerosis. Neurology 2008; 71(13):1033–5.

33. Waubant EM, Mowry EM, Krupp LB, et al. Infections with CMV and, in those HLA-DRB1*15 positive, HSV-1, are associated with a lower risk of MS. Neurology, in press.

34. Mikaeloff Y, Caridade G, Tardieu M, et al. Parental smoking at home and the risk of childhood-onset multiple sclerosis in children. Brain 2007;130(Pt 10):2589–95.

35. Mowry EM, Krupp LB, Milazzo M, et al. Vitamin D status is associated with relapse rate in pediatric-onset multiple sclerosis. Ann Neurol 2010;67(5): 618–24.

36. Boiko AN, Gusev EI, Alekseenkov AD, et al. Association and linkage of juvenile MS with HLA-DR2(15) in Russians. Neurology 2002;58(4):658–60.

37. Hahn JS, Pohl D, Rensel M, et al. Differential diagnosis and evaluation in pediatric multiple sclerosis. Neurology 2007;68(16 Suppl 2):S13–22.

38. Pohl D, Rostasy K, Treiber-Held S, et al. Pediatric multiple sclerosis: detection of clinically silent lesions by multimodal evoked potentials. J Pediatr 2006;149(1): 125–7.

39. Yeh EA, Weinstock-Guttman B, Ramanathan M, et al. Magnetic resonance imaging characteristics of children and adults with paediatric-onset multiple sclerosis. Brain 2009;132:3392–400.

40. Dale RC, de Sousa C, Chong WK, et al. Acute disseminated encephalomyelitis, multiphasic disseminated encephalomyelitis and multiple sclerosis in children. Brain 2000;123(Pt 12):2407–22.

41. Tenembaum S, Chamoles N, Fejerman N. Acute disseminated encephalomyelitis: a long-term follow-up study of 84 pediatric patients. Neurology 2002; 59(8):1224–31.

42. Banwell B, Ghezzi A, Bar-Or A, et al. Multiple sclerosis in children: clinical diagnosis, therapeutic strategies, and future directions. Lancet Neurol 2007;6(10): 887–902.

43. Chabas D, Castillo-Trivino T, Mowry EM, et al. Vanishing MS T2-bright lesions before puberty: a distinct MRI phenotype? Neurology 2008;71(14):1090–3.

44. Atzori M, Battistella PA, Perini P, et al. Clinical and diagnostic aspects of multiple sclerosis and acute monophasic encephalomyelitis in pediatric patients: a single centre prospective study. Mult Scler 2009;15(3):363–70.
45. Stark W, Huppke P, Gärtner J. Paediatric multiple sclerosis: the experience of the German Centre for Multiple Sclerosis in Childhood and Adolescence. J Neurol 2008;255(Suppl 6):119–22.
46. Sindern E, Haas J, Stark E, et al. Early onset MS under the age of 16: clinical and paraclinical features. Acta Neurol Scand 1992;86(3):280–4.
47. Ghezzi A, Pozzilli C, Liguori M, et al. Prospective study of multiple sclerosis with early onset. Mult Scler 2002;8(2):115–8.
48. Gorman MP, Healy BC, Polgar-Turcsanyi M, et al. Increased relapse rate in pediatric-onset compared with adult-onset multiple sclerosis. Arch Neurol 2009;66(1):54–9.
49. Ruggieri M, Iannetti P, Polizzi A, et al. Multiple sclerosis in children under 10 years of age. Neurol Sci 2004;25(Suppl 4):S326–35.
50. Simone IL, Carrara D, Tortorella C, et al. Course and prognosis in early-onset MS: comparison with adult-onset forms. Neurology 2002;59(12):1922–8.
51. Boyd JR, MacMillan LJ. Multiple sclerosis in childhood: understanding and caring for children with an "adult" disease. Axone 2000;22(2):15–21.
52. Amato MP, Goretti B, Ghezzi A, et al. Cognitive and psychosocial features of childhood and juvenile MS. Neurology 2008;70(20):1891–7.
53. Thannhauser JE. Grief–peer dynamics: understanding experiences with pediatric multiple sclerosis. Qual Health Res 2009;19(6):766–77.
54. Thannhauser JE, Mah JK, Metz LM. Adherence of adolescents to multiple sclerosis disease-modifying therapy. Pediatr Neurol 2009;41(2):119–23.
55. Kaufman J, Birmaher B, Brent D, et al. Schedule for Affective Disorders and Schizophrenia for Schoo-Age Children-Present and Lifetime Version (K-SADS-PL): initial reliability and validity data. J Am Acad Child Adolesc Psychiatry 1997;36(7):980–8.
56. Weisbrot DM, Ettinger AB, Gadow KD, et al. Psychiatric comorbidity in pediatric patients with demyelinating disorders. J Child Neurol 2010;25(2):192–202.
57. Varni JW, Burwinkle TM, Szer IS. The PedsQL Multidimensional Fatigue Scale in pediatric rheumatology: reliability and validity. J Rheumatol 2004;31(12): 2494–500.
58. MacAllister WS, Christodoulou C, Troxell R, et al. Fatigue and quality of life in pediatric multiple sclerosis. Mult Scler 2009;15(12):1502–8.
59. Banwell BL, Anderson PE. The cognitive burden of multiple sclerosis in children. Neurology 2005;64(5):891–4.
60. MacAllister WS, Belman AL, Milazzo M, et al. Cognitive functioning in children and adolescents with multiple sclerosis. Neurology 2005;64(8):1422–5.
61. Bobholz JA, Rao SM. Cognitive dysfunction in multiple sclerosis: a review of recent developments. Curr Opin Neurol 2003;16(3):283–8.
62. MacAllister WS, Christodoulou C, Milazzo M, et al. Longitudinal neuropsychological assessment in pediatric multiple sclerosis. Dev Neuropsychol 2007; 32(2):625–44.
63. Amato M, Goretti B, Ghezzi A, et al. Cognitive and psychosocial features of childhood and juvenile multiple sclerosis: a reappraisal after 2 years. Neurology 2010;75(13):1134–40.
64. Till C, Broche B, Ghassemi R, et al. Corpus callosum area and thalamic volume as predictors of cognitive impairment in children and adolescents with MS. Neurology 2010;74(Suppl 2):A507.

65. Benedict RH, Ramasamy D, Munschauer F, et al. Memory impairment in multiple sclerosis: correlation with deep grey matter and mesial temporal atrophy. J Neurol Neurosurg Psychiatry 2009;80(2):201–6.
66. Edwards SG, Liu C, Blumhardt LD. Cognitive correlates of supratentorial atrophy on MRI in multiple sclerosis. Acta Neurol Scand 2001;104(4):214–23.
67. Ozturk A, Smith SA, Gordon-Lipkin EM, et al. MRI of the corpus callosum in multiple sclerosis: association with disability. Mult Scler 2010;16(2):166–77.
68. Pohl D, Rostasy K, Reiber H, et al. CSF characteristics in early-onset multiple sclerosis. Neurology 2004;63(10):1966–7.
69. Chabas D, Castillo–Trivino T, Mowry EM, et al. Vanishing MS T2—bright lesions before puberty: a distinct MRI phenotype? Neurology 2008;71(14):1090–3.
70. Hynson JL, Kornberg AJ, Coleman LT, et al. Clinical and neuroradiologic features of acute disseminated encephalomyelitis in children. Neurology 2001; 56(10):1308–12.
71. Mikaeloff Y, Suissa S, Vallée L, et al. First episode of acute CNS inflammatory demyelination in childhood: prognostic factors for multiple sclerosis and disability. J Pediatr 2004;144(2):246–52.
72. Frohman E, Costello F, Zivadinov R, et al. Optical coherence tomography in multiple sclerosis. Lancet Neurol 2006;5(10):853–63.
73. Mikaeloff Y, Adamsbaum C, Husson B, et al. MRI prognostic factors for relapse after acute CNS inflammatory demyelination in childhood. Brain 2004;127(Pt 9): 1942–7.
74. Callen DJ, Shroff MM, Branson HM, et al. Role of MRI in the differentiation of ADEM from MS in children. Neurology 2009;72(11):968–73.
75. Neuteboom RF, Boon M, Catsman Berrevoets CE, et al. Prognostic factors after a first attack of inflammatory CNS demyelination in children. Neurology 2008; 71(13):967–73.
76. Chitnis T, Pirko I. Sensitivity vs specificity: progress and pitfalls in defining MRI criteria for pediatric MS. Neurology 2009;72(11):952–3.
77. Giovannoni G, Comi G, Cook S, et al. A placebo-controlled trial of oral cladribine for relapsing multiple sclerosis. N Engl J Med 2010;362(5):416–26.
78. Comi G, O'Connor P, Montalban X, et al. Phase II study of oral fingolimod (FTY720) in multiple sclerosis: 3-year results. Mult Scler 2010;16(2):197–207.
79. Pliskin NH, Hamer DP, Goldstein DS, et al. Improved delayed visual reproduction test performance in multiple sclerosis patients receiving interferon beta-1b. Neurology 1996;47(6):1463–8.
80. Weinstein A, Schwid SR, Schiffer RB, et al. Neuropsychologic status in multiple sclerosis after treatment with glatiramer. Arch Neurol 1999;56(3):319–24.
81. Cohen JA, Barkhof F, Comi G, et al. Oral fingolimod or intramuscular interferon for relapsing multiple sclerosis. N Engl J Med 2010;362(5):402–15.
82. Kappos L, Radue E-M, O'Connor P, et al. A placebo-controlled trial of oral fingolimod in relapsing multiple sclerosis. N Engl J Med 2010;362(5):387–401.
83. Mikaeloff Y, Moreau T, Debouverie M, et al. Interferon-beta treatment in patients with childhood-onset multiple sclerosis. J Pediatr 2001;139(3):443–6.
84. Banwell B, Reder AT, Krupp L, et al. Safety and tolerability of interferon beta-1b in pediatric multiple sclerosis. Neurology 2006;66(4):472–6.
85. Bykova OV, Kuzenkova LM, Maslova OI. [The use of beta-interferon-1b in children and adolescents with multiple sclerosis]. Zh Nevrol Psikhiatr Im S S Korsakova 2006;106(9):29–33 [in Russian].
86. Tenembaum SN, Segura MJ. Interferon beta-1a treatment in childhood and juvenile-onset multiple sclerosis. Neurology 2006;67(3):511–3.

87. Pohl D, Rostasy K, Gärtner J, et al. Treatment of early onset multiple sclerosis with subcutaneous interferon beta-1a. Neurology 2005;64(5):888–90.

88. Ghezzi A, Amato MP, Capobianco M, et al. Treatment of early-onset multiple sclerosis with intramuscular interferonbeta-1a: long-term results. Neurol Sci 2007;28(3):127–32.

89. Ghezzi A. Immunomodulatory treatment of early onset multiple sclerosis: results of an Italian Co-operative Study. Neurol Sci 2005;26(Suppl 4):S183–6.

90. Mikaeloff Y, Caridade G, Tardieu M, et al. Effectiveness of early beta interferon on the first attack after confirmed multiple sclerosis: a comparative cohort study. Eur J Paediatr Neurol 2008;12(3):205–9.

91. Kornek B, Bernert G, Balassy C, et al. Glatiramer acetate treatment in patients with childhood and juvenile onset multiple sclerosis. Neuropediatrics 2003; 34(3):120–6.

92. Ghezzi A, Amato MP, Capobianco M, et al. Disease-modifying drugs in childhood-juvenile multiple sclerosis: results of an Italian Co-operative Study. Mult Scler 2005;11(4):420–4.

93. Huppke P, Stark W, Zürcher C, et al. Natalizumab use in pediatric multiple sclerosis. Arch Neurol 2008;65(12):1655–8.

94. Ghezzi A, Pozzilli C, Grimaldi LM, et al. Safety and efficacy of natalizumab in children with multiple sclerosis. Neurology 2010;75(10):912–7.

95. Yeh E, Krupp L, Ness J, et al. Breakthrough disease in pediatric MS patients: a pediatric network experience. Annual Meeting of the American Academy of Neurology. Seattle (WA), May 1, 2009.

96. Karenfort M, Kieseier BC, Tibussek D, et al. Rituximab as a highly effective treatment in a female adolescent with severe multiple sclerosis. Dev Med Child Neurol 2009;51(2):159–61.

97. Makhani N, Gorman MP, Branson HM, et al. Cyclophosphamide therapy in pediatric multiple sclerosis. Neurology 2009;72(24):2076–82.

98. Kuntz NL, Chabas D, Weinstock-Guttman B, et al. Treatment of multiple sclerosis in children and adolescents. Expert Opin Pharmacother 2010;11(4):505–20.

99. Lukban MB, Rosales RL, Dressler D. Effectiveness of botulinum toxin A for upper and lower limb spasticity in children with cerebral palsy: a summary of evidence. J Neural Transm 2009;116(3):319–31.

100. Gooch JL, Patton CP. Combining botulinum toxin and phenol to manage spasticity in children. Arch Phys Med Rehabil 2004;85(7):1121–4.

101. Beers SR, Skold A, Dixon CE, et al. Neurobehavioral effects of amantadine after pediatric traumatic brain injury: a preliminary report. J Head Trauma Rehabil 2005;20(5):450–63.

102. Hurst DL, Lajara-Nanson W. Use of modafinil in spastic cerebral palsy. J Child Neurol 2002;17(3):169–72.

103. Stankoff B, Waubant E, Confavreux C, et al. Modafinil for fatigue in MS: a randomized placebo-controlled double-blind study. Neurology 2005;64(7): 1139–43.

104. Wingerchuk DM, Benarroch EE, O'Brien PC, et al. A randomized controlled crossover trial of aspirin for fatigue in multiple sclerosis. Neurology 2005; 64(7):1267–9.

105. Schwid SR, Petrie MD, McDermott MP, et al. Quantitative assessment of sustained-release 4-aminopyridine for symptomatic treatment of multiple sclerosis. Neurology 1997;48(4):817–21.

106. Bever CT, Judge SI. Sustained-release fampridine for multiple sclerosis. Expert Opin Investig Drugs 2009;18(7):1013–24.

107. Goodman AD, Brown TR, Krupp LB, et al. Sustained-release oral fampridine in multiple sclerosis: a randomised, double-blind, controlled trial. Lancet 2009; 373(9665):732–8.

108. Kachuck NJ. Sustained release oral fampridine in the treatment of multiple sclerosis. Expert Opin Pharmacother 2009;10(12):2025–35.

109. Geny C, Nguyen JP, Pollin B, et al. Improvement of severe postural cerebellar tremor in multiple sclerosis by chronic thalamic stimulation. Mov Disord 1996; 11(5):489–94.

110. Schulder M, Sernas TJ, Karimi R. Thalamic stimulation in patients with multiple sclerosis: long-term follow-up. Stereotact Funct Neurosurg 2003;80(1–4):48–55.

111. Kilic N, Balkan E, Akgoz S, et al. Comparison of the effectiveness and side-effects of tolterodine and oxybutynin in children with detrusor instability. Int J Urol 2006;13(2):105–8.

112. Rodriguez M, Warrington AE, Pease LR. Invited article: human natural autoantibodies in the treatment of neurologic disease. Neurology 2009;72(14): 1269–76.

113. Sim FJ, Zhao C, Penderis J, et al. The age-related decrease in CNS remyelination efficiency is attributable to an impairment of both oligodendrocyte progenitor recruitment and differentiation. J Neurosci 2002;22(7):2451–9.

114. Zhao C, Li WW, Franklin RJ. Differences in the early inflammatory responses to toxin-induced demyelination are associated with the age-related decline in CNS remyelination. Neurobiol Aging 2006;27(9):1298–307.

115. Mina R, Brunner HI. Pediatric lupus–are there differences in presentation, genetics, response to therapy, and damage accrual compared with adult lupus? Rheum Dis Clin North Am 2010;36(1):53–80, vii–viii.

116. Baumann RJ, Robertson WC Jr. Neurosarcoid presents differently in children than in adults. Pediatrics 2003;112(6 Pt 1):e480–6.

117. Duzova A, Bakkaloglu A. Central nervous system involvement in pediatric rheumatic diseases: current concepts in treatment. Curr Pharm Des 2008;14(13): 1295–301.

118. Goo HW, Weon YC. A spectrum of neuroradiological findings in children with haemophagocytic lymphohistiocytosis. Pediatr Radiol 2007;37(11):1110–7.

119. Marais BJ, Gie RP, Schaaf HS, et al. The spectrum of disease in children treated for tuberculosis in a highly endemic area. Int J Tuberc Lung Dis 2006;10(7): 732–8.

120. Van Rie A, Harrington PR, Dow A, et al. Neurologic and neurodevelopmental manifestations of pediatric HIV/AIDS: a global perspective. Eur J Paediatr Neurol 2007;11(1):1–9.

121. Kastrup O, Wanke I, Maschke M. Neuroimaging of infections of the central nervous system. Semin Neurol 2008;28(4):511–22.

122. Shah I, Chudgar P. Progressive multifocal leukoencephalopathy (PML) presenting as intractable dystonia in an HIV-infected child. J Trop Pediatr 2005;51(6):380–2.

123. Mygland A, Ljostad U, Fingerle V, et al. EFNS guidelines on the diagnosis and management of European Lyme neuroborreliosis. Eur J Neurol 2010;17(1): 8–16, e1–4.

124. Oschmann P, Dorndorf W, Hornig C, et al. Stages and syndromes of neuroborreliosis. J Neurol 1998;245(5):262–72.

125. Fernandez RE, Rothberg M, Ferencz G, et al. Lyme disease of the CNS: MR imaging findings in 14 cases. AJNR Am J Neuroradiol 1990;11(3):479–81.

126. Bitnun A, Ford-Jones E, Blaser S, et al. Mycoplasma pneumoniae ecephalitis. Semin Pediatr Infect Dis 2003;14(2):96–107.

127. Louis ED, Lynch T, Kaufmann P, et al. Diagnostic guidelines in central nervous system Whipple's disease. Ann Neurol 1996;40(4):561–8.
128. Chamberlain MC, Glantz M, Groves MD, et al. Diagnostic tools for neoplastic meningitis: detecting disease, identifying patient risk, and determining benefit of treatment. Semin Oncol 2009;36(4 Suppl 2):S35–45.
129. Chamberlain MC, Johnston SK, Van Horn A, et al. Recurrent lymphomatous meningitis treated with intra-CSF rituximab and liposomal ara-C. J Neurooncol 2009;91(3):271–7.
130. Fattapposta F, Restuccia R, Pirro C, et al. Early diagnosis in cerebral autosomal dominant arteriopathy with subcortical infarcts and leukoencephalopathy (CADASIL): the role of MRI. Funct Neurol 2004;19(4):239–42.
131. Callen DJ, Shroff MM, Branson HM, et al. MRI in the diagnosis of pediatric multiple sclerosis. Neurology 2009;72(11):961–7.
132. Kaye EM. Update on genetic disorders affecting white matter. Pediatr Neurol 2001;24(1):11–24.
133. Sasaki M, Sakuragawa N, Takashima S, et al. MRI and CT findings in Krabbe disease. Pediatr Neurol 1991;7(4):283–8.
134. Shapiro EG, Lockman LA, Knopman D, et al. Characteristics of the dementia in late-onset metachromatic leukodystrophy. Neurology 1994;44(4):662–5.
135. van der Knaap MS, Kamphorst W, Barth PG, et al. Phenotypic variation in leukoencephalopathy with vanishing white matter. Neurology 1998;51(2):540–7.
136. Pridmore CL, Baraitser M, Harding B, et al. Alexander's disease: clues to diagnosis. J Child Neurol 1993;8(2):134–44.
137. Wallace DC. Mitochondrial diseases in man and mouse. Science 1999;283(5407): 1482–8.
138. Kalb RC, DiLorenzo TA, La Rocca NG, et al. The impact of early-onset multiple sclerosis on cognitive and psychosocial indices. International Journal of MS Care 1999;1(1):2–17.
139. Weisbrot DM, Ettinger AB, Gadow KD, et al. Psychiatric comorbidity in pediatric patients with demyelinating disorders. J Child Neurol 2010;25(2):192–202.
140. MacAllister WS, Krupp LB, Christodoulou C, et al. Progressive cognitive decline in pediatric MS. Neurology 2005;64(6):A322.

Cognitive Functioning in Multiple Sclerosis

Laura J. Julian, PhD

KEYWORDS

- Multiple sclerosis • Cognitive • Supportive care

Cognitive deficits as a result of multiple sclerosis (MS) have been documented since the earliest clinical descriptions of MS[1]; yet cognitive decline was not fully acknowledged as a prevalent and disabling consequence of MS until more recently.[2] Since the 1990s we have seen a steady increase of research evaluating cognitive complications of MS.[3] Currently, it is well understood that approximately half of patients with MS will develop cognitive impairment as a result of their disease. Despite great variability in assessment methodology, prevalence rates of cognitive impairment in MS have remained remarkably consistent and fall in the range of 40% to 65% of persons with MS across 5 decades of study (**Table 1**). Similar to epidemiology studies in other conditions, prevalence rates of cognitive dysfunction are generally higher within clinical settings, ranging from 53% to 65%,[4–14] and slightly lower in community studies, at about 45%.[15,16]

Recent advances in neuroimaging have provided clues to the relationship of cognitive functioning to overall disease burden in MS, and specific neuropathological substrates have been highlighted as especially relevant for the development of cognitive decline in MS. The clinical presentation of cognitive impairment in MS is somewhat variable and can range from relatively mild cognitive impairment to a rarer presentation of severe impairment resembling dementia.[17] For most patients with MS, the cognitive loss represents a decline in comparison with their previous level of functioning and has great potential to impair a range of functional domains including social, occupational, and educational functioning. In the clinic, cognitive dysfunction that is milder in severity, yet very troublesome to the patient and detrimental to his or her daily function, is commonly encountered. Further, these cognitive problems are frequently present even when other signs and symptoms of MS are absent on the neurologic examination. Mild levels of cognitive impairment are not easily detectable in the general clinical encounter, prompting a push toward the development of reliable and valid screening

This work was supported by grant No. MH072724 from the National Institute of Mental Health. The author has nothing to disclose.
Department of Medicine, University of California San Francisco, 3333 California Street, STE 270, San Francisco, CA 94143-0920, USA
E-mail address: laura.julian@ucsf.edu

Neurol Clin 29 (2011) 507–525
doi:10.1016/j.ncl.2010.12.003
0733-8619/11/$ – see front matter © 2011 Elsevier Inc. All rights reserved.

| Table 1 | | | |
| Prevalence of cognitive impairment in MS | | | |
Sample Characteristics	N	% Impaired	References
Clinic	17	65	4
Clinic	18	64	5
Clinic	64	60	6
Clinic	22	55	7
Clinic	100	56	8
Clinic	44	64	9
Clinic	46	65	10
Clinic	30	60	11
Clinic	52	54	12
Community	100	43	15
Community	147	46	16
Clinic	291	60	13
Clinic	160	53	14
Community	84	48	39

Data from Amato MP, Zipoli V, Portaccio E. Multiple sclerosis-related cognitive changes: a review of cross-sectional and longitudinal studies. J Neurol Sci 2006;245(1–2):41–6.

measures to evaluate cognitive dysfunction in MS. Neuropsychological assessment can quantify the nature and severity of cognitive deficits not easily detected in the conventional clinical encounter, can be used to track the course of cognitive functions longitudinally, and can help determine the efficacy or adverse effects of specific therapeutic approaches on cognition. We recommend the use of neuropsychology as a component of a multidisciplinary clinical evaluation, not only because mild deficits cannot always be detected in the conventional clinic visit, but also because subjective patient complaints of cognitive decline are not always associated with objective performance on neuropsychological testing. This discordance among patient reports of cognitive dysfunction and performance on neuropsychological testing may stem from several sources, including the influence of psychological distress (eg, depression),[18] the impact of fatigue, and the relatively poor sensitivity of conventional bedside cognitive screening measures to subtle alterations in cognition.[19]

MS generally affects individuals in the prime years of their work life, and cognitive dysfunction can be quite debilitating and costly from the perspectives of both the individual and society.[20,21] It is well understood that cognitive problems have the potential to not only diminish an individual's overall quality of life,[22] but can confer specific effects on daily function, including decreased capacity in medical decision making[23] driving abilities,[24,25] and can be an important contributor to work loss.[26,27]

Overall, empirically validated treatments for cognitive dysfunction in MS are lacking. The US Food and Drug Administration has no approved agents for the treatment of cognitive dysfunction in MS, and almost no randomized clinical trials have been designed specifically to determine the efficacy of treatments for cognitive manifestations in MS. However, the consideration of treatments for cognitive deficits in MS is in the earliest stages of development and both pharmacologic and behavioral interventions hold promise as potential therapeutic options to treat these debilitating symptoms of MS.

In this article, the nature and course of cognitive dysfunction in MS are reviewed, particularly in the context of recent advances in our understanding of the diffuse nature of neuropathology in MS, and in the context of specific factors that may confer risk or protection for the development of cognitive impairment. In addition, assessment and screening approaches of MS-related cognitive dysfunction are discussed. MS is a condition not only restricted to the adult population, and this article includes a brief description of cognition in pediatric-onset MS. Finally, promising intervention approaches to treat cognitive problems in MS are summarized.

NATURE OF COGNITIVE IMPAIRMENT IN MS

Early assumptions about cognitive impairment in MS included (1) the belief that cognitive impairment appears late in the disease course, several years after disease onset; and (2) the belief that cognitive impairment occurs only after the onset of substantial physical disability. These notions have been largely refuted and it is well understood that cognitive dysfunction can present very early in the MS disease process, even at the stage of a clinically isolated syndrome (CIS). More than two-thirds of patients with CIS who also have abnormal MRI findings convert to a diagnosis of MS.[28–30] Although few studies have been conducted evaluating cognition in CIS, cognitive dysfunction is often observed at this early stage in the disease.[31–35] Additionally, some patients appear to present with initial cognitive problems and the absence of other neurologic signs and symptoms,[36] and are later determined to have MS.

With respect to MS disease subtypes, many studies find that patients with primary progressive MS (PPMS) or secondary progressive MS (SPMS) appear to have greater degrees of cognitive impairment when compared with patients with relapsing-remitting MS (RRMS) or CIS.[8,37–39] Importantly, in studies comparing SPMS and RRMS, not all studies have controlled for age, which thereby attenuates the conclusions one can make from these studies, given other age-related neurodegenerative processes. Overall, results of studies comparing SPMS and PPMS subtypes have varied and there is no clear conclusion as to whether one subtype has a clear cognitive disadvantage.[14,40–42]

Well-controlled longitudinal studies investigating the course of cognitive impairment in MS are needed, but difficult to carry out. Such studies are commonly weakened by bias in attrition rates, short follow-up periods, practice effects, and variable assessment methods. In general, cognitive dysfunction can vary over time, but an important subset of patients show progressive longitudinal decline. Important risk factors for progressive cognitive decline appear to be signs of cognitive deterioration at disease onset[43] and radiographic evidence of neocortical gray matter volume loss.[44] Amato and colleagues[45,46] have conducted perhaps most comprehensive prospective studies of cognitive functioning in MS. Although sample sizes were relatively small, Amato and colleagues found that after a period of 10 years, the proportion of patients observed to have cognitive impairment increased from 26% to 56%, with a subset of these patients showing a marked decline in severity of cognitive dysfunction over time.[46]

DOMAINS OF COGNITIVE IMPAIRMENT IN MS

Cognitive manifestations in MS range from the commonly observed deficits in processing speed and episodic memory to more unusual case reports of aphasia[47] and amnestic syndromes.[48,49] The most frequently observed domain of impairment observed in MS appears to be speeded processing, which refers to the speed with which one can process any modality of information (eg, verbal, visual).[50–54] Slowed processing can be observed independent of other domains of impairment, but also influences the development of impairment in cognitive domains, including working memory, executive functioning, memory, and retrieval. Working memory is also frequently impaired in patients with MS,[55–57] and is often defined as the cognitive process of temporary storage and the manipulation of information necessary for such complex cognitive tasks.[58,59] Verbal and visual episodic memory closely follow working memory with respect to prevalence of impairment in this domain, and in some studies these cognitive functions emerge as the most commonly affected domain of functioning.[13] In addition, impairments are also commonly observed in the broad range of executive functions.[60–66] A recent meta-analysis broadly evaluating neuropsychiatric symptoms (mood and psychological status, motor functioning, and cognitive domains) in RRMS (n = 2042) versus healthy controls (n = 1849) observed large effect sizes for depression, episodic verbal memory (recall), and motor functioning.[3] Moderate effect sizes were observed for all other cognitive domains, including overall cognitive ability, attention and executive functions, perception, memory and learning, verbal functions and language, and construction.[3]

Cognitive function is often only modestly correlated with traditional measures of MS-related disability, generally measured by Kurtzke's Expanded Disability Status Scale (EDSS).[67] It is commonly observed that persons with MS suffer significant cognitive dysfunction despite relatively low overall disability scores,[68–71] but given the reliance of the EDSS on ambulation and spinal cord involvement, the lack of a relationship between these two domains is not entirely unexpected. More recent evidence has observed that some aspects of cognitive functions may mirror disease progression in other domains. For example, one study found an association between speeded processing and overall change in disability (EDSS); whereas, memory decline appeared to progress independently of markers of disease activity and disability, including relapse rate and EDSS progression.[72] In response to the need for a more robust measure of overall disease burden, the MS Functional Composite (MSFC) was developed,[73] which includes a screening measure of cognitive functioning (discussed in greater detail later in this article, in the context of screening measures). In recent years, there has been a greater appreciation overall of the individual differences in disease manifestations across patients with MS. As a result, we may see relevant patterns of disease manifestations that co-occur with cognitive functions as a broader range of manifestations are more systematically evaluated.

RELATIONSHIPS AMONG COGNITIVE IMPAIRMENT AND NEUROIMAGING

In the past several years, improvements in imaging practices have broadened our appreciation of the range of neuropathology observed in MS. MS has long been characterized by demyelinating white matter lesions visible by conventional magnetic resonance imaging (MRI) techniques such as T2-MRI. Although correlations between T2-MRI lesion volume and cognitive functioning in MS are improving, the strength of these relationships remains modest.[65,74–78]

MS is increasingly appreciated as a diffuse disease of the central nervous system. Improved visualization of the range of neuropathology in MS has catalyzed new studies that have increasingly observed robust relationships between cognitive functioning and underlying structural alterations in both cortical and subcortical brain regions. Global and regional measures of atrophy have been shown to be more strongly correlated with cognition as compared with lesion volume, and may prove to be sensitive markers to help identify patients at risk for cognitive impairment.[79–84] Other structural abnormalities, including changes in "normal-appearing white matter" visible on such techniques as diffusion tensor imaging may be closely tied to important clinical outcomes including cognitive functioning and disability.[85,86] There is increasing attention on the neocortex in relation to cognitive functions in MS, with studies citing relationships among cortical thinning[87] and cortical lesions[88,89] in association with cognitive dysfunction in MS.

Recently, we have seen a rapid emergence of new tasks and experimental paradigms for functional MRI studies evaluating cognitive functions in MS. As a result, functional neuroimaging is advancing our knowledge not only of the relationships among cognitive functioning and disease burden in MS, but is also providing unique insights into neuroplasticity and specific neural mechanisms that may serve to compensate for reduced cortical efficiencies. In general, research to date has observed that individuals with MS show increased activation in brain regions not observed to be activated in controls. Individuals with MS also show an increased magnitude of activation compared with controls in the expected task-specific regions.[90] Suggested sources of this new and/or increased activation include cerebral reorganization and compensatory recruitment of other brain regions to maintain cognitive performance.[91,92]

In the past, modest correlations between brain MRI metrics and cognitive outcomes have left us searching for other etiologies for cognitive compromise in MS. However, with improvements in MRI, we are increasingly identifying important brain–behavior connections in MS. These advances support our understanding of the etiology of cognitive impairment in MS. Finally, these advances show that cognitive impairment is a sensitive clinical outcome associated with important neuropathological and neurodegenerative changes.

RISK AND PROTECTIVE FACTORS FOR COGNITIVE DYSFUNCTION IN MS

Like other neurodegenerative diseases, there is an increased interest in the identification of specific risk and protective factors for cognitive and neurodegenerative decline in MS. This area of inquiry in MS is in the earliest stages, but with a greater appreciation of both biologic (eg, genetic) and environmental (eg, smoking, vitamin insufficiencies) risk and protective factors for other disease manifestations in MS, we are coming closer to a better understanding of potentially modifiable factors that may either confer risk or protection against cognitive decline in MS. To date, the primary known risk factors are concomitant manifestations of MS that either directly or indirectly confer effects on cognition (eg, psychiatric distress, fatigue). Protective factors are just beginning to be evaluated in experimental studies, and other factors known to be protective in other neurodegenerative conditions, like cognitive reserve, are a target of ongoing investigations in MS.

RISK FACTORS
Psychiatric Distress

Depression, another common syndrome associated with MS, is known to have a negative impact on cognition, specifically speeded processing and executive functioning.[93–96] In longitudinal studies of patients without the presence of a clinical depressive disorder, the presence of negative affect at baseline was independently predictive of cognitive decline over 1 year in a cohort of persons with MS.[97] The relationships among depression and cognitive impairment are likely complex and interactive. Cognitive dysfunction results from depressive symptomatology (eg, lack of concentration, attentional problems, reduced effortful processing); however, both depression and cognitive function may originate from damage to similar neuropathological pathways. Lesion-depression relationships have been identified in MS,[98,99] and the presence of cognitive impairment has been shown to identify patients with MS who have responded poorly to conventional antidepressant therapies.[100] Further studies to better understand these neural pathways potentially contributing to both depression and cognitive impairment in MS are warranted.

Although relatively understudied, anxiety also confers significant effects for poorer cognitive functioning,[101] and in some cases predicts cognition independent of depression.[93] In sum, although neuropathology has the propensity to precipitate both symptoms of psychiatric distress (eg, depression, anxiety) and cognitive impairment, it is also known that these psychiatric syndromes constitute an independent factor predictive of cognitive impairment and should be considered in the context of any bedside screening evaluation and/or formal neuropsychological evaluation.

Pain

Headache, spasticity, neuropathic pain, and paroxysmal symptoms can all lead to pain in MS. MS-related pain is also not always easily remediated through medication, physical therapy, or other relief strategies. Pain has a well-established direct and indirect effect on cognitive functioning. Chronic or acute pain affects attention, processing speed, and difficulties with encoding.[102] Indirectly, pain can also produce changes in mood, including depression, and medications (eg, benzodiazepines) that are used to treat pain frequently have adverse impacts on cognitive functioning.[103]

Fatigue

Fatigue is the most common clinical symptom of MS and a decline in cognitive function can be a result of physical as well as cognitive fatigue. Cognitive fatigue is defined as a decline in cognitive performance over brief period of time, such as a neuropsychological testing session or part of a workday. Although the patient is not participating in any physically fatiguing activities, this decline is often still observed. Krupp and Elkins[104] found that patients with MS demonstrate clear declines in performance on measures of verbal memory and executive functioning over a 4-hour session. In contrast, medically healthy controls demonstrated improvement in memory and executive functioning over the same period, an observation likely attributable to practice effects. Therefore, it is recommended that patients with MS pace themselves adequately, particularly when performing tasks that are cognitively demanding, to keep fatigue to a minimum.

PROTECTIVE FACTORS

An important area of exploration is the role of cognitive reserve as a moderator of a range of adverse outcomes in MS, including cognitive decline. Cognitive reserve refers to the notion that intellectual enrichment is associated with cerebral efficiency and therefore the neuropsychological expression of a neurologic condition is thereby attenuated among persons with higher intellectual enrichment. Preliminary studies evaluating these constructs have found that when patients with MS were stratified by proxies for intellectual enrichment (eg, education, markers of premorbid intelligence), patients with increased enrichment were better able to withstand MS-related neuropathology and these effects may be protective against some aspects of cognitive decline.[105–107] Although these studies have some limitations with respect to sample size and assessment measures, they have prompted new investigation into the role of cognitive reserve as a potential buffer against cognitive problems in MS.

ASSESSMENT AND SCREENING METHODS FOR COGNITIVE IMPAIRMENT IN MS

A routine cognitive evaluation would be beneficial for most patients with MS. There are many reasons why this option is not always readily available, including issues related to access to neuropsychological services, costs of comprehensive neuropsychological evaluations, and time. However, given the prevalence of cognitive impairment in MS and impact on daily functioning, systematic approaches to identifying patients with cognitive impairment are necessary.

Although a range of assessment techniques and batteries have been used, there are a relatively small number of assessment approaches that appear to be the most commonly used and the most sensitive for the detection of cognitive impairment in MS (**Table 2**). The Neuropsychological Screening Battery for MS (NSBMS) was developed in collaboration with the Cognitive Function Study Group of the National Multiple Sclerosis Society in the United States.[15] This battery includes several measures assessing the most commonly observed deficits in MS, including measures of processing speed, working memory, episodic verbal and visual memory, and fluency. Later, to accommodate repeat testing, the Brief Repeatable Neuropsychological Battery (BRNB) (Rao SM, Manual for the Brief, Repeatable Battery of Neuropsychological Tests in Multiple Sclerosis, unpublished manuscript, 1991) was developed from the NSBMS with some modifications. The BRNB has been adapted for use in several countries and is a commonly used instrument for studies evaluating neuropsychological outcomes over time.[108–110]

A second approach is the Minimal Assessment of Cognitive Function in MS (MAC-FIMS) battery developed in 2001 by an expert panel composed of neuropsychologists and psychologists convened by the Consortium of MS Centers.[111] This consensus panel identified a neuropsychological test battery requiring approximately 90 minutes to administer and appears to be a reliable and valid method for detecting cognitive impairment in MS.[13] The MACFIMS battery is composed of 7 neuropsychological tests assessing 5 cognitive domains commonly impaired in MS (processing speed/working memory, learning and memory, executive function, visual-spatial processing, and word retrieval). Further, regression-based normative data have been developed for this battery accounting for important demographic variables including age, sex, and education.[112]

The addition of a neuropsychological measure to the more recently developed measure of functional disability, the MSFC, represented the improved appreciation of cognitive dysfunction as a prevalent manifestation and relevant to the overall

Table 2
Commonly used cognitive screening batteries for MS

	Minimal Assessment of Cognitive Function in MS (MACFIMS)	Brief Repeatable Neuropsychological Battery (BRNB)
Processing speed/working memory	Paced Auditory Serial Addition Test	Paced Auditory Serial Addition Test
	Symbol Digit Modalities Test	Symbol Digit Modalities Test
Learning and memory	California Verbal Learning Test–II	Selective Reminding Test
	Brief Visuospatial Memory Test–Revised	10/36 Spatial Recall Test
Visual perception/spatial processing	Judgment of Line Orientation Test	
Executive functions	Delis-Kaplan Card Sorting Test	
Language/Other	Controlled Oral Word Association Test	Controlled Oral Word Association Test

picture of functional disability among patients with MS. The MSFC is a 3-part instrument evaluating arm, leg, and cognitive functions: (1) the 9-Hole Peg Test to measure arm and hand disability; (2) the 25-foot Walk to measure leg dysfunction and ambulation difficulties, and (3) the Paced Auditory Serial Addition Test (PASAT3, 3-second version).[73] The PASAT3 is a modification of the original PASAT designed to provide an estimate of speeded processing and working memory. This task requires the examinee to sustain attention to single digits while performing simultaneous mental calculations.[113] Although the PASAT3 has shown sensitivity in some domains relevant for MS,[114] utility of the PASAT is limited by the presence of strong practice effects and poor sensitivity in predicting MS-related disease progression.[115,116] These findings point to the more recent conclusions that PASAT3 may not be sufficient for use in an assessment battery designed for repeated assessments, and it may be best to replace this measure in future revisions of the MSFC or similar instruments of function in MS.

Both the BRNB and MACFIMS represent reasonable intermediate assessment approaches, are comparable in their overall sensitivity to detect cognitive compromise in MS,[117] and strike a compromise between a single-measure screening test and a comprehensive neuropsychological evaluation. As a field, we continue to seek very brief but sensitive approaches to detect cognitive impairment at the bedside. Conventional bedside mental status screening examinations are lacking in sensitivity to detect cognitive impairment profiles typical of MS.[118] Therefore, other screening techniques that may facilitate the identification of patients with cognitive impairment that are feasibly administered during the course of routine clinical care are needed. One promising tool is the Symbol Digit Modalities Test[119] (SDMT), a test of processing speed that takes approximately 2 minutes to administer, and has minimal practice effects.[120] Using the SDMT, a total score of 55 or lower accurately categorized 72% of MS patients with cognitive impairment, yielding sensitivity of 0.82 and specificity of 0.60.[121]

Another approach to detecting cognitive impairment in MS has been to use self-report or informant-report questionnaires that evaluate the patient's perception of cognitive impairment. The Multiple Sclerosis Neuropsychological Screening Questionnaire (MSNQ)[122] and the Perceived Deficits Questionnaire (PDQ)[123] from the MS Quality of Life Inventory (MSQLI) are two commonly used self-report measures of cognitive functioning in MS. These measures are correlated with cognitive impairment in MS, and have been associated with vocational disability and findings on MRI.[13] Importantly, these self-report measures are often more strongly correlated with severity of depressive symptoms than with performance on neuropsychological tests, and these contaminating factors must be considered when administering self-report measures of cognitive function.[18]

Despite these limitations, self-report and informant-report measures have a role in clinical practice, and patient reports of cognitive impairment should be considered as clinically meaningful. These measures provide an evaluation of the patient's perception of their cognitive abilities, and have the potential to indicate very mild cognitive changes noticeable to the patient but not yet detected on the examination. In addition, a comparison of these measures to informant-based measures and objective neuropsychological testing can provide important information about a patient's insight into his or her own functioning.[124] In sum, using measures of perceived cognitive impairment in conjunction with a depressive symptom severity scale may help to identify patients who would benefit from a more comprehensive neuropsychological examination and/or a mental health screening examination.

OTHER FACTORS IMPLICATED IN COGNITIVE DYSFUNCTION: PEDIATRIC MS AND NEUROPSYCHOLOGY

Two percent to 5% of persons with MS develop the condition in childhood[125,126] and relatively little is known about the cognitive sequelae of MS in children. Children with MS may be especially prone to cognitive impairment given that the neuropathologic processes of MS, including inflammation, blood–brain barrier permeability, atrophy, and demyelination that occur simultaneous to many aspects of brain development.[127] Most studies of cognitive dysfunction in MS are based on single case reports or small clinical series.[45,128–131] Therefore, these studies are limited by small sample sizes, lack of control groups, and variability of assessment techniques. Overall, it is estimated that at least one-third of children and adolescents with MS develop cognitive dysfunction.[130–134] The cognitive profile appears to parallel the known profile in adult-onset MS, including involvement of memory functions, complex attention and processing speed, and aspects of executive functions. However, the breath of deficits in childhood-onset MS may also be somewhat broader and may encompass other cognitive domains including language functions and overall intelligence. For example, marked language deficits have been observed in children with MS, a domain that is relatively spared in adults with MS.[135]

Very few longitudinal studies have been conducted evaluating cognitive function in children and adolescents with MS. In one study by MacAllister and colleagues,[136] 12 children and adolescents with MS underwent 2 neuropsychological assessments, separated by a mean inter-assessment duration of 8 months. At baseline, all but 2 participants demonstrated impairment on at least 1 neuropsychological task. At follow-up, the frequency of impairments increased on several tasks. An association was also observed between baseline EDSS score and increasing cognitive impairment. An Italian cohort of children with MS were also observed over the course of 2 years,[137] with preliminary results suggesting a deterioration of neuropsychological functions in most (ie, 70%) of the cohort that was predominantly treated with disease-modifying therapies and had relatively stable MRI course.

In pediatric MS, large-scale systematic studies with a longitudinal design are needed. It is critical to determine the overall course of cognitive functioning as well as the relationships of cognitive change with the expected trajectory of cognitive development.

Unlike in adults, cognitive impairment in children with MS appears to be associated with overall disability scores and the number of relapses a child has experienced.[136] It is unknown how MS disease processes will impede or interrupt normal cognitive development in children or how vocational and educational functioning may be affected by cognitive compromise. Multisite pediatric MS clinical research studies are currently under way to improve our understanding of this disease in children.

TREATMENT OF COGNITIVE DYSFUNCTION IN MS

For the treatment of cognitive dysfunction in MS, several approaches have been considered, including both pharmacologic and nonpharmacologic methods. The use of disease-modifying therapies (DMT) for the improvement of cognitive functions in MS has been a target of investigation for several years. DMT therapy may improve cognitive function through the prevention of new lesions or potentially through the deceleration of neurodegeneration. All of these investigations have been conducted via post hoc analyses of DMT randomized clinical trials (RCT) designed to determine the effect of DMT on the appearance of new lesions, reductions in relapse rate, and time to disability, and were not designed for the assessment of cognitive outcomes (eg, patients were not selected for cognitive impairment). An initial study in this area was conducted by Fischer and colleagues,[138] who conducted a post hoc analysis of cognitive data from a 24 month RCT of interferon beta–1a (IFNβ1a). Compared with untreated patients, treated individuals were observed to have improved cognitive functions in some areas, and a lack of deterioration in others. Trials investigating interferon beta–1b (IFNβ1b) also showed some improvements in cognitive functioning.[139,140] So far, studies of glatiramer acetate were largely negative with respect to the improvement of cognitive functions.[141] Kappos and colleagues found improvements on the PASAT in a group of patients with CIS and MS treated early with IFNβ1b, and these effects appeared to be maintained after 1 to 3 years of open-label follow-up.[142] Most recently, an uncontrolled study of 39 patients treated with natalizumab observed improvements across a number of cognitive measures; however, this study is limited by lack of RCT methodology.[143] Overall, findings related to studies investigating MS DMTs on cognitive function must be interpreted with caution, as they are conducted as secondary analyses of RCTs and therefore designed (and powered) for other outcomes, they did not select patients based on cognitive status, or were conducted as an uncontrolled trial. One observational study, the Cognitive Impairment in Multiple Sclerosis (COGIMUS) study was conducted to compare DMT-naive patients treated with intramuscular subcutaneous IFNβ1a 22 μg 3 times weekly (40.5%), IFNβ1a 44 μg 3 times weekly (42.9%), intramuscular IFNβ1a (11.6%), or subcutaneous IFNβ1b (4.9%). In this study, all groups remained relatively stable cognitively over the course of 3 years, and some improvement was observed in the subcutaneous IFNβ1a, with a slightly more pronounced effect among patients prescribed a higher dose. Again, with the lack of an experimental control group, it is difficult to make conclusions other than the tenuous suggestion that DMTs may also be protective against cognitive decline in MS.

In addition to the DMT findings, a number of studies have explored the benefits of agents known to improve cognitive status in other neurodegenerative conditions. First, donepezil, an acetylcholinesterase inhibitor approved to treat dementia, has been studied in MS. Christodoulou and colleagues[144] hypothesized that because of MS lesions intersecting specific neural pathways, cholinergic deficits may also emerge in MS. Preliminary RCTs investigating the effects of donepezil for cognitive dysfunction in MS have yielded some promising findings, both on objective neuropsychological tests and on patient and physician ratings of improvement.[144,145] Memantine is a N-methyl D-aspartate (NMDA, glutamate) receptor antagonist that is approved for use in Alzheimer's disease. Because glutamate transport has been observed to be altered in MS, Lovera and colleagues[146] hypothesized that memantine would be an effective means to facilitate the signal transduction of neurons and abate abnormally high levels of extracellular glutamate leading to neurotoxicity. This group conducted an RCT using memantine in 114 persons with MS, with no findings of clinical improvement in cognitive functions at least in this short-term study duration of 12 weeks. *Ginkgo biloba* is an herb that has been a target of interest in other neurodegenerative disorders and, in a small RCT for cognitive function in MS, showed some limited effects for some measures of inhibition and processing speed.[147] In addition, medications for attentional problems (single-dose methylphenidate) and fatigue (amantadine and pemoline) have also been studied in RCTs with moderate effects.[148–150] The study of pharmacologic agents approved for other cognitive disorders remains promising. So far, these studies have largely followed comparable methodology used in other studies of cognition in neurodegenerative disease, particularly those characterized by a more rapid decline in functioning (eg, Alzheimer's disease). Given the relatively slower progression of disease and related cognitive deficits in MS, future RCTs investigating these agents over a longer RCT duration (eg, 2–3 years) or among patients early in their disease could provide novel insights into the use of these agents both as remediators of cognitive dysfunction, but also as neuroprotective agents to slow cognitive decline.

NONPHARMACOLOGIC APPROACHES

Effective rehabilitation and cognitive remediation techniques are in need to address cognitive problems in MS. Like pharmacologic trials, few RCTs investigating cognitive rehabilitation in MS have been conducted. Early studies are hindered by methodological problems including the lack of controlled trials, the presence of baseline group differences, and reliance on case studies that generally produced mixed results. More recent studies using targeted interventions for cognitive functions that are vulnerable to decline in MS have yielded more promising results.[151] One RCT in a group of 20 patients living in a skilled nursing facility found no effects from a "memory book" intervention. This study is somewhat weakened by the nonspecific intervention and the lack of patient selection for cognitive problems. Solari and colleagues,[152] implementing a computer-aided intervention for remediation of memory and attention, found no significant differences between the active treatment group and the control group. Chiaravalloti and colleagues[151] conducted an RCT of the modified "story memory technique" to improve learning and memory and found a significant treatment effect, particularly for MS patients with memory impairment of at least moderate severity. This trial by Chiaravalloti and colleagues is an improvement on prior studies for several reasons: first, this study uses an RCT quantitative design; second, the experimental intervention had theoretical appeal and demonstrated efficacy in other populations (eg, traumatic brain injury); and third, patients were recruited based on the presence of specific cognitive deficits. As reviewed by O'Brien,[153] the field of cognitive remediation for MS is in the earliest stages, but this field also holds promise. Future studies using similar rigorous methodology practices are needed before we can fully appreciate the utility of this therapeutic approach in MS. In addition, the few controlled studies to date have examined memory and learning difficulties, whereas other commonly occurring domains of impairment, including speeded processing, have not been studied. Finally, it will be important to consider long-term maintenance of gains; and like pharmacologic trials, it will be important to consider extending trial durations to fully appreciate the potential applicability of these therapies in clinical practice.

SUMMARY

In recent years, we have seen an increased appreciation of the debilitating consequences of cognitive dysfunction in MS. Novel neuroimaging technologies have catalyzed research evaluating important brain-behavior relationships in MS, both in terms of neurodegenerative properties, but also in terms of potential compensatory processes that can help compensate for brain injury. Currently, studies are under way to better understand potentially modifiable risk and protective factors that can be used to identify patients who are at risk for cognitive impairment and perhaps intervene to protect patients from developing cognitive decline. Finally, although large, well-controlled randomized clinical trials targeting cognitive symptoms in MS have yet to be completed, there are a number of pharmacologic and nonpharmacologic alternatives that hold promise and have the potential to benefit a large number of persons with MS.

REFERENCES

1. Charcot JM. Lectures on diseases of the nervous system. London: New Sydenham Society; 1877.

2. Butler MA, Corboy JR, Filley CM. How the conflict between American psychiatry and neurology delayed the appreciation of cognitive dysfunction in multiple sclerosis. Neuropsychol Rev 2009;19:399–410.
3. Prakash RS, Snook EM, Lewis JM, et al. Cognitive impairments in relapsing-remitting multiple sclerosis: a meta-analysis. Mult Scler 2008;14(9):1250–61.
4. Parsons OA, Stewart KD, Arenberg D. Impairment of abstracting ability in multiple sclerosis. J Nerv Ment Dis 1957;125(2):221–5.
5. Surridge D. An investigation into some psychiatric aspects of multiple sclerosis. Br J Psychiatry 1969;115:749–64.
6. Staples D, Lincoln B. Intellectual impairment in multiple sclerosis and relation to functional abilities. Rheumatol Rehabil 1979;18(3):153–60.
7. Bertrando P, Maffei C, Ghezzi A. A study of neuropsychological alterations in multiple sclerosis. Acta Psychiatr Belg 1983;83(1):13–21.
8. Heaton RK, Nelson LM, Thompson DS, et al. Neuropsychological findings in relapsing-remitting and chronic-progressive multiple sclerosis. J Consult Clin Psychol 1985;53(1):103–10.
9. Rao SM, Hammeke TA, McQuillen MP, et al. Memory disturbance in chronic progressive multiple sclerosis. Arch Neurol 1984;41(6):625–31.
10. Medaer R, De Smedt L, Swerts M, et al. Use of rating scales to reflect cognitive and mental functioning in multiple sclerosis. Acta Neurol Scand Suppl 1984;101: 65–7.
11. Lyon-Caen O, Jouvent R, Hauser S, et al. Cognitive function in recent-onset demyelinating diseases. Arch Neurol 1986;43(11):1138–41.
12. Peyser JM, Edwards KR, Poser CM, et al. Cognitive function in patients with multiple sclerosis. Arch Neurol 1980;37(9):577–9.
13. Benedict RH, Cookfair D, Gavett R, et al. Validity of the minimal assessment of cognitive function in multiple sclerosis (MACFIMS). J Int Neuropsychol Soc 2006;12(4):549–58.
14. Potagas C, Giogkaraki E, Koutsis G, et al. Cognitive impairment in different MS subtypes and clinically isolated syndromes. J Neurol Sci 2008;267(1/2): 100–6.
15. Rao SM, Leo GJ, Bernardin L, et al. Cognitive dysfunction in multiple sclerosis. I. Frequency, patterns, and prediction [see comments]. Neurology 1991;41(5): 685–91.
16. McIntosh-Michaelis SA, Roberts MH, Wilkinson SM, et al. The prevalence of cognitive impairment in a community survey of multiple sclerosis. Br J Clin Psychol 1991;30(Pt 4):333–48.
17. Stoquart-ElSankari S, Périn B, Lehmann P, et al. Cognitive forms of multiple sclerosis: report of a dementia case. Clin Neurol Neurosurg 2010;112(3): 258–60.
18. Julian L, Merluzzi NM, Mohr DC. The relationship among depression, subjective cognitive impairment, and neuropsychological performance in multiple sclerosis. Mult Scler 2007;13(1):81–6.
19. Leritz E, Brandt J, Minor M, et al. "Subcortical" cognitive impairment in patients with systemic lupus erythematosus. J Int Neuropsychol Soc 2000; 6(7):821–5.
20. Rao SM, Leo GJ, Ellington L, et al. Cognitive dysfunction in multiple sclerosis. II. Impact on employment and social functioning [see comments]. Neurology 1991; 41(5):692–6.
21. Smith MM, Arnett PA. Factors related to employment status changes in individuals with multiple sclerosis. Mult Scler 2005;11(5):602–9.

22. Glanz BI, Healy BC, Rintell DJ, et al. The association between cognitive impairment and quality of life in patients with early multiple sclerosis. J Neurol Sci 2010;290(1/2):75–9.
23. Basso MR, Candilis PJ, Johnson J, et al. Capacity to make medical treatment decisions in multiple sclerosis: a potentially remediable deficit. J Clin Exp Neuropsychol 2010;32(10):1050–61.
24. Schultheis MT, Garay E, DeLuca J. The influence of cognitive impairment on driving performance in multiple sclerosis. Neurology 2001;56(8):1089–94.
25. Marcotte TD, Rosenthal TJ, Roberts E, et al. The contribution of cognition and spasticity to driving performance in multiple sclerosis. Arch Phys Med Rehabil 2008;89(9):1753–8.
26. Beatty WW, Blanco CR, Wilbanks SL, et al. Demographic, clinical, and cognitive characteristics of multiple sclerosis patients who continue to work. J Neurol Rehabil 1995;9:167–73.
27. Julian LJ, Vella L, Vollmer T, et al. Employment in multiple sclerosis. Exiting and re-entering the work force. J Neurol 2008;255(9):1354–60.
28. Brex PA, Ciccarelli O, O'Riordan JI, et al. A longitudinal study of abnormalities on MRI and disability from multiple sclerosis. N Engl J Med 2002;346(3):158–64.
29. Morrissey SP, Miller DH, Kendall BE, et al. The significance of brain magnetic resonance imaging abnormalities at presentation with clinically isolated syndromes suggestive of multiple sclerosis. A 5-year follow-up study. Brain 1993;116(Pt 1):135–46.
30. Tintoré M, Rovira A, Río J, et al. Baseline MRI predicts future attacks and disability in clinically isolated syndromes. Neurology 2006;67(6):968–72.
31. Feuillet L, Reuter F, Audoin B, et al. Early cognitive impairment in patients with clinically isolated syndrome suggestive of multiple sclerosis. Mult Scler 2007; 13(1):124–7.
32. Achiron A, Barak Y. Cognitive impairment in probable multiple sclerosis. J Neurol Neurosurg Psychiatry 2003;74(4):443–6.
33. Callanan MM, Logsdail SJ, Ron MA, et al. Cognitive impairment in patients with clinically isolated lesions of the type seen in multiple sclerosis. A psychometric and MRI study. Brain 1989;112(Pt 2):361–74.
34. Feinstein A, Youl B, Ron M. Acute optic neuritis: a cognitive and magnetic resonance imaging study. Brain 1992;115(5):1403–15.
35. Feinstein A, Kartsounis LD, Miller DH, et al. Clinically isolated lesions of the type seen in multiple sclerosis: a cognitive, psychiatric, and MRI follow-up study. J Neurol Neurosurg Psychiatry 1992;55(10):869–76.
36. Staff NP, Lucchinetti CF, Keegan BM. Multiple sclerosis with predominant, severe cognitive impairment. Arch Neurol 2009;66(9):1139–43.
37. Denney DR, Sworowski LA, Lynch SG. Cognitive impairment in three subtypes of multiple sclerosis. Arch Clin Neuropsychol 2005;20(8):967–81.
38. Gaudino EA, Chiaravalloti ND, DeLuca J, et al. A comparison of memory performance in relapsing-remitting, primary progressive and secondary progressive, multiple sclerosis. Neuropsychiatry Neuropsychol Behav Neurol 2001;14(1):32–44.
39. Smestad C, Sandvik L, Landrø NI, et al. Cognitive impairment after three decades of multiple sclerosis. Eur J Neurol 2009;17(3):499–505.
40. Huijbregts SC, Kalkers NF, de Sonneville LM, et al. Cognitive impairment and decline in different MS subtypes. J Neurol Sci 2006;245(1/2):187–94.
41. Wachowius U, Talley M, Silver N, et al. Cognitive impairment in primary and secondary progressive multiple sclerosis. J Clin Exp Neuropsychol 2005; 27(1):65–77.

42. Kraus JA, Schütze C, Brokate B, et al. Discriminant analysis of the cognitive performance profile of MS patients differentiates their clinical course. J Neurol 2005;252(7):808–13.

43. Kujala P, Portin R, Ruutiainen J. The progress of cognitive decline in multiple sclerosis. A controlled 3-year follow-up. Brain 1997;120(2):289–97.

44. Amato MP, Portaccio E, Goretti B, et al. Association of neocortical volume changes with cognitive deterioration in relapsing-remitting multiple sclerosis. Arch Neurol 2007;64(8):1157–61.

45. Amato MP, Ponziani G, Pracucci G, et al. Cognitive impairment in early-onset multiple sclerosis. Pattern, predictors, and impact on everyday life in a 4-year follow-up. Arch Neurol 1995;52(2):168–72.

46. Amato MP, Ponziani G, Siracusa G, et al. Cognitive dysfunction in early-onset multiple sclerosis: a reappraisal after 10 years. Arch Neurol 2001;58(10): 1602–6.

47. Arnett PA, Rao SM, Hussain M, et al. Conduction aphasia in multiple sclerosis: a case report with MRI findings. Neurology 1996;47(2):576–8.

48. Vighetto A, Charles N, Salzmann M, et al. Korsakoff's syndrome as the initial presentation of multiple sclerosis. J Neurol 1991;238(6):351–4.

49. Zarei M, Chandran S, Compston A, et al. Cognitive presentation of multiple sclerosis: evidence for a cortical variant. J Neurol Neurosurg Psychiatry 2003;74(7): 872–7.

50. Archibald CJ, Fisk JD. Information processing efficiency in patients with multiple sclerosis. J Clin Exp Neuropsychol 2000;22(5):686–701.

51. DeLuca J, Johnson SK, Natelson BH. Information processing efficiency in chronic fatigue syndrome and multiple sclerosis. Arch Neurol 1993;50(3):301–4.

52. Demaree HA, DeLuca J, Gaudino EA, et al. Speed of information processing as a key deficit in multiple sclerosis: implications for rehabilitation. J Neurol Neurosurg Psychiatry 1999;67(5):661–3.

53. Denney DR, Lynch SG, Parmenter BA. A 3-year longitudinal study of cognitive impairment in patients with primary progressive multiple sclerosis: speed matters. J Neurol Sci 2008;267(1/2):129–36.

54. DeLuca J, Chelune GJ, Tulsky DS, et al. Is speed of processing or working memory the primary information processing deficit in multiple sclerosis? J Clin Exp Neuropsychol 2004;26(4):550–62.

55. Foong J, Rozewicz L, Davie CA, et al. Correlates of executive function in multiple sclerosis: The use of magnetic resonance spectroscopy as an index of focal pathology. J Neuropsychiatry Clin Neurosci 1999;11:45–50.

56. Ruchkin DS, Grafman J, Krauss GL, et al. Event-related brain potential evidence for a verbal working memory deficit in multiple sclerosis. Brain 1994;117(Pt 2): 289–305.

57. Wishart H, Sharpe D. Neuropsychological aspects of multiple sclerosis: a quantitative review. J Clin Exp Neuropsychol 1997;19(6):810–24.

58. Baddeley A. Exploring the central executive. Q J Exp Psychol 1996;49A(1): 5–28.

59. Baddeley AD, Hitch GJ. Working memory. In: Bower GH, editor. The psychology of learning and motivation. San Diego: Academic Press; 1974. p. 47–90.

60. Rao S. Neuropsychology of multiple sclerosis: a critical review. J Clin Exp Neuropsychol 1986;8(5):503–42.

61. Beatty WW, Goodkin DE, Beatty PA, et al. Frontal lobe dysfunction and memory impairment in patients with chronic progressive multiple sclerosis. Brain Cogn 1989;11(1):73–86.

62. Thornton AE, Raz N. Memory impairment in multiple sclerosis: a quantitative review. Neuropsychology 1997;11(3):357–66.
63. Zakzanis K. Distinct neurocognitive profiles in multiple sclerosis subtypes. Arch Clin Neuropsychol 2000;15(2):115–36.
64. Basso MR, Beason-Hazen S, Lynn J, et al. Screening for cognitive dysfunction in multiple sclerosis. Arch Neurol 1996;53:980–4.
65. Rovaris M, Filippi M, Falautano M, et al. Relation between MR abnormalities and patterns of cognitive impairment in multiple sclerosis. Neurology 1998;50: 1601–8.
66. DeLuca J, Barbieri-Berger S, Johnson SK. The nature of memory impairments in multiple sclerosis: acquisition versus retrieval. J Clin Exp Neuropsychol 1994; 16:183–9.
67. Kurtzke JF. Rating neurologic impairment in multiple sclerosis: an expanded disability status scale (EDSS). Neurology 1983;33(11):1444–52.
68. Haase CG, Tinnefeld M, Lienemann M, et al. Depression and cognitive impairment in disability-free early multiple sclerosis. Behav Neurol 2003;14(1/2): 39–45.
69. Haase CG, Lienemann M, Faustmann PM. Neuropsychological deficits but not coping strategies are related to physical disability in multiple sclerosis. Eur Arch Psychiatry Clin Neurosci 2008;258(1):35–9.
70. Ruggieri RM, Palermo R, Vitello G, et al. Cognitive impairment in patients suffering from relapsing-remitting multiple sclerosis with EDSS < or = 3.5. Acta Neurol Scand 2003;108(5):323–6.
71. Franklin GM, Heaton RK, Nelson LM, et al. Correlation of neuropsychological and MRI findings in chronic/progressive multiple sclerosis. Neurology 1988; 38:1826–9.
72. Duque B, Sepulcre J, Bejarano B, et al. Memory decline evolves independently of disease activity in MS. Mult Scler 2008;14(7):947–53.
73. Cutter GR, Baier ML, Rudick RA, et al. Development of a multiple sclerosis functional composite as a clinical trial outcome measure. Brain 1999;122(Pt 5): 871–82.
74. Tiemann L, Penner IK, Haupts M, et al. Cognitive decline in multiple sclerosis: impact of topographic lesion distribution on differential cognitive deficit patterns. Mult Scler 2009;15(10):1164–74.
75. Rao SM, Leo GJ, Haughton VM, et al. Correlation of magnetic resonance imaging with neuropsychological testing in multiple sclerosis. Neurology 1989; 39(2 Pt 1):161–6.
76. Swirsky-Sacchetti T, Mitchell DR, Seward J, et al. Neuropsychological and structural brain lesions in multiple sclerosis: a regional analysis. Neurology 1992; 42(7):1291–5.
77. PAArnett, Rao SM, Bernardin L, et al. Relationship between frontal lobe lesions and Wisconsin Card Sorting Test performance in patients with multiple sclerosis. Neurology 1994;44(3 Pt 1):420–5.
78. Foong J, Rozewicz L, Quaghebeur G, et al. Executive function in multiple sclerosis. The role of frontal lobe pathology. Brain 1997;120(1):15–26.
79. Benedict R, Bakshi R, Simon JH, et al. Frontal cortex atrophy predicts cognitive impairment in multiple sclerosis. J Neuropsychiatry Clin Neurosci 2002;14(1): 44–51.
80. Parmenter BA, Zivadinov R, Kerenyi L, et al. Validity of the Wisconsin Card Sorting and Delis-Kaplan Executive Function System (DKEFS) Sorting Tests in multiple sclerosis. J Clin Exp Neuropsychol 2007;29(2):215–23.

81. Lazeron RH, de Sonneville LM, Scheltens P, et al. Cognitive slowing in multiple sclerosis is strongly associated with brain volume reduction. Mult Scler 2006; 12(6):760–8.

82. Brass SD, Benedict RH, Weinstock-Guttman B, et al. Cognitive impairment is associated with subcortical magnetic resonance imaging grey matter T2 hypointensity in multiple sclerosis. Mult Scler 2006;12(4):437–44.

83. Zivadinov R, Sepcic J, Nasuelli D, et al. A longitudinal study of brain atrophy and cognitive disturbances in the early phase of relapsing-remitting multiple sclerosis. J Neurol Neurosurg Psychiatry 2001;70(6):773–80.

84. Amato MP, Bartolozzi ML, Zipoli V, et al. Neocortical volume decrease in relapsing-remitting MS patients with mild cognitive impairment. Neurology 2004;63(1):89–93.

85. Fink F, Eling P, Rischkau E, et al. The association between California Verbal Learning Test performance and fibre impairment in multiple sclerosis: evidence from diffusion tensor imaging. Mult Scler 2010;16(3):332–41.

86. Tedeschi G, Lavorgna L, Russo P, et al. Brain atrophy and lesion load in a large population of patients with multiple sclerosis. Neurology 2005;65(2):280–5.

87. Calabrese M, Rinaldi F, Mattisi I, et al. Widespread cortical thinning characterizes patients with MS with mild cognitive impairment. Neurology 2010;74(4): 321–8.

88. Calabrese M, Agosta F, Rinaldi F, et al. Cortical lesions and atrophy associated with cognitive impairment in relapsing-remitting multiple sclerosis. Arch Neurol 2009;66(9):1144–50.

89. Roosendaal SD, Moraal B, Pouwels PJ, et al. Accumulation of cortical lesions in MS: relation with cognitive impairment. Mult Scler 2009;15(6):708–14.

90. Chiaravalloti ND, DeLuca J. Cognitive impairment in multiple sclerosis. Lancet Neurol 2008;7(12):1139–51.

91. Filippi M, Rocca MA. Cortical reorganisation in patients with MS. J Neurol Neurosurg Psychiatry 2004;75(8):1087–9.

92. Wishart HA, Saykin AJ, McDonald BC, et al. Brain activation patterns associated with working memory in relapsing-remitting MS. Neurology 2004;62(2):234–8.

93. Julian LJ, Arnett PA. Relationships among anxiety, depression, and executive functioning in multiple sclerosis. Clin Neuropsychol 2009;23(5):1–11.

94. Arnett PA. Speed of presentation influences story recall in college students and persons with multiple sclerosis. Arch Clin Neuropsychol 2004;19(4):507–23.

95. Arnett PA, Higginson CI, Randolph JJ. Depression in multiple sclerosis: relationship to planning ability. J Int Neuropsychol Soc 2001;7(6):665–74.

96. Arnett PA, Higginson CI, Voss WD, et al. Depression in multiple sclerosis: relationship to working memory capacity. Neuropsychology 1999;13(4):546–56.

97. Christodoulou C, Melville P, Scherl WF, et al. Negative affect predicts subsequent cognitive change in multiple sclerosis. J Int Neuropsychol Soc 2009; 15(1):53–61.

98. Zorzon M, de Masi R, Nasuelli D, et al. Depression and anxiety in multiple sclerosis. A clinical and MRI study in 95 subjects. J Neurol 2001;248(5):416–21.

99. Zorzon M, Zivadinov R, Nasuelli D, et al. Depressive symptoms and MRI changes in multiple sclerosis. Eur J Neurol 2002;9(5):491–6.

100. Julian LJ, Mohr DC. Cognitive predictors of response to treatment for depression in multiple sclerosis. J Neuropsychiatry Clin Neurosci 2006;18(3):356–63.

101. Stenager E, Knudsen L, Jensen K. Multiple sclerosis: correlation of anxiety, physical impairment and cognitive dysfunction. Ital J Neurol Sci 1994;15(2): 97–101.

102. Hart RP, Martelli MF, Zasler ND. Chronic pain and neuropsychological functioning. Neuropsychol Rev 2000;10(3):131–49.
103. Brown RT, Zuelsdorff M, Fleming M. Adverse effects and cognitive function among primary care patients taking opioids for chronic nonmalignant pain. J Opioid Manag 2006;2(3):137–46.
104. Krupp LB, Elkins LE. Fatigue and declines in cognitive functioning in multiple sclerosis. Neurology 2000;55:934–9.
105. Sumowski JF, Chiaravalloti N, DeLuca J. Cognitive reserve protects against cognitive dysfunction in multiple sclerosis. J Clin Exp Neuropsychol 2009; 31(8):913–26.
106. Sumowski JF, Chiaravalloti N, Wylie G, et al. Cognitive reserve moderates the negative effect of brain atrophy on cognitive efficiency in multiple sclerosis. J Int Neuropsychol Soc 2009;15(4):606–12.
107. Sumowski JF, Wylie GR, Deluca J, et al. Intellectual enrichment is linked to cerebral efficiency in multiple sclerosis: functional magnetic resonance imaging evidence for cognitive reserve. Brain 2010;133(Pt 2):362–74.
108. Sepulcre J, Vanotti S, Hernández R, et al. Cognitive impairment in patients with multiple sclerosis using the Brief Repeatable Battery-Neuropsychology test. Mult Scler 2006;12(2):187–95.
109. Boringa JB, Lazeron RH, Reuling IE, et al. The brief repeatable battery of neuropsychological tests: normative values allow application in multiple sclerosis clinical practice. Mult Scler 2001;7(4):263–7.
110. Scherer P, Baum K, Bauer H, et al. Normalization of the Brief Repeatable Battery of Neuropsychological tests (BRB-N) for German-speaking regions. Application in relapsing-remitting and secondary progressive multiple sclerosis patients. Nervenarzt 2004;75(10):984–90 [in German].
111. Benedict R, Fischer JS, Archibald CJ, et al. Minimal neuropsychological assessment of MS patients: A consensus approach. Clin Neuropsychol 2002;16(3): 381–97.
112. Parmenter BA, Testa SM, Schretlen DJ, et al. The utility of regression-based norms in interpreting the minimal assessment of cognitive function in multiple sclerosis (MACFIMS). J Int Neuropsychol Soc 2010;16(1):6–16.
113. Strauss E, Sherman EMS, Spreen O. A compendium of neuropsychological tests: administration, norms, and commentary. 3rd edition. Oxford (UK): Oxford University Press; 2006.
114. Wim Van H, Guy N, Alexander L, et al. Correlation of cognitive dysfunction and diffusion tensor MRI measures in patients with mild and moderate multiple sclerosis. J Magn Reson Imaging 2010;31(6):1492–8.
115. Polman CH, Rudick RA. The multiple sclerosis functional composite: a clinically meaningful measure of disability. Neurology 2010;74(Suppl 3):S8–15.
116. Bosma L, Kragt JJ, Brieva L, et al. Progression on the Multiple Sclerosis Functional Composite in multiple sclerosis: what is the optimal cut-off for the three components? Mult Scler 2010;16(7):862–7.
117. Strober L, Englert J, Munschauer F, et al. Sensitivity of conventional memory tests in multiple sclerosis: comparing the Rao Brief Repeatable Neuropsychological Battery and the Minimal Assessment of Cognitive Function in MS. Mult Scler 2009;15(9):1077–84.
118. Aupperle RL, Beatty WW, Shelton Fde N, et al. Three screening batteries to detect cognitive impairment in multiple sclerosis. Mult Scler 2002;8(5):382–9.
119. Smith A. Symbol Digit Modalities Test (SDMT). Manual (revised). Los Angeles (CA): Western Psychological Services; 1982.

120. Benedict RH, Duquin JA, Jurgensen S, et al. Repeated assessment of neuro-psychological deficits in multiple sclerosis using the Symbol Digit Modalities Test and the MS Neuropsychological Screening Questionnaire. Mult Scler 2008;14(7):940–6.

121. Parmenter BA, Weinstock-Guttman B, Garg N, et al. Screening for cognitive impairment in multiple sclerosis using the Symbol Digit Modalities Test. Multiple Sclerosis 2007;13(1):52–7.

122. Benedict RH, Cox D, Thompson LL, et al. Reliable screening for neuropsychological impairment in multiple sclerosis. Mult Scler 2004;10(6):675–8.

123. Sullivan JJL, Edgley K, Dehoux E. A survey of multiple sclerosis. Part 1: Perceived cognitive problems and compensatory strategy use. Can J Rehabil 1990;4:99–105.

124. Marrie RA, Chelune GJ, Miller DM, et al. Subjective cognitive complaints relate to mild impairment of cognition in multiple sclerosis. Mult Scler 2005;11(1): 69–75.

125. Duquette P, Murray TJ, Pleines J, et al. Multiple sclerosis in childhood: clinical profile in 125 patients. J Pediatr 1987;111(3):359–63.

126. Ghezzi A, Deplano V, Faroni J, et al. Multiple sclerosis in childhood: clinical features of 149 cases. Mult Scler 1997;3(1):43–6.

127. Fields RD. White matter in learning, cognition and psychiatric disorders. Trends Neurosci 2008;31(7):361–70.

128. Bye AM, Kendall B, Wilson J. Multiple sclerosis in childhood: a new look. Dev Med Child Neurol 1985;27(2):215–22.

129. Dale RC, de Sousa C, Chong WK, et al. Acute disseminated encephalomyelitis, multiphasic disseminated encephalomyelitis and multiple sclerosis in children. Brain 2000;123(Pt 12):2407–22.

130. Banwell BL, Anderson PE. The cognitive burden of multiple sclerosis in children. Neurology 2005;64(5):891–4.

131. MacAllister WS, Belman AL, Milazzo M, et al. Cognitive functioning in children and adolescents with multiple sclerosis. Neurology 2005;64(8):1422–5.

132. Semel E, Wiig EH, Secord WA. Clinical evaluation of language fundamentals - 3. San Antonio (TX): Psychological Corporation a Pearson Brand; 1995.

133. Amato MP, Goretti B, Ghezzi A, et al. Cognitive and psychosocial features of childhood and juvenile MS. Neurology 2008;70(20):1891–7.

134. Portaccio E, Goretti B, Lori S, et al. The brief neuropsychological battery for children: a screening tool for cognitive impairment in childhood and juvenile multiple sclerosis. Mult Scler 2009;15(5):620–6.

135. Kaplan EF, Goodglass H, Weintraub S. The Boston Naming test. 2nd edition. Philadelphia: Lea & Febiger; 1983.

136. MacAllister WS, Christodoulou C, Milazzo M, et al. Longitudinal neuropsychological assessment in pediatric multiple sclerosis. Dev Neuropsychol 2007; 32(2):625–44.

137. Amato MP, Goretti B, Ghezzi A, et al. Cognitive and psychosocial features in childhood and juvenile MS: two-year follow-up. Neurology 2010;75(13): 1134–40.

138. Fischer JS, Priore RL, Jacobs LD, et al. Neuropsychological effects of interferon beta-1a in relapsing multiple sclerosis. Multiple Sclerosis Collaborative Research Group. Ann Neurol 2000;48(6):885–92.

139. Barak Y, Achiron A. Effect of interferon-beta-1b on cognitive functions in multiple sclerosis. Eur Neurol 2002;47(1):11–4.

140. Pliskin NH, Hamer DP, Goldstein DS, et al. Improved delayed visual reproduction test performance in multiple sclerosis patients receiving interferon beta-1b. Neurology 1996;47(6):1463–8.
141. Weinstein A, Schwid SR, Schiffer RB, et al. Neuropsychologic status in multiple sclerosis after treatment with glatiramer. Arch Neurol 1999;56:319–24.
142. Kappos L, Freedman MS, Polman CH, et al. Long-term effect of early treatment with interferon beta-1b after a first clinical event suggestive of multiple sclerosis: 5-year active treatment extension of the phase 3 BENEFIT trial. Lancet Neurol 2009;8(11):987–97.
143. Mattioli F, Stampatori C, Bellomi F, et al. Natalizumab efficacy on cognitive impairment in MS. Neurol Sci 2010;1–3.
144. Christodoulou C, Melville P, Scherl WF, et al. Effects of donepezil on memory and cognition in multiple sclerosis. J Neurol Sci 2006;245(1/2):127–36.
145. Krupp LB, Christodoulou C, Melville P, et al. Donepezil improved memory in multiple sclerosis in a randomized clinical trial. Neurology 2004;63(9):1579–85.
146. Lovera JF, Frohman E, Brown TR, et al. Memantine for cognitive impairment in multiple sclerosis: a randomized placebo-controlled trial. Mult Scler 2010; 16(6):715–23.
147. Lovera J, Bagert B, Smoot K, et al. *Ginkgo biloba* for the improvement of cognitive performance in multiple sclerosis: a randomized, placebo-controlled trial. Mult Scler 2007;13(3):376–85.
148. Harel Y, Appleboim N, Lavie M, et al. Single dose of methylphenidate improves cognitive performance in multiple sclerosis patients with impaired attention process. J Neurol Sci 2009;276(1/2):38–40.
149. Geisler MS, Sliwinski M, Coyle PK, et al. The effects of amantadine and pemoline on cognitive functioning in multiple sclerosis. Arch Neurol 1996;53:185–8.
150. Cohen RA, Fisher M. Amantadine treatment of fatigue associated with multiple sclerosis. Arch Neurol 1989;46(6):676–80.
151. Chiaravalloti ND, DeLuca J, Moore NB, et al. Treating learning impairments improves memory performance in multiple sclerosis: a randomized clinical trial. Mult Scler 2005;11(1):58–68.
152. Solari A, Filippini G, Gasco P, et al. Physical rehabilitation has a positive effect on disability in multiple sclerosis. Neurology 1999,52:57–62.
153. O'Brien CP. Review. Evidence-based treatments of addiction. Philos Trans R Soc Lond B Biol Sci 2008;363(1507):3277–86.

Index

Note: Page numbers of article titles are in **boldface** type.

A

N-Acetylaspartate, in MS, MRS of, 365
ACTH. See *Adrenocorticotropic hormone (ACTH)*.
Acupuncture, for MS, 466–467
Acute disseminated encephalomyelitis (ADEM), in children, MS related to, 482
ADEM. See *Acute disseminated encephalomyelitis (ADEM)*.
Adrenocorticotropic hormone (ACTH), for MS, 412, 414
Alemtuzumab, for MS, 415–416, 438–440
Alternative medicine, defined, 466
Antioxidant(s), in MS management, 469
APCs, in MS, 269
Atrophy, brain, in MS, MRI of, 347–348, 358
Autologous hematopoietic stem cell transplantation, for MS, 415
Axonal damage, in MS, 269–271

B

B cell–mediated CNS damage, in MS, 265–267
Bee venom therapy, for MS, 467–468
Behavior(s), health-related, in modifying disease course in MS, 304–305
BG-12, for MS, 441
Biology, as factor in RRMS, 285–287
Birth month, as risk factor in MS, 210–211
Birth place, as risk factor in MS, 209
Bladder, neurogenic, in MS patients, 449–450
Bowel, neurogenic, in MS patients, 450–451
Brain atrophy, in MS, MRI of, 347–348, 358
"Breakthrough disease," definitions of, 351, 416–417

C

CAM. See *Complementary and alternative medicine (CAM)*.
CD6 gene, 224
CD58 gene, 221–222
CD226 gene, 225
Central nervous system (CNS), B cell–mediated damage to, in MS, 265–267
Cerebrospinal fluid (CSF) analysis, in MS diagnosis, 383–384
    in children, 495
Children, MS in, 302–303, **481–505**
    academic consequences of, 494
    ADEM and, 482
    clinical course of, 485, 492

Neurol Clin 29 (2011) 527–538
doi:10.1016/S0733-8619(11)00018-1
0733-8619/11/$ – see front matter © 2011 Elsevier Inc. All rights reserved.

neurologic.theclinics.com

Printed and bound by CPI Group (UK) Ltd, Croydon, CR0 4YY

03/10/2024

01040457-0013

Moving?

Make sure your subscription moves with you!

To notify us of your new address, find your **Clinics Account Number** (located on your mailing label above your name), and contact customer service at:

Email: journalscustomerservice-usa@elsevier.com

800-654-2452 (subscribers in the U.S. & Canada)
314-447-8871 (subscribers outside of the U.S. & Canada)

Fax number: 314-447-8029

Elsevier Health Sciences Division
Subscription Customer Service
3251 Riverport Lane
Maryland Heights, MO 63043

Moving?

Make sure your subscription moves with you!

To notify us of your new address, find your Clinics Account number (located on your mailing label above your name), and contact customer service at:

Email: journalscustomerservice-usa@elsevier.com

800-654-2452 (subscribers in the U.S. & Canada)
314-447-8871 (subscribers outside of the U.S. & Canada)

Fax number: 314-447-8029

Elsevier Health Sciences Division
Subscription Customer Service
3251 Riverport Lane
Maryland Heights, MO 63043

To ensure uninterrupted delivery of your subscription, please notify us at least 4 weeks in advance of move.